T0220250

The Body Bears the Burden

When *The Body Bears the Burden* made its debut in 2001, it changed the way people thought about trauma, PTSD, and the treatment of chronic stress disorders. Now in its third edition, this revered text offers a fully updated and revised analysis of the relationship between mind, body, and the processing of trauma. Here, clinicians will find detailed, thorough explorations of some of neurobiology's fundamental tenets, the connections between mind, brain, and body, and the many and varied ways that symptoms of traumatic stress become visible to those who know to look for them.

Robert Scaer, MD, has practiced neurology and rehabilitation for 36 years. His three books, *The Body Bears the Burden*, *The Trauma Spectrum*, and *8 Keys to Brain–Body Balance*, address the intimate relationship between life trauma and chronic disease, the ubiquitous association of modern society with intrinsic sources of trauma, and the role of somatic techniques for healing trauma.

The Body Bears the Burden

Trauma, Dissociation, and Disease

Third Edition

ROBERT SCAER

Routledge
Taylor & Francis Group

NEW YORK AND LONDON

Third edition published 2014
by Routledge
711 Third Avenue, New York, NY 10017

and by Routledge
27 Church Road, Hove, East Sussex BN3 2FA

© 2014 Robert Scaer

Routledge is an imprint of the Taylor & Francis Group, an informa business

First edition published by The Haworth Press, Inc. 2001
Second edition published by The Haworth Press, Inc. 2007

Library of Congress Cataloging-in-Publication Data
Scaer, Robert C.
The body bears the burden : trauma, dissociation, and disease / Robert Scaer.—3rd
  edition.
    pages cm
  Includes bibliographical references and index.
  1. Post-traumatic stress disorder—Treatment.   2. Bioenergetic psychotherapy.
3. Mind and body therapies.   4. Somatoform disorders—Treatment.   I. Title.
  RC552.P67S2236 2014
  616.85′21—dc23
  2013024486

ISBN: 978-0-415-64151-7 (hbk)
ISBN: 978-0-415-64152-4 (pbk)
ISBN: 978-0-203-08182-2 (ebk)

Typeset in Minion
by Apex CoVantage, LLC

Contents

Foreword

About a century ago, scientists became aware of the existence of memories that are different from the memories of everyday experience. Ordinarily, events are remembered as stories that change over time and that do not evoke intense emotions and sensations. However, since time immemorial there have been records of people being tormented by memories that fill them with feelings of irreparable loss, and sensations of fright and horror. The neurologists and psychiatrists at the end of the nineteenth century elucidated the nature of posttraumatic conditions and showed that elements of the past were relived with an immediate sensory and emotional intensity that makes victims feel as if it were occurring all over again. While trauma related emotions and sensations endured, however, conscious knowledge of the event itself was sometimes absent. They discovered that, paradoxically, even though vivid elements of the trauma intrude insistently in the form of flashbacks and nightmares, many traumatized people have a great deal of difficulty relating precisely what has happened.

They often experience sensory elements of the trauma without being able to make sense out of what they are feeling or seeing. These mysterious combinations of remembering emotions and sensations, while forgetting the origin and the content, were called "repression" and "dissociation." These early scientists hypothesized that these amnesias and intrusive reexperiences were the result of severely paralyzing fears in response to terrifying life events. For example: the "father of neurology," Jean-Martin Charcot, noted that: "The patient ... does not preserve any recollection, or he preserves it in a vague manner. Questions addressed to him upon this point are attended with no result. He knows nothing or almost nothing." These early students of the effects of fear-related trauma noted that the loss of memory is not merely an inability to recall the specific event, but, more relevant, a lack of capacity for sustained thought, and for continued application to work. These patients had problems with attention, and were easily fatigued. They also noted that traumatic memories are intricately connected with one's sense of "self" and "self-awareness," and that, when the fear, fright, and hyperarousal that accompany trauma interfere with forming a well-defined, verbal memory of events, people lose their sense of themselves, start feeling helpless, and look to others for reassurance.[1] At the beginning of the past century, the great physiologist Walter Cannon proposed that traumatic emotions constitute phases of physiological mobilization in an internal environment that is perpetually striving to adjust itself, through the actions of the sympathetic nervous system and the endocrines, to changes and challenges in the organism's external environment: "[T]he bodily changes which occur in the intense emotional states—such as fear and fury—occur as results of sympathetic discharges, and are in the highest degree serviceable to the organism in the struggle for existence. Thus are the body's reserves—the stored adrenalin [*sic*], and the accumulated sugar—called forth for instant service; thus is the blood shifted to nerves and muscles that may have to bear the brunt of struggle; thus is the heart set rapidly beating to speed the circulation; and thus also, are the activities of the digestive organs for the time abolished" (Cannon 1914:275). Cannon pointed out how sometimes what starts out as a survival mechanism (mobilization) is transformed into its opposite to such a degree that it may even lead to "'Voodoo' Death."[2] When people develop PTSD, the replaying of the trauma leads to sensitization: With every replay of the trauma there is an increasing level of distress. In those individuals, the traumatic event, which started out as a social and interpersonal process, develops secondary biological consequences that are hard to reverse once they become entrenched. Because these patients have intolerable sensations and feelings, their tendency is to actively avoid them. Mentally, they split off or "dissociate" these feelings; physically, their bodies tighten and brace against them. They seem to live under the assumption that if they feel those sensations and feelings, they will overwhelm them forever. These are patients who rely on medications, drugs, and alcohol to make these sensations and feelings go away, because they have lost confidence that they can learn to tolerate them without outside help. The fear of being consumed by these "terrible" feelings leads them to believe that only not feeling them will make them go away.

Allan Young has pointed out that implicit traumatic memories, avoidance, and helplessness challenge two core foundations of the Western consciousness: free will and self-determination. The emotional dependency of traumatized people, and their inability to utilize the help offered, in turn, evokes frustration, contempt, and even sadism in those to whom the victims turn for help.[3]

Most whiplash victims have emotional symptoms: They may feel numb or detached, while experiencing anxiety related to automobile travel. This may progress to actual panic attacks when other cars drive too closely, approach rapidly behind them, or when they drive by the scene of their accident. Many suffer from flashbacks of the accident. Many also suffer from exaggerated startle responses to loud noises. Bright lights and loud or unpleasant noises may become intolerable, and cause anxiety and "overload." They may wake up in the middle of the night with severe anxiety, sometimes accompanied by memories of nightmares. If enough of these symptoms appear, they may receive the diagnosis of post-traumatic stress disorder (PTSD), although most of them suffer from only a few of these symptoms. Traditionally, the symptoms of traumatic brain injury have been ascribed to injury to the brain and the tissues of the head. Post-concussion syndrome, however, tends to follow minor brain injury much more often than more severe brain injury. Ironically, the long-term disability after six to twelve months post-accident is greater in mild concussion than in moderate brain injury in which the patient does not remember the accident. The mechanisms of minor traumatic brain injury are generally thought to be due to the tearing or stretching of axons (axonal shearing) due to forces related to excessive changes in velocity of the head during the acceleration/deceleration of the head during the movement of whiplash. However, studies have shown, on the one hand, that actual head impact is not necessary to cause axonal shearing and, on the other, that there is a remarkable consistency in the cognitive symptoms of the traumatized patients, regardless of the specific impact.

As with other traumatized patients described over the past years, traumatic brain injury patients suffer from a reduced rate of information processing, increased reaction time, and problems with divided attention. They are distracted, and have problems with concentration. They will forget events, appointments, and things they have said to other people. One of the most persistent and debilitating symptoms is pervasive fatigue: They "shut down." All of these symptoms are compatible with the abnormalities found in neuroimaging studies of traumatized patients. In this book, Scaer proposes to discard the concept of physical and structural injuries to the spine, jaw, and brain as the model for whiplash-based injury, and instead proposes that the whiplash experience is a model of traumatization, with long-standing and at times permanent neurophysiological and neurochemical changes in the brain that are experience-based, rather than injury-based. Scaer proposes that these changes are triggered by a cascade of neural impulses and neurotransmitters precipitated by a continuous state of intense arousal alternating with recurrence of the freeze response resulting in turn from an unresolved perceived life threat in a state of relative helplessness. The depth of memory is a function of the arousal or emotional content of the experience that accompanied the event. The brain readily forms procedural memories of intense emotional events. These are acquired and stored without the necessary involvement of conscious memory centers serving declarative memory, such as the hippocampus and prefrontal cortex. The basic premise is that whiplash injury is a traumatic experience that represents a threat to the very survival of the individual. In this definition, the meaning of the event may be as important to the traumatized person as what actually physically happens to that person.

This is a dramatic departure from the long-standing and traditional concept of whiplash as spinal injury. It presents, however, a compelling and logical theory, bringing together the diverse elements of the whiplash syndrome into a cohesive whole. To understand and properly treat these symptoms clinicians need to appreciate what happens to a body frozen in fear. Post-concussion syndromes need to be understood as representing disassociated imprints of traumatic experience—physical sensations, panic, and helplessness—that have overwhelmed these patients. Fighting against and/or hiding from unpleasant or painful sensations and feelings will generally make things worse. The more feelings need to be avoided, the more energy is spent on keeping them at bay—energy that should have been used for feeling alive and open to new experiences. What is not felt remains unchanged or gains in inward pressure, which forces people to step up their methods of avoidance. This is the sort of vicious cycle that trauma creates. Abandoned feelings call out for attention from the growing shadow of existence. Treatment must aim at putting these disjointed sensations together. Doing this involves coaxing them gently to begin to feel and tolerate the sensations that once overwhelmed them.

Bessel A. van der Kolk, MD
Medical Director, the Trauma Center
Professor of Psychiatry
Boston University School of Medicine

Notes

1. van der Kolk, B.: Post-traumatic stress disorder and the nature of trauma. *Dialogues in Clinical Neuroscience*, 2000, pp. 2, 7–22.
2. van der Kolk, B., McFarlane, A., Weisaeth, L. (Eds.).: *Traumatic Stress: The Effects of Overwhelming Experience on Mind, Body, and Society.* New York: Guilford Press, 1996.
3. Young, A.: *The Harmony of Illusions: Inventing Post-Traumatic Stress Disorders.* Princeton, NJ: Princeton University Press, 1998.

Preface

When Beth first came to my office, she brought her best friend, a nurse, to interpret for her, and clearly also to provide moral support. Beth was quite guarded, almost suspicious, with wide, frightened eyes. She sat with her arms held tightly at her side, gripping a handkerchief. Her head was canted forward, and her shoulders elevated and tense. Her forehead was furrowed, and at twenty-five, she looked closer to forty. She said that she had suffered whiplash in an accident, and wasn't getting any better. A friend had referred her to me because of my interest in motor vehicle accident-related injuries. Her insurance company was beginning to question her treatment, since the accident had occurred at speeds of 5 to 10 mph. No damage occurred to either car, and the driver of the other car suffered no injuries. Beth, on the other hand, continued to suffer from terrible neck and shoulder pain, numbness of her right arm, disabling headaches, and grinding of her teeth at night. Six months of chiropractic treatment and massage therapy brought her only temporary relief from pain, and a nighttime dental splint only slightly helped her morning headaches. Recently she developed severe pain in her right hip and buttock, with the pain radiating down the back of her leg. X-rays and MRIs failed to show any cause for her spinal or leg pain.

Beth had also experienced worsening problems of distractibility and an inability to concentrate. She made frequent errors in her checkbook. Her memory was terrible, and she would frequently misplace things and go somewhere but forget what she had intended to do when she got there. She had recently started to drive again, and would travel to some familiar place in town, and on arriving, realize that she could not remember the route she took. She would stumble over words, say the wrong word for what she meant, and then feel stupid. She even had developed a strange stutter whenever stressed.

Since the accident, she had become panicky when traveling in a car, especially as a passenger. Her heart would pound for no reason. She had become edgy and irritable, and jumped at every loud sound. Thoughts and images of the accident kept popping into her mind, producing distraction and anxiety. Although she finally was able to fall asleep without drugs, she kept waking fully aroused, sometimes with a racing heart, sometimes with dreams of the accident or of being threatened with no means of escape. She was exhausted by every physical and mental effort, and had dropped out of her master's program in clinical social work. Her extreme sensitivity to almost any stimulus had resulted in her isolation from almost all of her prior social activities.

Beth had also developed many neurological symptoms. She felt dizzy when she moved her head too quickly, kept losing her balance and bumping into things, and noticed that her vision blurred whenever she moved her focus from one object to another. Reading caused blurring of vision and a headache. Only an MRI of her brain reassured her that she had no brain disease or damage.

As I do with all of my motor vehicle accident (MVA) patients, I asked her in detail about past traumatic life experiences, especially as a child. Similar to many of my patients, she was very open and candid and willing to share with me what must have been a hellish nightmare of her childhood. She was supported in this discussion by the confidante and friend who had accompanied her. From the ages of six through twelve, she was visited several times a week after bedtime by her brother, who was older by seven years. As if by ritual, he would painfully twist her right arm behind her back as she lay in bed on her stomach, pull down her panties, and rape her. Any sound by her would result in his beating her, or covering her head with a pillow as he abused her. She never told her parents for fear of punishment by her verbally abusive alcoholic father. At age nineteen, her brother ran away from home and the abuse stopped. During college, memories and panic related to the abuse resurfaced, and she underwent years of counseling, which enabled her to "put it all behind her." She obtained her degree, and, prior to the accident, had been pursuing a graduate degree with the goal of becoming a social worker.

When I examined Beth, she was quite guarded and defensive. Her dramatic response to strength and sensory perception could be described as "exaggerated pain behavior." She manifested "give-away" weakness of her right arm and leg, and diminished sensation to pin prick of these extremities and over the entire right side of her head and face. These were all findings that doctors have long considered to be "psychological" or "hysterical." Remarkably, however, her right hand was slightly cooler to touch than the left, and patterns of hair growth revealed subtle but definite thinning over the right half of her scalp. Her neck was quite resistant to passive movement, and bending her neck back immediately caused her to become nauseated. Tightness, tenderness, and trigger points were prominent in her neck, jaw, and shoulder girdle muscles, and raising of her right leg while lying on her back caused pain in her hip and tingling of her right foot.

The story of Beth's whiplash experience is a compilation of symptoms seen consistently in thousands of my patients who have suffered injuries in MVAs. These unusual symptoms, encompassing many areas of the body and mind, are so universal and consistent from patient to patient that they either constitute a vast medico-legal conspiracy to defraud the auto insurance industry, or a remarkably consistent and reproducible clinical syndrome. The whiplash syndrome has been a source of controversy, confusion, derision, and misunderstanding for most of its described existence. It is indeed a syndrome, a diagnosis defined as "The aggregate of signs and symptoms associated with any morbid process, and constituting together the picture of the disease."[1]

The "picture of the disease" in this case is a diverse constellation of symptoms consisting of pain, neurologic symptoms, cognitive impairment, and emotional complaints. Each specific symptom and group of symptoms is remarkably similar from person to person, suggesting a unique and common cause. The legal defense bar and a substantial number of physicians would assert that this remarkable similarity is related to the phenomenon of secondary gain, and the sophisticated coaching of the plaintiff bar. Doubt is cast upon this assertion by the fact that few of these patients seem to recover after settlement of their case, even for substantial sums of money. The "green poultice" (the healing power of lots of settlement money) is more myth than reality.

A real dilemma in assessing the cause and validity of this syndrome, however, is the fact that it frequently occurs in a setting of an insufficient velocity and force of collision to logically cause bodily injury. Another major dilemma is the diffuse and diverse nature of the symptoms. The whiplash syndrome seems to affect a great portion of the victim's conscious existence. It impairs the mind (cognitive and attention deficits), the body (severe and widespread pain, vertigo, visual impairment, numbness and tingling), and the spirit (anxiety, insomnia, depression, loss of sense of self). Indeed, one of the most poignant complaints I heard is that the patient has "lost who I once was." And years later, although much healing may have taken place, most patients feel permanently and irrevocably changed by their experience. No amount of financial reward cures them of their recurrent episodes of unexplained pain or their altered sense of self. Even relatively minor life conflicts and stresses seem to throw them back into the distraction and confusion, the jitteriness and arousal, and the familiar tightening and spasm of the same groups of neck, shoulder, and low back muscles they know so well.

For years I have struggled with the inconsistencies between the physical injuries and the resulting diffuse and disabling symptoms experienced by patients after MVAs. I have searched the scientific literature on whiplash, much of which seeks to explain the injuries to ligaments, discs, muscles, nerves, and brain cells and axons from a biomechanical standpoint. In courtroom testimony, I have struggled to justify the fact that an individual could have suffered permanent injuries to the brain and spine from a 10-mph rear-end collision, in the face of contrary testimony by accident reconstruction engineers and the powerful weight of common sense. How could one person, knocked unconscious for an hour in a football game, be left with no measurable cognitive impairment three years later, while another, rear-ended at 10 mph, with damage only to the bumper, be effectively cognitively disabled in the same time frame? Why are professional race car and demolition derby drivers not disabled early in their careers from whiplash or brain injury?

Certainly the recent documentation of permanent damage to brain neurons with repetitive blows to the head in football merits consideration in auto accident concussions, but in that case we are talking about dozens, even hundreds of relatively high-velocity blows to the head.

The first clue, I believe, lies in the meaning of the event during which the injury occurred. One tends not to develop the diverse and disabling symptoms described previously unless the injury occurs in a state of relative helplessness. A second clue lies in the life history of specific traumatic events, especially those experienced in childhood. I have found that the severity of a person's whiplash-related symptoms strongly correlates with his or her cumulative load of traumatic life experiences before the accident occurred. These experiences may be incredibly varied. They will be discussed in more detail in Chapter 10.

Another clue lies in the fact that all of the symptoms commonly seen in the whiplash syndrome may occur with remarkable similarity in other severely traumatic events not associated with physical injury. Examples include natural disasters, exposure to warfare, and social trauma (assault, kidnapping, rape). Symptoms following these traumatic events are generally attributed to post-traumatic stress disorder (PTSD), a purely psychiatric diagnosis. Much of the medical literature tends to ignore the often dramatic physical symptoms, including bowel disorders, myofascial pain, and cognitive impairment that accompany PTSD in a fashion often identical to that experienced in the whiplash syndrome. Many soldiers returning from multiple tours of duty in the Middle East suffer from a constellation of physical symptoms quite similar to whiplash. We therefore seem to be dealing with a syndrome affecting all aspects of a person's being, including body, brain, and mind.

This post-traumatic syndrome is produced by a threat, shock, or injury that occurred in a state of helplessness. The combination of a life threat in a state of helplessness causes all of the sensory and motor experiences to be stored in a person's unconscious body-based procedural memory in a cumulative manner, along with other such life experiences. These past unconscious memories will then tend to recur with any environmental cues to the trauma. Accumulation of traumatic life experiences, especially beginning in childhood, then leads to a condition of increasing vulnerability and decreasing resiliency to further trauma.

The somatic and emotional consequences of traumatic stress are generally misunderstood by members of the mainstream medical profession, who refer to the resulting constellation of symptoms as psychosomatic or psychological, yet it is clear that this syndrome is common. Research suggests that it is probably well represented in all societies. It may well account for many of the unexplained and poorly managed chronic illnesses that afflict us, and perhaps constitute the major source of visits to the physician's office. Indeed, it may well account for the worldwide epidemic of unexplained back and neck pain that fills the medical literature.

The journey that led to this book began when Marcus Kurek, one of the physical therapists in the chronic pain treatment program that I directed in the 1990s, referred me to the writings of Peter Levine, psychologist and trauma specialist. Levine developed his model of treatment of traumatized individuals from his observations of animals in the wild, noting that prey animals, although repeatedly threatened, did not seem to develop behaviors similar to traumatized human beings. He noted that when prey animals are no longer able to flee or fight, they enter the freeze, or immobility, response. During this period of relative "suspended animation," all of the chemical, neurological events associated with the fight/flight response persist. This produces a high state of activation of the emotional brain, the limbic system, and both sympathetic and parasympathetic parts of the autonomic nervous system. If the prey animal survives, it will arouse, and then seem to "discharge" the fight/flight energy through shaking or trembling in a manner that replicates the physical behavior of the last act of self-defense. This trembling, perspiring, and deep breathing, effectively "completes" the somatic and autonomic activities associated with flight. In doing so, it essentially erases the brain's unconscious memory for what the body tried to do to protect the animal. Without the discharge, the recurrent emergence of these body-based memories triggered by internal or environmental cues to the event produces all of the emotional and physical experiences of trauma/PTSD.

Levine noted that humans, although frequently freezing in the face of threat, seldom go through this "discharge" of retained fight/flight energy. This may be related to our highly developed cognitive brain centers that tend to suppress many instinctual behaviors because of our acquired patterns of acculturation. Dramatic shaking all over is "unseemly" or "hysterical," and tends to be suppressed in advanced Western cultures. Abnormal storage of this intense state of arousal, and what the body unsuccessfully tried to do to survive is stored in selected brain centers. It will then tend to emerge in the future with any environmental cues to the trauma, even as simple as the whiplash victim getting into a car. This process leads to the syndrome of trauma that he describes in his writings.[2]

I realized at the time that the behavior, perceptions, and sensations preceding the freeze response typified the immediate post-accident experience of my whiplash patients—a state of shock, numbing, immobility, and even depersonalization. I realized that the mental state called dissociation very likely represents what humans consciously experience while in the freeze. The time it took the brain to incorporate all of the physical, autonomic, and emotional experiences into unconscious procedural/body-based memory explained the significant delay of several days in the onset of pain, cognitive impairment, and emotional symptoms seen in many of my patients. It also explained why many of my patients began to deteriorate weeks and even months after the accident. Finally, it explained why symptoms did not improve and disappear, but rather kept returning after hundreds of therapy treatments; why imaging studies seldom explained the cause of spinal soft tissue pain; and why so few of my patients recovered after their litigation was settled. The so-called green poultice of legal settlement money was basically a myth.

Since that moment of enlightenment, I have seen hundreds of victims of MVAs in a new light, taken detailed trauma histories, and begun to prescribe treatment programs emphasizing trauma therapy whenever possible. I have taken my ideas to the major auto insurance companies to enlist support in this area of treatment and in research, and have received a predictably negative reception. In this process, I also began to examine and study victims of trauma with a new perspective, and started to correlate physical symptoms and syndromes with the burgeoning literature on the physiology of the brain in PTSD. Viewed in this context, I recognized subtle but consistent physical changes in my patients who have been labeled with the diagnosis of somatization, conversion, hysteria, and secondary gain. The consistency of these findings among patients and their startling correlation with concepts of altered brain/autonomic physiology has led me to the inescapable conclusion that clinical syndromes previously categorized as "malingering," "non-physiological," "psychosomatic," or "functional" are based on altered brain physiology secondary to trauma. These in turn may cause subtle but observable changes in the symptomatic body region involved in the trauma. I now realize that the concept of whiplash remains only one small example of the pervasive physical, mental, and emotional devastation of traumatic stress. Although the brain and body is often damaged in auto accidents, the complex but reproducible symptoms of whiplash represent a physiological rewiring within neurons and their connections in the brain more than an injury of the body. The burgeoning literature on brain plasticity in the past few decades has provided powerful support for the concept of life experiences producing structural changes in the brain and its function. Whiplash syndrome in this scenario represents an example of negative neuroplasticity within the brain, not physical damage to the body or to the brain itself.

I realize that I am treading on the dangerously thin divide separating the slippery slopes of the brain and the mind; time may prove that I have slipped a few times. But the research in brain plasticity I believe has strongly supported the concept of the brain changing the body and experiences of the body changing the brain. As a neurologist, pursuing the topic of a psychiatric illness has presented a dilemma and a challenge. In presenting my evolving theories to my medical colleagues, I have predictably been met with skepticism by physicians that a dramatic physical syndrome with numerous, apparently disparate features could have its roots solely in a change in brain and body function produced by an experience. Colleagues in the field of behavioral science have been more receptive, but have still struggled with my contention that the physical manifestations of conversion hysteria have a distinct neurophysiological origin, and are not solely expressions of impaired psychological dynamics.

Despite the medical community giving increasing lip service to rejecting Cartesian dualism (the functional separation of the mind from the body), current allopathic and even many holistic physicians continue to consider "exaggerated" emotional states and "non-physiological" physical symptoms and findings to be derived from psychological causes. Descartes, in fact, was probably not the author of our current concept of mind/body dualism.[3] In his treatise, *Meditation VI, Of the Existence of Material Things, and of the Real Distinction Between the Soul and the Body of Man*, he argues that the soul in relationship to the body is "very closely united to it, and so to speak so intermingled with it that . . . [they] seem to compose . . . one whole."[4] In addition, in *The Passions of the Soul*, Descartes attributes a series of states of the mind to physical alterations of the body preceding or accompanying these mental states. However, in *Passions*, Descartes indeed proposes that anger, joy, and other intense emotional states may be a consequence of somatic or material physical states, but not a cause of them (p. 326).[5] This specific theoretical departure from his contemporary colleagues may well have destined Descartes to be the scapegoat for the evolution of the concept of separation of mind and body in contemporary medicine.

As a result, Descartes has been blamed for a concept and language placing emotional and unexplainable somatic complaints in the intangible category of psychological events, and those symptoms and signs that we can measure by our tangible physiological images and measures in the category of physiological diseases.

Although we have come to accept that prolonged emotional distress appears to have adverse health effects on the body, our rigid application of the scientific method to our relatively primitive science of medicine has tended to blind us to the subtleties of somatic manifestations of emotional states. In the absence of sophisticated imaging studies and laboratory measures, the early pioneers of medical science relied on keen senses of observation, and the necessity of deriving their diagnoses from the history and physical examination alone. They derived their insights and wisdom from case studies and experience, and the cumulative knowledge taught to them by their patients. Many of the insights presented in this book also derive from clinical observations that patients alone can provide, built on a base of knowledge gleaned from the neurophysiological literature on traumatic stress. The result is not an affirmation of the mind/body connection, but of the mind/brain/body continuum.

Finally, through this journey, my belief that patient education is a powerful therapeutic tool has been greatly enhanced. Altering the threat of the unknown by informing and educating the patient changes the body's stress response and promotes healing. Many whiplash victims suffer almost as much from the dismissal and invalidation by the medical and insurance industries as they do from the effects of the accident itself. Providing them with a rational and comprehensive explanation for their symptoms is strong medicine. The obvious enlightenment experienced by my patients, the gratitude expressed, and the improved response to therapy resulting from detailed education, have inspired and strengthened me in writing this book.

I purposely geared the first edition of this book to general professionals in the fields of rehabilitation, psychotherapy, patient care, and general medical practice in the hope that it would prove to be valuable to their understanding of this challenging group of patients. I provided copious references to show my medical colleagues that I had done my homework. I found, however, that many lay individuals and patients have bought and read the book. Because of its medical complexity, many found it to be formidable reading. In the second and third editions, I have attempted to simplify more complex medical terminology, to add explanatory notes, and to soften the somewhat pedantic prose that often typifies medical articles and textbooks. I have significantly restructured several chapters to resolve some issues of redundancy, and have drastically rewritten the chapter on trauma therapy to include new concepts and ideas that I have developed since the first edition. In the third edition, I have added a chapter on the burgeoning evidence for brain plasticity, a concept giving great hope for the healing of trauma, and justifying much of my theoretical foundation. I hope that the third edition will provide readers with a more user-friendly route through the complexities of trauma and its brain physiology.

Notes

1. *Stedman's Medical Dictionary:* Twenty-Fourth Edition. Baltimore: Williams &Wilkins, 1982. p. 1382.
2. Levine, P.: *Waking the Tiger: Healing Trauma.* Berkeley, CA: North Atlantic Press, 1997.
3. Brown, T.: Cartesian dualism and psychosomatics. *Psychosomatics,* 1989; 30(3):322–331.
4. Descartes, R.: Meditation IV (1641). In *The Philosophical Works. Volume 1.* Translated by Haldane, E., Ross, D., New York/Dover, 1955, p. 2. In Brown, T.: Cartesian dualism and psychosomatics. *Psychosomatics,* 1989; 30(3):322–331, p. 325.
5. Descartes. R.: The Passions of the Soul (1649). In *The Philosophical Works. Volume 1.* Translated by Haldane, E., Ross, D., New York/Dover, 1955. p. 2. In Brown, T.: Cartesian dualism and psychosomatics. *Psychosomatics,* 1989; 30(3):322–332, pp. 325–326.

Acknowledgments

In 1996 I came across the writings of psychologist and traumatologist Peter Levine. I recognized in his description of the phenomenon of the freeze response in animals many of the symptoms and features of my whiplash victims immediately after an accident. The persisting symptoms in my patients who failed to recover after prolonged treatment matched in remarkable detail the late effects of trauma described by Levine. I would specifically refer the reader to his book, *Waking the Tiger: Healing Trauma* (North Atlantic Press, 1997), for a detailed discussion of Dr. Levine's theories and treatment method for trauma. These ideas led me to redefine symptoms of the whiplash syndrome, and ultimately to my exploration of the somatic syndromes associated with trauma. I am grateful to Dr. Levine for writing the foreword to my second book, *The Trauma Spectrum*. We have remained close friends and colleagues.

I am also indebted to the studies of numerous researchers in the field of trauma. The books and review articles of psychiatrist and traumatologist, Bessel A. van der Kolk, and his personal advice about this book have been especially helpful. His extensive review articles on the psychobiology of stress and trauma reenactment provided a wealth of background information.

The seminal book, *Affect Development and the Origin of the Self* (Lawrence Erlbaum Associates, 1994), by Allan Schore, provided powerful support for concepts of the neurobiology of experience-based development of the brain in the newborn infant, with resulting alteration of brain chemistry and circuitry, a central thesis for this book. Through our personal interaction and his writings, Dr. Schore has been a mentor and a rich source of information.

A book exploring auto accident-related PTSD, *After the Crash* (American Psychological Association Press, 1997), by psychologists Edward Blanchard and Edward Hickling, validated my own strong impressions that the experience and neurophysiology of trauma accounts for most of the emotional and physical symptoms related to mild to moderate motor vehicle accidents (MVAs). This book also underscored the fact that MVAs are a substantial and relatively poorly appreciated cause of societal traumatic stress. I have also learned a great deal from the writings of the many experts in the field of traumatic stress, and am very grateful to them for facilitating my travels in search of knowledge.

I could not have even approached this topic and written the first edition of the book without the dedicated help of Connie Cencich-Myers, medical librarian at Boulder Community Hospital. Her tireless assistance in my pursuit of the literature addressing the rapidly emerging field of the neurophysiology of trauma was invaluable. It allowed me to expedite my education and to formulate my own theories of trauma on a sound foundation of knowledge of the literature.

Finally, I perhaps am most grateful to my patients, whose stories, insights, and courage in the face of terrible pain have taught me a great deal of what this book is about. They have taught me that if physicians permit patients to tell them everything they have to say, then physicians are likely to know everything there is to know. The many case studies that fill the pages of this book are all true and accurate, although names have been changed throughout, and the stories modified to protect anonymity.

one
Concepts of Traumatization: The Role of Boundaries

Jane came into my office clearly in a state of distraction and fear. She had been involved in a relatively low-speed auto accident two months before, and instead of improving, she had begun to experience worsening cognitive and emotional symptoms. She had begun to misplace things frequently, had spells of severe physical weakness, had fallen several times, and had developed a stutter. At other times she felt agitated and fearful, and was intolerant of any stimulus, including noises, bright lights, and even simple conversation with family and friends. Even brief exposure to these seemingly minor stimuli produced confusion, anxiety, and ultimately exhaustion. When I examined her, she visibly jumped, and then pulled her arms tightly around herself when I walked around the back of the exam table to examine her spine. When asked, she stated that she felt extremely anxious and uncomfortable when I stood behind her out of her field of vision, even with a female chaperone in the room. Her past social history revealed that she had experienced a physically traumatic rape at age sixteen. She acknowledged that she had always been uncomfortable when she was in a crowd with people behind her whom she could not see. In a classroom, a theater, or at a party, she usually positioned herself with her back to the wall.

* * *

The benchmark for psychiatric diagnoses, the *Diagnostic and Statistical Manual of Mental Disorders, Fourth Edition* (DSM–IV), defines trauma as, "The person experienced, witnessed, or was confronted with an event or events that involved actual or threatened death or serious injury, or a threat to the physical integrity of self or others." In addition, trauma requires that "the person's responses involved intense fear, helplessness, or horror"[1] (pp. 427, 428).* In earlier editions, the DSM was more vague, defining trauma in part as "a stressful occurrence that is outside the range of usual human experience"[2] (p. 236).** The critical change in this definition is the addition to the concept of trauma that involves "threatened death or serious injury." In other words, this concept now implies that trauma is an event or experience that threatens the survival of the individual.

Examples of traumatic events that the DSM–IV lists include "military combat, violent personal assault (sexual assault, physical attack, robbery, mugging) . . . kidnapping . . . being taken hostage, terrorist attack, torture, POW, natural or man-made disasters, severe MVA's . . . life-threatening illnesses"[3] (p. 424).* For children, "developmentally inappropriate sexual experiences without violence" may be traumatic[3] (p. 424).* Actually viewing these types of traumatic events or seeing a dead body may be traumatic. Learning about these types of events occurring to a family member or close personal friend also may be defined as trauma[3] (p. 424).* When the trauma is inflicted by another person, it is especially intense, or when the traumatized person is extremely close to the trauma, the severity of the trauma and its symptoms may be especially profound.

These definitions of trauma and its causes are useful, and much more specific than earlier concepts of sources of trauma as representing "stressful events outside the usual range of human experience." However, they still do not approach the basic premise that in all cases, a traumatic experience in its intrinsic sense is one that represents a threat to the very survival of the individual. In this definition, the meaning of the experience may be as important to the traumatized person as what actually physically happens to that person.

Being kidnapped, mugged, raped, involved in warfare, or in a severe MVA are all life-threatening experiences, and therefore potentially traumatizing. Photographs of survivors of tornadoes, floods, or other natural disasters clearly reflect the shock, grief, and suffering associated with shocking and life-threatening natural events. Witnessing a graphically violent event could be perceived as shocking and traumatizing, especially if the event had personal meaning or involved another human being. Childhood trauma is perhaps the easiest to understand, given the intrinsic vulnerability of the developing child to all types of experiences. Even learning second hand about a severe traumatic event involving a loved one generally is a source of shock to a person. How all of these events may represent a threat to one's survival is less clear unless one considers the concept more carefully. We can basically say that trauma is an experience that is perceived to be a threat to life in the face of helplessness. And helplessness may in fact be the defining element that generates the neurophysiology of trauma itself.

---

* Reprinted with permission from the *Diagnostic and Statistical Manual of Mental Disorders,* Fourth Edition (DSM–IV) (Copyright 1994). American Psychiatric Association.
** Reprinted with permission from the *Diagnostic and Statistical Manual of Mental Disorders,* Third Edition (DSM–III) (Copyright 1981). American Psychiatric Association.

The Concept of Boundaries

We all live in a small and safe world of our own defined by invisible but very real perceptual barriers, or boundaries. These boundaries are formed by our collective experiences with the world around us, some of which are positive or rewarding, some negative or punishing. Negative experiences are associated with pain, which may be as obvious as physical discomfort, or as subtle as withdrawal of a reward. Perhaps one of the earliest pains that we are likely to experience is the disapproving frown of our mother to our irritating infantile behavior. The mother's negative response produces shame, and creates perhaps the first boundary in the perception of the infant-mother connection. All of our senses—smell, vision, hearing, vestibular input, taste, touch, nociception (sense of pain) and proprioception (sense of joint motion)—contribute to the formation of these boundaries that eventually tell us where we end as a perceptual entity, and where the rest of the world begins. Our unconscious awareness of these boundaries allows us to move about in the world without literally impacting obstacles that are not part of our own self. We receive positive or negative information as a developing infant and child from sensory experiences that contribute to our unconscious perception of our safe boundaries. Painful or unpleasant feedback leads us to avoid moving beyond the boundary created by that experience, whereas positive feedback stimulates us to explore the area within that expanded boundary more. This sensory feedback loop continuously helps form and reform our boundaries based on ongoing life experiences and the sensory messages associated with them. We are able to develop a very specific awareness of how safely we may challenge the world around us. This perceptual concept of our boundaries theoretically could be a significant part of our sense of self. The more positive our ongoing life experience and the more intense the associated positive sensory experience, the more solid our personal sense of boundary will become. The more solid our boundaries, the more safe, secure, and effective we will be in dealing with the world outside us. In many respects, this concept of boundary envisions a tangible, physiological, and perceptual entity.

The Role of Boundaries in Trauma

How does this discussion of esoteric and invisible boundaries relate to concepts of trauma and threats to our survival? We identify from our very beginnings those objects in our environment that are essential to our survival through the process of boundary definition. Obviously the first persons we identify with are our caregivers, particularly our mothers, through attunement between the infant and mother. We hopefully receive more rewarding experiences from these critical figures in our early childhood than we will ever again receive in our lives. We are able to expand our boundaries with our caregivers far beyond our perceived physical selves. Before the sense of shame is inevitably introduced, we are literally without a sense of boundary between our maternal caregiver and ourselves. But the early maternal-child bond is temporary, and boundaries must be formed for survival of the growing child. This is accomplished through the introduction of shame as a boundary-forming tool. Shame is usually first experienced by the infant in response to their own behavior that is felt to be excessive by the mother.[4] She signals displeasure through a negative facial expression—the "blank-faced mother"—in response to the infant's behavior, instilling in the infant its first sense of boundary definition. She then automatically restores the connection through approval with a smile and vocal reassurance. In a healthy caregiver and family environment, the growing child will experience a sense of expansive and generous boundaries. The child's sense of self may range widely and freely without risk of traumatic impact. The caregiver is always there to address the hurt, discharge the threat, and, in effect, rebuild the safe boundary. At the same time, a solid sense of where the infant indeed does impact the rest of the world is instilled in gradual ways through subtle negative maternal feedback. A strong sense of self and of safe boundaries separating us from the world around us gives us unique resilience to deal with perceived threats to survival that we inevitably experience in our daily lives. Using this concept of boundary allows us to understand why all of the relatively disparate examples of trauma in the DSM–IV have in common the specific concept of threats to survival.

Violent physical assault in any form needs no rationalization to qualify as a survival-threatening event. The sense of safe separation between the assaulted person and the real world is shattered, especially if associated with physical pain and injury. Although a life-threatening illness presents a less physically tangible assault on one's sense of self, the safe haven of our body is ruptured and redefined. Once again, witnessing a violent event involving life-threatening bodily injury or death may redefine what constitutes a safe boundary for us, may shrink that boundary, and therefore constitute a threat to our survival.

Boundaries and Childhood

A child whose boundaries are evolving, ebbing, and flowing with new life experiences is especially vulnerable to traumatic stress. We are taught from infancy by means of word, inference, or simple behavior that our sexual expression constitutes the most private and central part of our self, and therefore represents the most vulnerable zone of our boundary awareness. It is quite reasonable that "developmentally inappropriate sexual experiences without . . . violence" might still constitute a threat to survival of the vulnerable child[3] (p. 424).* In addition, the child's caregiver(s) and immediate family provide the child with his or her intrinsic sense of self, and create the child's initial sense of safe boundary with the world. Death, critical illness or injury, or even the threat of these events happening to those important individuals seen as caregivers represent to children a threat to their own existence. The meaning of those individuals to our survival

---

* Reprinted with permission from the *Diagnostic and Statistical Manual of Mental Disorders*, Fourth Edition (DSM–IV) (Copyright 1994). American Psychiatric Association.

always persists, and threats to the existence of our former caregivers remain a threat to us throughout our adulthood.

The most devastating form of traumatic stress therefore clearly occurs when caregivers, our intrinsic safe haven, the providers of our basic sense of boundaries, become the existential threat. When the maternal caregiver at times is also the raging and alcoholic abuser, when the loving father is also the source of incest, molestation, or physical/psychological abuse, there is no safe haven and no safe boundary between the child and the external world. The child's perception of self will constrict and shrink, with little residual buffer between what is perceived as a safe, bounded space and the unknowable threats of the external environment. A much smaller or less intense threat in the world outside the home may create traumatic stress for such a child when the source of the original threat has been a caregiver. In the absence of a generous boundary, the child will lose resilience and the ability to test the world, to take risks in order to establish a healthy sense of self-perception. As this child approaches adulthood, stresses and threats that might be considered trivial tend to assume the proportions of threats to survival. This compromise in boundary perception is probably the main factor in the well-known phenomenon of vulnerability to trauma in adults who have experienced abuse as children.

The next line of defense, the next presumably safe line of boundary formation, lies within the expanding network of other members of our human species. The pivotal importance of those members of our human society to maintain our safe boundary perception gradually diminishes as one moves from less immediate family members, through close friends, neighborhoods, tribes, cultures, religions, and nations. Eventually human members of other tribes, religions, or nations may represent mortal threats. Nevertheless, those members of the human species apart from our immediate caregivers whom we still perceive to be closely related to us represent a significant source of safe boundary perception. Therefore, trauma may be especially severe when inflicted by another human being. Trauma resulting from rape, assault, and torture is known to be especially devastating, probably because all of these acts represent a loss of sense of safety or boundary between individuals and members of their own species.

Defining trauma as a perceived life threat in the face of helplessness, however, opens up a host of life experiences that may be perceived as being traumatic. In addition, I would propose that regions of one's boundary, or perceptual surround, might be altered by the experience of a traumatic event. This concept implies that such an area of altered perception will be vulnerable to negative stimuli from the environment—that is, sensitive to perceived threat. The case of Jane at the beginning of this chapter is illustrious of this concept. Having been sexually attacked from behind, her perceptual boundary behind her was impaired, or ruptured, resulting in relatively benign stimuli perceived from this area causing arousal, fear, and panic. The area of the perceptual surround where a severe traumatic event occurred will predictably create a region of subliminal perceived threat that would constitute a boundary rupture. This has huge implications for trauma and its deleterious effects on emotions, and on the body itself. This will be discussed in detail in subsequent chapters.

Conclusion

From a conceptual standpoint, then, I am defining trauma, or a traumatic event, as anything that represents a threat to our survival as a human being—"threatened death or serious injury"—as defined in the DSM–IV (p. 424).* But I will maintain that the implied threat is based more on its meaning to the individual based on prior traumatic experiences than its intrinsic severity. The mechanism by which traumatic stress occurs is by impinging upon, or rupturing, that intangible but very real perceptual boundary that separates our safe sense of self from the world around us. Although this, of course, is a theoretical model, it explains why the severity of trauma is worst with experiencing, less with witnessing, and least with learning about it; in other words, the physically closer and more intimate the traumatic experience, the worse the damage. The boundary model explains why even lesser degrees of trauma inflicted by another person may be a mortal threat if that person represents a vital resource in the formation of our safe sense of self. Finally, it illustrates the reasons why trauma is most devastating when it comes from persons or events surrounding those persons who are the primary source of our safe boundary formation: our primary caregivers. We are basically left without adequate boundary perception throughout the lifespan if boundaries have not been developed in childhood. Under those circumstances, life may be perceived as a continuous fingernail scratch on a chalkboard, with a possible presence of a threat around any corner.

I specifically did not address the issue of the person's response to a traumatic event, although as we shall see, that response—whether it is to fight, flee, or freeze—is critical to how the individual's brain and body react to that trauma, and how it affects one's resulting well-being. I suggest that the experience of terror or horror in the face of a traumatic event represents a state of helplessness, which I also maintain is the pivotal state on which trauma is based. Terror and horror represent the state of impending freeze. The chemical and physical responses of the brain to trauma in a state of perceived helplessness—i.e., the freeze response—form the thesis for this book. As we will see, the concept of boundaries is also central to that thesis.

Notes

1. American Psychiatric Association: *Diagnostic and Statistical Manual of Mental Disorders*. Fourth Edition (DSM–IV). Washington, DC: American Psychiatric Association, 1994. pp. 427–428.
2. American Psychiatric Association: *Diagnostic and Statistical Manual of Mental Disorders*. Third Edition (DSM–III). Washington, DC: American Psychiatric Association, 1981. p. 136.
3. American Psychiatric Association: *Diagnostic and Statistical Manual of Mental Disorders*. Fourth Edition (DSM–IV), p. 424.
4. Schore. A: *Affect Regulation and the Origin of the Self*. Hillsdale, NJ: Lawrence Erlbaum Associates, 1994.

---

* Reprinted with permission from the *Diagnostic and Statistical Manual of Mental Disorders*, Fourth Edition (DSM–IV) (Copyright 1994). American Psychiatric Association.

two
Trauma, Instinct, and the Brain: The Fight/Flight/ Freeze Response

"When I was a kid living on the farm, I woke up one morning to a weird sound, almost like a baby crying. I went outside, and in the yard was an opossum, lying there crying and gasping for breath. He had a broken bottle around his neck that was choking him. He must have gotten it stuck around his neck when he was young, and as he grew it eventually began to choke him. So I got a towel and wrapped him in it so he wouldn't bite me, and he went limp and unconscious. I cracked the bottleneck with a hammer, unwrapped him, and he just lay there for a few minutes. Then he began to shake all over on the ground, and after about a minute, got up and staggered off."

This story was told to me by a patient who had been injured in an auto accident, and who had experienced a similar physical event, the discharge of a freeze response, that he had observed in the opossum as a child.

* * *

The Neurophysiology of Trauma

A number of theories concerning the biological response of the body to acute and chronic stress have developed over the past century. They have clarified the intricate and interrelated responses of the brain, the autonomic and hormonal system, and behavior involved in stress and trauma. Cannon presented the concept of the sympathetic-adrenal stress response, linking the role of the adrenal medulla and epinephrine to the body's adaptation to emergencies.[1] Selye introduced the theory of a general adaptation syndrome (GAS) in response to prolonged stress, characterized by three phases: alarm, resistance, and exhaustion.[2] His concept addressed not only the acute fight/flight response, but also the sustained self-protective effort of the body in the face of ongoing stress. The following text presents a simplified and abbreviated review of how the brain and body respond to such a life threat.

The brain's pathways for the acute response to a threat are primarily located in the right half of the brain (Figure 2.1). They receive messages primarily from the sensory organs located in the head related to sight, smell, taste, hearing, and vestibular sense (balance). This process of sensory scanning of the environment is called the orienting response, a physical act of side-to-side head movement that brings all of the sensory organs of the head and neck into play. These messages are then sent to the thalamus, a relay center in the middle of the brain. This sensory information is then routed by the thalamus to appropriate areas of the cerebral cortex that involve perceiving sensation and initiating movement. It is also sent by the thalamus to the limbic system (the emotional brain), particularly the amygdala, the nucleus, or center, for arousal. The amygdala is the brain's alarm system and storehouse of emotion-linked memory. It basically evaluates the emotional content of the sensory messages, particularly whether they represent danger.

Input from the sensory organs of the head and neck are also sent to the locus ceruleus, a cluster of cells in the reptilian brainstem that is the most primitive early warning system of the brain for arousal. The locus ceruleus also sends messages directly to the right amygdala through the neurotransmitter—norepinephrine—and this input ups the ante for that arousal. Olfaction (sense of smell) accesses the amygdala directly without traversing the filter of the thalamus, suggesting the role of smell as the primary message system of survival in many mammals.

The amygdala then sends information to the right hippocampus, the brain nucleus/center for processing conscious memory, where a cognitive and conscious structure for the threat-based information is first formed. The hippocampus, along with other limbic structures, also plays a role in modulating the threat response. Every brain nucleus is balanced by other modulating brain centers, a system of checks and balances routinely fine-tuning the brain's responses. The hippocampus then sends this revised information to the right orbitofrontal cortex (the OFC) for the purpose of further information and memory processing, and for further modulation of the amygdala.[3]

The OFC evaluates the threat for its severity, and either ramps up or tones down any further survival behavior through its influence on the amygdala. If the threat is meaningful, the OFC organizes physical motor defensive behavior (fight or flight) as well as autonomic and hormonal responses to this threat[4] (Figure 2.1). Another limbic system center, the anterior cingulate, also plays a role in modulating and regulating the signals sent throughout the limbic system by the amygdala. In concord with the OFC, the cingulate gyrus inhibits the amygdala if the threat is perceived as being relatively minor. As we'll see, the cingulate also shares with the OFC a role in facilitating maternal-infant and societal bonding.

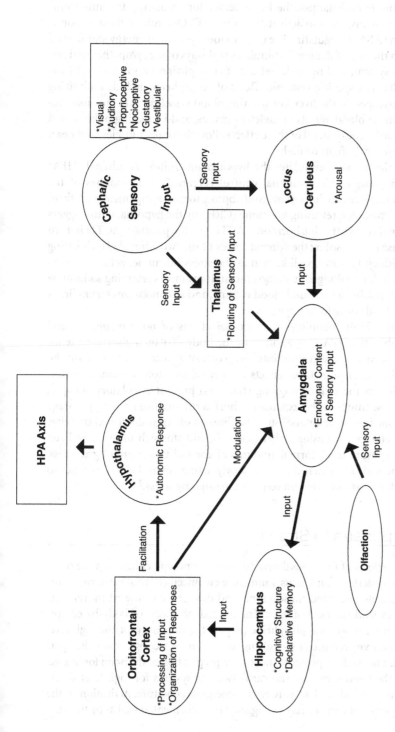

FIGURE 2.1 Theoretical diagram of pathways for arousal and memory mechanisms in the brain in response to a threat. Sensory input is transmitted directly to the brainstem locus ceruleus, and routed through the thalamus, except for olfaction, which is transmitted directly to the locus ceruleus and amygdala. Input from these information resources is routed to the right amygdala, where it is evaluated for its emotional content. Related information from the amygdala is then routed to the hippocampus, the center for declarative memory, where a cognitive structure for the information is developed. This information is then transmitted to the right orbitofrontal cortex where it is processed, and a behavioral and autonomic response to the threat is organized.

Centers in the hypothalamus, the brain center for regulating the autonomic and endocrine systems, are also activated by the OFC. One role of the autonomic nervous system (ANS) is regulating the unconscious systems of energy storage and expenditure. In the face of danger, it stimulates pathways of the sympathetic (fight/flight) nervous system, leading to the release of epinephrine, or adrenaline, by the adrenal medulla. The specific systemic effects of epinephrine include mobilizing glucose from glycogen in the liver, constricting blood vessels in skin and abdominal organs, dilating blood vessels in skeletal muscles, and increasing pulse, blood pressure, and cardiac output. All of these effects allow the brain, muscles, and heart to operate efficiently in fight or flight.

The hypothalamus also stimulates the hypothalamic/pituitary/adrenal (HPA) axis, the brain pathway for hormonal control (Figure 2.2). Hormones of the body's endocrine system are important contributors to managing threat and stress. Release of corticotrophic releasing hormone (CRH) by the hypothalamus triggers release of adrenal corticotrophic hormone (ACTH) by the pituitary. ACTH in turn facilitates release of cortisol by the adrenal cortex of the two adrenal glands sitting astride each kidney. Cortisol, well known as the stress hormone, actually acts to prepare the body for prolonged sustained threat. It promotes retaining sodium by the body, which results in increased blood volume, and also mobilizes serum lipids and increases blood sugar for energy use.

Cortisol also inhibits ongoing brain arousal effects of norepinephrine, and selectively inhibits the HPA axis, another of the body's balancing servo-systems. So although it seems a little counterintuitive, cortisol also acts as a brake on the brain's arousal mechanisms. Later effects of cortisol promote sustained cardiovascular stability in the face of ongoing stress and prevent circulatory collapse. It does all of these things at the expense of short-term sacrifice of energy storage and diffuse tissue injury, or catabolism. The diseases of stress described by Selye, including diabetes, hypertension, atherosclerosis, and stomach ulcers have been attributed to exposure to abnormal amounts of cortisol under prolonged stress. Some researchers also feel that the more slowly acting cortisol effect may act to promote avoidance conditioning in response to ongoing stress.[5]

Brain Responses to Stress

The immediate effects of the arousal neurotransmitter norepinephrine on the brain include increased alertness and focus, immediate enhancement of short-term memory, dilatated pupils, increased muscle tone, and divergence (outward movement) of the eyes to expand the field of view. The immediate effects of body-based epinephrine and brain-based norepinephrine prepare the organism for the high-level neuromuscular activity required for ensuring survival in the face of threat—the fight/flight response. These effects promote short-term preparation of the brain for intense alertness, and the neuromuscular and cardiovascular systems for high-level short-term skeletal muscle and cardiac activity and energy expenditure. Activation of the fight/flight response, of course, may be triggered by excitement as well as by threat.

Threat/Stress

Hypothalamus
[CRH, AVP]

Stimulate

Stimulate

Inhibit

Anterior Pituitary
[ACTH]

Adrenal Cortex
[Cortisol]

Modulates,
Inhibits HPA
Axis

Long-Term
Mediation

- Cardiovascular adaptation
- Increased arousal, vigilance
- Decreased vegetative function
  (Catabolism)
- Immune suppression
- Growth suppression

FIGURE 2.2 Hypothalamic/pituitary/adrenal axis. Sensory input signaling stress or threat (see Figure 2.1) activates the hypothalamus, triggering release of corticotropin-releasing hormone (CRH) and arginine vasopressin (AVP). These promote release of cortisol from the adrenal medulla. Cortisol inhibits further release of ACTH, modulates the basic noradrenergic arousal response, and mediates the long-term stress adaptation response to stress.

The basic physiological sympathetic nervous system response of the prey in response to threat is mirrored by that of the predator as it prepares for attack. Pregame jitters, stage fright, sexual arousal, and the thrill of the roller coaster ride all reflect the physical sensations associated with arousal in the face of threat. What separates the experience of the fight/flight response from that of anticipatory excitement, of course, is the meaning of the event to the participant. This piece of information processing takes place in the hippocampus (comparison of new information with past associative memories), and the orbitofrontal cortex (problem solving and planning).[4] Whether the animal or human then assumes the role of predator or prey based on this higher level cognitive process, the end result of epinephrine-based arousal is similar—the initiation of intense muscular activity and exertion. Excitatory neurotransmitters and hormones fuel both the attack of the predator and the flight of the prey, initiating a high-level energy expenditure response in both creatures.

Many species operate both as prey and predator in the pecking order of eating and being eaten throughout the animal kingdom, and mobilize epinephrine at both ends of the spectrum. Adrenaline is an equal opportunity energizer, and whether the weasel is catching a mouse, or being caught by a hawk, the initial physiological effects of both predation and flight are similar in many respects, and contribute to the function of resisting, escaping, or attacking. Very soon, however, the meaning of the arousal sequence assumes an important role in subsequent events involving the brain and hormonal systems. Mason has introduced the role of "psychological" meaning into the stress response equation, disputing Selye's avoidance of cognitive mediation of the stress response. Under Mason's concepts, a more complex interaction of cortical/hypothalamic/pituitary circuitry is involved in the stress, or flight response, and allows for a broader range of behavioral response to threat or arousal. Mason maintains that the neurological and hormonal events of predation and defense diverge and lead to quite different behavioral and physiological responses.[6]

Other brain neurotransmitter systems also contribute to the effectiveness of the fight/flight response. Norepinephrine, as we have noted, facilitates alerting mechanisms and transmission of messages throughout the brain's central sympathetic pathways. Endorphins, the brain's pain-modulating neurotransmitters, are also released, accounting for the well-documented increased pain threshold in acute arousal.[7,8] The obvious function served by endorphins includes blunting of pain reflexes and inhibition of conscious and unconscious self-protective responses that might interfere with effective survival behavior. For example, with the aid of the analgesic effects of endorphins released with fight/flight arousal, the injured soldier is able to complete the physical activity necessary for his survival without the interference of debilitating pain. The wounded prey animal is able to continue its fight/flight behavior without instinctively tending to its wounds.

Release of endorphins as part of arousal also has interesting implications concerning brain reward mechanisms in human behavior. Since arousal related to predation or excitement is also linked to endorphin release, it is easy to appreciate the reward involved in high-risk recreational activities associated with the "adrenaline rush," because this experience also involves the pleasurable reward of endorphins. Risk-taking thrills seem unique to the human species, and it is clear that certain personality traits may predispose to this kind of behavior. Some evidence suggests that this trait may be apparent in childhood. At any rate, one does not see weasels jumping into the talons of hawks just to experience the thrill of the wild ride.

Once again, the meaning of the event that triggers the relatively stereotyped initial neurological and chemical contributions to the fight/flight response likely has a marked effect on later similar behavior. Risk taking and the human element related to reward from endorphins in arousal may well contribute to the peculiar tendency for trauma reenactment in PTSD, as explored in Chapter 9.

Fighting, Fleeing, or Freezing

Animals and humans cycle in and out of varying states of arousal many times a day in response to thousands of widely varying stimuli. This cycle takes place between the *ergotropic*, or energy-spending activity of the sympathetic nervous system, and the *trophotropic*, or energy storing activity of the parasympathetic nervous system.[9] The main effects of activation of the parasympathetic nervous system, mediated by the neurotransmitter acetylcholine, include slowing of the heart, lowering the blood pressure, shunting of blood away from the muscles and to the abdominal viscera, activation of the digestive process, and storage of nutrients. It is also the state in which the acquisition of information through declarative memory, with the storage of facts and events best takes place. However, high levels of norepinephrine may interfere with certain types of memory storage,[10] resulting in declarative memory associated with high arousal being permanent, but often inaccurate. Although the parasympathetic nervous system is relatively inactivated in arousal, it does play a role in the freeze, or immobility response, the third and least understood or appreciated part of the fight/flight/freeze sequence.

The Animal Model

Those of us fascinated by animal behavior in the wild love to watch shows on TV devoted to observations of animals in this setting. Many of these TV specials relate to the prey/predator experience, and sometimes display this in graphic and even grisly detail, at least to our civilized eye. If one closely watches the details of pursuit of the prey by the predator, one will see that the fleeing prey may sometimes collapse and become limp even before being seized by the predator. An example is a film involving a gazelle pursued and run to the ground by a cheetah. At the moment that the cheetah caught the gazelle, it struck the gazelle lightly on the flank, at which point the gazelle collapsed and lay inert on the ground in the freeze or immobility response. In another example, after fighting off a pride of lions for more than half an hour, the lone water buffalo was knocked off its feet, at which point it became limp, immobile, and frozen. In other words, when fleeing and fighting are no longer physically possible, and the prey animal is in a state of helplessness, it will frequently enter the freeze, or immobility state, a totally instinctual and unconscious reflex. This reflexive behavior is common in most species including insects, reptiles, birds, and mammals. Since most such reflexes have evolved as a means of perpetuating the species, the freeze response clearly is of critical importance for survival.

In a surprising number of cases, the attack of the predator may be triggered by the instinctual response to movement of the prey rather than by hunger. In such a case, the freeze response of the prey may abort the attack of the predator and result in survival of the prey. The freeze response mimics death, sometimes fooling the predator enough to leave the scene of its "kill" and gather its offspring without delivering the tooth and claw coup de grâce, thereby allowing the prey to recover and escape, as in "playing 'possum." In addition, the freeze response, which is analogous to the state of dissociation in humans, is associated with additional release of endorphins, rendering the animal relatively analgesic. Another purpose of freeze analgesia may be to inhibit self-ministering activities, such as wound licking, which could impede escape of the prey animal in the case of arousal from the freeze.

The basic laboratory model of the freeze response utilizes the method of inescapable shock (IS).[11] Although acute IS in the previously unexposed animal initially induces a state of acute arousal and defensive postures, subsequent IS produces a consistent freeze in the face of threat, resulting in manifest, or "learned," helplessness. In escapable shock (ES), the animal will quickly discover the means of escape through trial and error, and may never experience a freeze. By definition, that option does not exist in IS, where trial and error escape techniques are to no avail. In the face of continued shock/threat in the face of helplessness, the animal will eventually freeze. Animals who have experienced IS with freezing sufficiently in the past will continue to exhibit passive immobility and continued freeze in the face of repetitive IS, even if presented with a new possibility of escape.[12] They seem to have lost their ability to problem solve and learn, not to mention to fight or flee, having faced shock in the past without means of escape. Perpetuation or frequent experiencing of the freeze response clearly creates a learned tendency to freeze in the face of even minor threat.

In addition, animals exposed to several episodes of IS linked in time with neutral stimuli will begin to exhibit freezing in the face of the neutral conditioned stimuli presented independently.[13] A freeze response triggered by a traumatic event may become linked to ambient environmental cues through conditioning. Just as Pavlov's dog "learned" to salivate to the sound of a bell if it were paired with food, so environmental cues, although intrinsically benign, may similarly serve as traumatic stimuli if they occurred at the time of a traumatic experience. Finally, attempts to break through freezing from IS by administering shock as a punishing stimulus result in relative increase in freeze behavior rather than triggering escape behavior.[14] These findings therefore suggest that repetitive exposure to IS seems to impair basic storage of memory and information. IS conditions the freeze response to benign but trauma-related cues and assures that freezing will eventually follow trauma even if escape is feasible. Comparison of these animal behaviors has led van der Kolk and colleagues to postulate that IS may be a biological model for PTSD.[15] Such observations have also led Nijenhuis, Vanderlinden, and Spinhoven to draw a parallel between animal defensive traits that are triggered by severe life threat, such as freezing, and the characteristics of dissociative states in patients with major dissociation.[16] Trauma therefore may be classified as learned helplessness.

Assumption of the immobility response is associated with a dramatic change in the state of autonomic equilibrium, along with the release of endorphins. An animal in a state of high sympathetic tone—fighting or fleeing—for a period of time at the onset of the freeze, theoretically may have an autonomic nervous system in a state of having both "accelerator and the brake on" simultaneously during the freeze. However, I believe that it is more likely that rapid and exaggerated sympathetic/parasympathetic oscillation characterizes the freeze. As you will see, this unstable autonomic state may predispose the trauma victim to many of the diseases of trauma involving the viscera—the organs of the chest and abdomen, the digestive and circulatory systems.

With onset of the freeze, the racing heart will slow to a crawl, blood pressure will drop, and tense muscles become flaccid. The bowel and bladder sphincters may relax, resulting in involuntary defecation and urination. These effects are produced by the dramatic influence of the dorsal vagal nucleus, a brain center in the reptilian hindbrain, or medulla. The dorsal vagal nucleus regulates the functions of the viscera—the organs of the chest and abdominal cavities, including the heart and the blood vessels of the body. It essentially is the engine of the parasympathetic nervous system, and enforces the body's responses not only in resting and digesting, but also in freezing.

In this state of the freeze, the focused and alert mind becomes numb and dissociated, at least in part due to high levels of endorphins. Memory access and storage are impaired, and amnesia may be expected for at least some of the events occurring during the freeze. The frozen animal—or person—is in a state of suspended animation, with high levels of parasympathetic activity and endorphins, with variable residuals of the preceding state of high sympathetic arousal.[17] This state represents a distinct departure from the usual homeostatic equilibrium between sympathetic and parasympathetic systems. In mammals, the freeze response is indeed a perilous and unstable state.

The Freeze Discharge

In most cases, the frozen prey animal does not need to deal with the relatively unhealthy state of the freeze response—it becomes another animal's meal. High levels of epinephrine and endorphins apparently do not affect taste. In some cases, however, the frozen prey animal survives the period of immobility without being killed. Subsequent events in this case are of critical importance to the thesis of this book. In virtually all such instances, at some point, the animal will arouse and begin to tremble. This may be as imperceptible as a shudder, or as dramatic as a grand mal seizure. In some cases analyzed by slow-motion video, the trembling will resemble the last act of the animal before freezing—the act of running.

The animal's behavior in what Levine has called the "freeze discharge" seems to resemble an unconscious attempt to complete the act of survival, as if the last protective motor or muscular activity is locked in unconscious procedural memory and needs to be released, or completed, perhaps as a means of "discharging" retained autonomic energy. This motor and autonomic response may persist for several minutes, and is usually terminated by a series of deep, sighing breaths, a means of "re-regulating" autonomic homeostasis. The animal at this point will usually arouse fully, regain its feet, often stagger a bit, shake itself, and then run off, apparently none the worse for its life-threatening experience. Long-term observations of such animals do not seem to show any harmful effects on behavior, health, or other measures of survival. It would appear from these observations that animals in the wild possibly possess an instinctual means of dissipating autonomic activity stored and accumulated in the freeze response.[18] Figuratively speaking, they seem to instinctually "complete" the act of escape within their unconscious memory through the freeze discharge. By this means, I feel that the discharge effectively extinguishes all of the unconscious procedural memories of what the body tried to do to escape the life-threatening event so that these body memories are relegated to past experience, and don't return to haunt them or induce another freeze whenever they experience cues to that event.

This remarkable phenomenon may occur in a much more subtle fashion, and may take place many times a day in the life of a prey animal. The gazelle may arouse to the scent of predators on many occasions, manifesting an alerting response with tensing of muscles, and with scanning movements of the head and eyes, an instinctual behavior called the orienting response common to all species. If they perceive that the threat is false, they usually then return to their calm grazing state, but usually only after a slight muscular shudder or trembling.[18] The bird that inadvertently flies into a window and is stunned will often remain immobile when picked up by the concerned homeowner and cradled in the hand. When placed on the ground, it will frequently arouse, shake, or tremble, and then fly away, having effectively discharged the stored autonomic energy of its freeze, and extinguished its arousing procedural sensorimotor memories.

A patient told me a story about saving a caged pet rabbit from a burning house. The rabbit appeared limp, unresponsive, and supposedly dead when found by the homeowner. Suddenly the rabbit "went into convulsions," after which it aroused and then appeared to be normal. What the patient interpreted as an episode of smoke inhalation in a rabbit was clearly a freeze response, with a healthy and life-affirming discharge of retained autonomic energy. This stereotyped neuromuscular reflex response in fact may have represented completion of the truncated act of flight within those parts of the brain that process and store conditioned survival-based memory.

The Human Anomaly

Very little literature addresses the freeze response in the human species. Even in the case of overwhelming threat and trauma, it is rare for a human being to actually collapse and appear unconscious without physical injury. Although some people will be shaky and tremulous after a shocking event, they seldom pursue the relatively stereotypical and involuntary physical behavior of the freeze discharge seen in animals. Rather, they will frequently relate that they felt as if they were "in shock." This is often related as a sense of detachment, numbing, and even confusion. Time often seems to stand still. Some patients report that they feel as if they are detached and removed from their body, occasionally reporting the events of the trauma as if they were seeing them as a third person—the "out of body" experience. Although some will relate that they were "full of adrenaline," many report the sensation as one of remarkable calm. Although serious injuries may have occurred, pain is usually not intense during this period, a state consistent with the role of endorphins in the freeze response. Psychologists commonly refer to these phenomena as dissociation, which is defined as "an unconscious process by which a group of mental processes is separated from the rest of the thinking processes, resulting in an independent functioning of these processes and a loss of the usual relationships, for example, a separation of affect from cognition."[19] Many researchers now feel that dissociation constitutes a major element of the freeze response, and people who report symptoms of shock and numbness after a traumatic event, and exhibit symptoms of dissociation, are actually in the freeze response at the time. In fact many of the posttraumatic symptoms that occur often for years after the unresolved trauma are characteristic of dissociation, or the recurrence of the feelings and perceptions of freezing. When cues in the environment mimic those messages related to old, severe trauma, the conditioned emergence of a failed act of self-defense may seem quite inappropriate, and has been called "conversion hysteria" by mental health professionals. We will discuss this in detail in the chapter on dissociation.

The salient point here is that human beings, at least in Western cultures, seldom go through this somatic and autonomic discharge after a traumatic event. One is tempted to consider the rarity of this phenomenon in humans as a positive adaptation to basic animal behavior as a result of the brain's evolving frontal neocortex which allows us to think, problem solve, and plan without the tyranny of primitive instinct. There is a real concern, however, that this apparent lack of physical "completion" of the traumatic experience in the human species may indeed not be a functionally adaptive mechanism. Instead, it may represent a dangerous suppression of instinctual reflex behavior, resulting in the imprinting of the traumatic experience in unconscious memory and arousal systems of the brain.

An answer to this dilemma may lie in observation of animal behavior. Levine describes a conversation that he had with African gamekeepers.[18] When they are captured, animals commonly enter a freeze, or immobility, response. After release, they will usually go through a form of reflex physical behavior typical of the freeze discharge. If they do not go through a period of shaking, however, the gamekeepers note that they will usually die after release into the wild. This fact might lead one to speculate that retaining the autonomic and procedural memories of the traumatic experience by these animals reduces their capacity to adapt to the threats and demands of existence in the wild. Basically, the freeze discharge may be a means of reversing/extinguishing fear conditioning, the prerequisite for trauma/PTSD. Clearly, self-protective skills in animals are likely to be inhibited if they are prone to experience states analogous to intermittent dissociation in humans, or if they are fear-conditioned.

In fact, evidence indicates that freeze discharge may also be inhibited in animals chronically maintained in captivity, such as domesticated and laboratory animals, as well as those imprisoned in zoos and circuses. Indeed, early studies of the stress response in laboratory animals were limited by the intrinsic arousal associated with handling them, leading to the freeze response, and subsequent "experimental neurosis." In fact, the necessity for laboratory and zoo animals to live in cages may intrinsically create learned helplessness and subsequent vulnerability to trauma.

Acculturation of the human species has resulted in an increasing pattern of urban living in closely confined habitats that intrinsically might inhibit the instinctual capability to flee or defend oneself under threat. This inhibition in turn might generate a state of helplessness, predisposing to the freeze response in humans under threat. The state of intense proximity and cultural interdependence may also act to inhibit the natural discharge of autonomic freeze energy in acculturated humans. The constraints and restrictions imposed on the populace of a complex culture by its institutions for the purpose of maintaining order may also intrinsically create a low-level state of helplessness. The suppression of the freeze discharge in humans may suggest that we also live in a cage, in our case a cultural cage. It may explain the prevalence of symptoms of trauma in complex modern cultures.

If we do not discharge or complete the freeze response, our brains will literally be fooled by environmental cues into thinking that the memories of the traumatic event that inevitably periodically re-emerge represent events that are actually in the present and not actually in the past. When they emerge, we go through all of the experiences of that event, emotional, cognitive, and autonomic as if it was actually happening again. Retention in procedural memory of this experience may serve as an internal cue for recurrent arousal patterns, alternating with numbing and dissociation, constituting the basically bipolar and self-perpetuating nature of PTSD. Until that act of flight or self-defense has been completed and its procedural memories extinguished; therefore, the "survival brain" may continue to perceive that the threat continues to exist, and is unable to relegate it to memory as a past experience. And emergence of that past memory in present consciousness is likely to trigger repeatedly the freeze/dissociation response.

Conclusion

The theory that human trauma has its roots in inhibition of the freeze discharge after surviving a mortal threat has important implications for treatment of physical and emotional disorders in victims of trauma. The neurophysiological and neurohormonal events involved in the fight/flight/freeze response clearly have profound effects on all organ systems of the body. The truncated freeze discharge appears to be the physiological event that initiates the central nervous system changes leading to post-traumatic stress disorder. I believe that the effects of the unresolved freeze response on the body and brain have important implications for concepts and treatment of human disease. Many of those chronic diseases that seem to be the most common, and which the field of allopathic medicine has been most ineffective in treating, may well have their roots in the insidious systemic effects of cumulative life trauma. In fact, I believe that the most common complaint in current medical practice, that of persistent and unexplained chronic pain, has its roots in the actual changes in brain circuitry associated with unresolved trauma. As we have noted, the patterns of defensive and protective movement at the time of a traumatic event are stored in procedural memory for the purpose of adaptation to future related threat. By the same token, the pain and other types of sensory messages associated with the same threat are also stored in conditioned procedural memory, leading to perpetuation of the pain experience as a dysfunctional survival tool.

As noted earlier, the bulk of my experience in human trauma is in MVA-related injuries, and the majority of these patients have the diagnosis of whiplash. The beauty of using the whiplash syndrome as a model for trauma is the fact that patients who have experienced this injury routinely present with a startlingly similar cluster of symptoms, many of which defy logical medical explanation. However, all of these varied symptoms involving many body systems are remarkably and logically explainable when viewed from the model of an aborted freeze discharge and its neurophysiological and behavioral implications, in the absence of tangible physical injury. Whiplash and its associated symptom complex represent a uniquely graphic depiction of the somatic consequences of trauma when viewed as a phenomenon of false procedural memory. The stereotyped and consistent replication of the sensory messages and motor responses of the body experienced in an accident are the primary symptoms of whiplash. Whiplash victims also have symptoms across the spectrum of experience—chronic somatic pain, cognitive, emotional, and neurological disability. In the face of an absent discharge/completion/extinction of these procedural memories, they will continue to emerge with any clue of the experience, involving the entire range of body sensations and motor defensive reflexes associated with the motor vehicle accident. Whiplash, as we shall see, is primarily based on trauma and procedural memory, and not primarily a physical injury.

Notes

1. Cannon, W.: The emergency function of the adrenal medulla and the major emotions. *American Journal of Physiology,* 1914; 33:356–372.
2. Selye, H.: *The Stress of Life.* New York: McGraw-Hill, 1956.
3. LeDoux. J.: *Mind and Bruin: Dialogues in Cognitive Neuroscience.* New York: Cambridge University Press, 1986.
4. van der Kolk, B.: The body keeps the score: Memory and the evolving psychobiology of posttraumatic stress. *Harvard Review of Psychiatry,* 1994; 1(5): 253–265.
5. Levine, P.: Stress. In Coles, M., Donchin, E., Porges. S. (Eds.). *Psychophysiology, Systems, Processes, and Application* (pp. 351–353). New York: Guilford Press, 1986.

6. Mason, J.: Confusion and controversy in the stress field. *Journal of Human Stress,* 1975; 1: 6–35.

7. van der Kolk, B., Greenberg, M., Orr, S., Pitman. R.: Endogenous opioids and stress-induced analgesia in post-traumatic stress disorder. *Psychopharmacological Bulletin,* 1989; 25: 108–112.

8. Pitman. R., van der Kolk, B., Orr. S., Greenberg, M.: Naloxone reversible stress-induced analgesia in post-traumatic stress disorder. *Archives of General Psychiatry,* 1990; 47: 541–547.

9. Hess. W.: *Das Zwischenhirn.* Basel, Switzerland: Schwahe, 1949.

10. McGaugh, J.: Involvement of hormonal and neuromodulatory systems in the regulation of memory storage. *Annual Review of Neuroscience,* 1989; 2: 255–287.

11. Seligman. M., Maier. S.: Failure to escape traumatic shock. *Journal of Experimental Psychology,* 1967; 74: 1–9.

12. Seligman, M.: Helplessness: On Depression, Development and Death. San Francisco: Freeman, 1975.

13. Bouton, M., Bolles, R.: Conditioned fear assessed by freezing and by the suppression of three different baselines. *Animal Learning and Behavior,* 1980; 429–434.

14. Fanselow, M., Lester, L: A functional behavioristic approach to aversively motivated behavior: Predatory imminence as a determinant of the topography of defensive behavior. In Bolles, R., Beecher, M. (Eds.). *Evolution and Learning* (pp. 185–212). Hillsdale, NJ: Lawrence Erlbaum Associates, 1988.

15. van der Kolk, B., Greenberg, M., Boyd, H., Krystal, J.: Inescapable shock, neurotransmitters and addiction to trauma: Toward a psychobiology of posttraumatic stress. *Biologic Psychiatry,* 1985; 20: 314–325.

16. Nijenhuis, E., Vanderlinden, L., Spinhoven, P.: Animal defense reactions as a model for trauma-induced dissociative reactions. *Journal of Traumatic Stress,* 1998; 11(2):243–260.

17. Gellhorn, E.: The tuning of the autonomic nervous system through the alteration of the internal environment (asphyxia). *Acta Neurologica,* 1960; 20:515–540.

18. Levine, P.: *Waking The Tiger: Healing Trauma.* Berkeley, CA: North Atlantic Press. 1997.

19. *Stedman's Medical Dictionary.* Twenty-Fourth Edition. Baltimore: Williams & Wilkins, 1982. p. 416.

three
The Whiplash Syndrome I: Symptoms in Search of a Meaning

"I dreamed last night that I was playing basketball with a pro team, and all of the players had knives strapped to their arms and legs. Pretty soon we were all cut up, and there was blood all over everyone, and all over the floor. The ball was so slippery that it kept slipping out of everyone's hands."

This was a dream related to me by a patient who had awakened during surgery in a state of complete awareness while strapped down, intubated, and paralyzed shortly after induction of anesthesia, and who remained in this state of existential helplessness throughout a ninety-minute surgical procedure. Her symptoms consisted of all of the symptoms of the whiplash syndrome described in the previous chapter, including myofascial pain, TMJ symptoms, visual impairment, vertigo, cognitive impairment, and of course, post-traumatic stress disorder.

* * *

The History of Whiplash

Recognized for over 100 years, criticized, analyzed, debated, defended, debunked, and generally misunderstood, the complex group of symptoms that follow velocity-related injuries in vehicles of conveyance continues to defy medical scientific explanation. With the advent of the railroad in the nineteenth century, a group of symptoms of chronic neck and back pain associated with severe emotional disturbance was described in association with train accidents. It was generally called "Railroad Spine," and was placed in the category of psychoneuroses.[1] With the invention of the automobile, reports of persisting neck pain after motor vehicle accidents (MVAs) began to appear as early as 1919.[2] The noted American author, Mark Twain, described the physical properties producing whiplash when he wrote about the skills of his hero, Huckleberry Finn, in beheading snakes by holding them by the tail, and snapping them like a whip.

The first use of the term "whiplash" in medicine occurred in an article in 1945.[3] In 1953, Gay and Abbott described the condition of "whiplash" in detail. They clearly stated the dilemma that has continued to plague physicians, patients, and insurance companies: "Characteristically, these patients were more disabled and remained handicapped for longer periods than was anticipated, considering the mild character of the accident."[4] Severy and colleagues further emphasized this dilemma in their 1955 study, observing, "unlike most injury-producing accidents, there is generally no visible sign of injury for the rear-end collision victim."[5] Because of this remarkable discrepancy seen in many whiplash patients, some doctors have gone to great lengths to discredit the concept that actual spinal injury could occur at speeds of 10 mph or less. Some have tested the forces of "perturbations of daily living," such as plopping into a chair, slapping on the back, and jumping off a step, and have found forces just as strong as a low velocity MVA.[6] Other physicians have considered the wide spectrum of symptoms occurring after a whiplash in addition to neck pain, and concluded that only compensation neurosis ("secondary gain") or other emotional factors could cause such a diversity of physical complaints.[7]

The Clinical Syndrome

Patients suffering from even a minor to moderate velocity rear-end MVA often suffer from a confusing variety of symptoms. Not only do they "have the typical complaints of headache and neck pain and stiffness, they also often complain of emotional symptoms, depression, and anxiety. Neurological complaints are common, ranging from dizziness and vertigo, ringing in the ears, blurred vision, fainting spells, and balance difficulties to remarkable problems with thinking, concentration, and memory. Rather than making a steady recovery like a comparable sports-related accident, whiplash patients often pursue a slow, unpredictable course. They often take several years to improve, with episodic periods of worsening that don't make sense when related to other types of soft tissue injuries. Long-term studies in whiplash patients in general show that a majority (70 to 80 percent) returned to normal activities in six months.[8,9,10] On the other hand, in other studies, persistent chronic pain has been noted in 18 percent of victims at three years[11] and up to 40 percent at eight to ten years.[12] It is understandable that certain segments of the insurance, legal, and medical communities express skepticism about the validity of many whiplash symptoms, and in fact the whole syndrome.

Physical Forces and Structural Injury

Physicians who sincerely believe the whiplash syndrome is a valid physical injury have gone to great lengths to prove it by exhaustively analyzing the forces brought to bear on the body in an MVA.[5,13,14,15] To their credit, they have shown that the forces on the head itself are three to four times greater than on the body with a sudden change in velocity due to the pendulum effect produced by the weight of the head supported by the stalk-like neck. We know that a body of mass tends to resist movement when a force is applied to it based on the laws of inertia. As a result, if a car is hit from behind and rapidly moved forward, the logical conclusion for years has been that the head will tend to resist movement, and therefore move backward in relation to the car. The head will then rebound forward as the car slows. Most whiplash patients, however, only recall the forward movement of their head.

Video re-enactment of crash dummies in whiplash surprisingly reveals that the backward and forward movement of the head is much less than was thought. The initial movement of the body is backward, as expected. However, because of relatively greater inertia of the ten-pound head, it will not move backward as quickly as the body, and will therefore assume a temporary position of forward flexion relative to the body. The initial head movement, in fact, is actually flexion of the chin, followed by the head moving up and slightly backward, followed by a rebound forward move. These studies suggest that a violent "whiplash" of the head backward and forward is probably less than was previously thought.[16] Despite this finding, the diagnosis almost always given to the neck pain after whiplash is "cervical strain." Stretching and tearing of the ligaments of the jaw joints and the posterior facet joints of the cervical spine, damage and rupture of the intervertebral discs, and compression of cervical nerve roots have all been attributed to these forces.[17,18] Acute cervical disc rupture with radiculopathy, or nerve injury, however, is a rare occurrence after whiplash, both in my experience and in the medical literature.

Other velocity-related injuries attributed to whiplash include minor traumatic brain injury with post-concussion syndrome. Shearing and tearing of axons related to rapid change in velocity of the semi-fluid brain is the generally accepted mode of damage to the brain.[19] This injury leads to a specific spectrum of cognitive symptoms, as well as vestibular (balance) and often visual complaints.[20,21] This entire spectrum of injuries has been based on theories dependent on at least a minimum force applied to the body. Despite numerous attempts at analysis, however, the complexity of automobile impacts makes accurate force determinations extremely difficult.

At impact speeds of 5 mph or less, a small cluster of patients present with the full-blown post-concussion syndrome described previously, making a justification for physical injury as a basis for the symptoms even more difficult. Perhaps the most remarkable fact is that the symptoms of the whiplash syndrome, regardless of the speed and velocity changes of the accident, are remarkably similar from patient to patient. This fact justifies the classification of whiplash as a syndrome. In fact, the remarkable experiencing of the same symptoms in thousands of whiplash victims suggests a common physiological cause, not a conspiracy to defraud the auto insurance industry.

The Pathophysiology of Whiplash

Physicians and chiropractors who believe that whiplash is a legitimate and quite real set of physical injuries generally believe that neck pain during the early period after a whiplash is due to tearing and stretching of the cervical ligaments, the tough tissues that hold bones together. Healing of ligaments and other soft tissues is generally considered to occur after about six to eight weeks based on experience in sports-related ligament tears. Other discrepancies also pose a challenge to the concept of prolonged cervical pain related to ligament injury in whiplash. The remarkably persistent pain and disability seen in many whiplash patients is seldom seen in recreational activities or sports in which the individual is subjected to velocity forces as severe as low to medium velocity MVAs.

Professional race car drivers throughout relatively long careers are usually subjected to similar forces several times in accidents involving impact, but seldom end their careers because of disabling pain. In fact, one study of demolition derby drivers who experienced an average of 52 collisions per event, with average speeds of 26 to 45 mph, showed that 80 percent experienced no neck pain whatsoever, and only 4 percent experienced neck pain longer than 3 months.[22] None experienced any of the neurological or emotional symptoms. Cervical injuries in sports involving contact, especially football, are relatively common and occasionally neurologically catastrophic. Recent studies of professional football players now show evidence in a startling number of cases of diffuse brain damage due to repetitive impacts. Chronic disabling cervical pain from ligament injuries, and neurological symptoms of post-concussion syndrome, however, are rare. Football as a sport would be impossible if persistent post-concussion syndrome, minor traumatic brain injury, cervical injury and pain occurred commonly at impact speeds or change of velocities of 5 to 10 mph.

Myofascial Pain

Much of the neck and shoulder pain persisting for six to eight weeks after a MVA is believed to be attributable to myofascial pain. Myofascial pain, of course, is a common condition found in many types of injuries, and also notably triggered by life stress. Common tension headaches are due to stress-related myofascial spasm in head and neck muscles. In fact, probably the most common cause for chronic headaches, neck, and low back pain is myofascial pain. In whiplash, it may persist for months and even years. Even after it subsides, it may recur in the same muscle groups with uncanny persistence with ordinary life stress. I have had the opportunity to follow a few patients over periods of fifteen years who experienced up to three MVAs during that time. Even after the third accident, patterns of myofascial pain, spasm, and trigger points related to the first accident continued to be prominent and apparently selective for the same group of muscles. Some practitioners of body therapy, such as chiropractors, physical therapists, and massage therapists call this "body memory."

Described by a number of researchers in the late nineteenth century and the early 1900s, myofascial pain was initially called fibrositis or myofibrositis.[23,24,25]

From its earliest descriptions, it has generally been attributed to a sudden violent strain of muscles, ligaments, or tendons, or in some cases to extended overuse of the muscle-tendon unit. Clinical features include tender areas in muscles that contain isolated taut bands of muscle fibers. One can actually feel hardness of a small area within these taut bands that is exquisitely painful. These areas of unique tenderness, when compressed, refer pain to a usually predictable distant site based on which muscle was being palpated. These painful spots were first called trigger points, and the name myofascial pain was applied to the condition in 1952.[26] Over the years, clinicians have discovered that injecting saline or a local anesthetic into these trigger points not only would consistently produce predictable referred pain to another specific area of the body, but often would "turn off" the trigger point and its associated muscle pain for variable periods of time. Autonomic characteristics of trigger points include constriction of blood vessels, sweating with increased electro-dermal response, pilomotor activity ("goose bumps"), and dermatographia (persisting redness when the skin was scratched). These findings suggest that autonomic regulation of blood vessels is distorted or impaired in the affected area, possibly leading to ischemia, or impaired circulation.

Early biopsies of trigger points reveal subtle changes in mitochondria or adenosine triphosphate (ATP) (cellular organs of energy), with mucopolysaccharide (complex sugars) deposition and sarcolemmal (muscle fiber) disruption. These findings were suggestive of deterioration of muscle fibers due to impaired blood supply, perhaps related to increased metabolic demand in the face of reduced circulation. In summary, these studies suggest the possibility of impaired circulation and altered autonomic control in the smallest blood vessels that supply nutrition to the affected muscles. Many of these findings have not been reproduced in subsequent studies, however.

Theories of causation have included, among others, an "energy crisis"[27] involving the muscle fiber, dysfunctional muscle stretch reflex fibers,[28] an abnormal attachment of spinal motor nerves,[29,30] abnormal stretch reflex nerve circuits[31] and abnormal nerve signals from movement detection nerve sensors in the muscle to the cerebellum, basal ganglia, and spinal cord.[32] In summary, these theories generally address abnormalities in the organization of motor reflexes within the spinal cord and unconscious reflex centers in the brain that control movement. These theories are guesswork at best. Myofascial pain appears to be a chronic, self-perpetuating condition that is remarkably resistant to treatment, is often regionally specific, and in some cases may last indefinitely. Many physicians believe that myofascial pain may be the most common reason for patients to seek medical attention.

Thoracic Outlet Syndrome (TOS)

With prolonged myofascial pain involving the neck and shoulders, the head will usually be pulled forward, and the shoulders protracted (drawn forward) and elevated. The patient usually is acutely aware of this posture but is unable to correct it or consciously sustain it. The resulting postural deformity results in narrowing of the space bounded by the clavicle, the scapula, and first few ribs—i.e., the thoracic outlet—leading to a postural or myofascial thoracic outlet syndrome.

The thoracic outlet is a space characterized by the hollow place on each side of the base of the neck. The brachial plexus, a bundle of nerves from the cervical spine to the arm, and the arteries and veins providing blood to the arm pass through this space. Narrowing the space would compress these structures. The softest, most compressible structures are the veins that carry cooler, deoxygenated blood back to the heart. One theory is that myofascial TOS results from relative venous congestion caused by impaired venous return to the heart caused by the head-forward posture just described. Pooling of cooler venous blood in the hands causes coolness and mild swelling of the hand, pain in the arm, and numbness of the hand due to relative hypoxia (impaired oxygen supply) to muscles and nerves of the arm. Sensory examination in these cases usually reflects mild numbness to pin prick in a "glove" distribution (involving the whole hand and fingers), suggesting the numbness is circulatory, not due to nerve injury. Since this is an intermittent phenomenon, objective documentation of impaired venous return that might indicate actual obstruction of venous blood flow has not been well documented.

Another theory attributes TOS in whiplash to myofascial involvement of the scalene muscles that form one border of the TOS. The scalene muscles attach to several of the cervical vertebrae and to the first two ribs. Shortening and spasm of the scalene muscles might not only narrow the available space for nerves and blood vessels by elevating these two ribs, but also might cause referred pain and numbness to the hand from scalene trigger points.[33] Paresthesias (tingling) of the hand in whiplash are unfortunately often confused with a cervical radiculopathy (nerve injury from a ruptured disc) or carpal tunnel syndrome. If such patients are found to have a coincidental and unrelated bulging disc on their MRI, they may be subjected to needless surgery on the assumption that the disc was compressing one of the cervical nerves. TOS is a vexing component of the whiplash syndrome that defies ready explanation.

Piriformis Syndrome

Low back myofascial pain is also common, often affecting the region of the sacroiliac joints, where the sacral base of the spine rests in a V-shaped notch in the pelvis. It also commonly affects the piriformis muscle, a muscle originating on the sacrum, and inserting on the greater tuberosity, a bony projection of the upper femur. The function of the piriformis is to externally rotate the femur, and to tighten the pelvic floor, as in the Kegel maneuver, the clenching exercise taught to strengthen the pelvic muscles after childbirth and also used to stop the stream of urine. The piriformis muscle is usually pierced by the sciatic nerve on its way from the lumbar spine through the pelvic outlet and down the back of the leg. Spasm and shortening of the piriformis muscle may compress the sciatic nerve and cause sciatica. This sciatica, unlike lumbosacral radicular (nerve-root) pain, encompasses referral patterns of both the L-5 and S-1 nerve roots, both spinal nerve segments contributing to the sciatic nerve. Conversely, a ruptured disc will usually compress only one spinal nerve.

Sciatica in piriformis syndrome is associated with numbness or tingling in the distribution of both L-5 and S-1 nerve roots, but with no motor symptoms or loss of the Achilles reflex, a finding seen when the S-1 root is damaged by a ruptured disc. Although the piriformis syndrome frequently responds to physical therapy, the patient may be at risk for an unnecessary operation if the MRI of the lumbar spine happens to show a coincidental bulging disc and the surgeon fails to detect the subtle differences between the piriformis syndrome and a disc rupture and pinched spinal nerve. A unique feature of the piriformis syndrome, seen primarily in women, is presented in Chapter 12.

Temporomandibular Joint Syndrome (TMJ)

Myofascial pain may affect the temporalis and masseter muscles of the jaw, causing jaw and tooth pain, headaches, and a feeling of congestion in the ear. Occasionally dizziness and tinnitus, or ringing in the ears may occur as well. The temporomandibular joint (TMJ) lies immediately in front of the middle ear, semicircular canals, and cochlea. The pain of TMJ often mimics an earache.

One theory relates post-whiplash TMJ dysfunction to traumatic forward dislocation of the joint disc cartilage. This might happen when the neck is hyperextended backward at the point of impact. The posteriorly attached disc ligament of the jaw could be stretched, leading to laxity and recurrent anterior disc displacement.[34,35] Bruxing, or unconscious grinding or clenching of the teeth, is a well-known symptom in whiplash-related TMJ syndrome, often leading to myofascial pain involving the muscle of mastication (chewing). Myofascial pain is probably the main source of pain that persists in whiplash-related TMJ syndrome.

Minor Traumatic Brain Injury (MTBI)

Impairment of cognition after a whiplash is usually attributed to minor traumatic brain injury (MTBI), or concussion. Documentation of the loss of consciousness formerly was a requirement to establish this diagnosis. It is now felt that any alteration of consciousness, such as stunning or confusion at the time of the injury, is adequate to diagnose MTBI in the presence of other criteria.[36] The mechanism of MTBI in whiplash is thought to be the tearing or stretching of axons (axonal shearing) as a result of relative changes in velocity of the head due to acceleration/deceleration during the movement of whiplash.[19,37] Studies have shown that actual head impact is not necessary to cause axonal shearing.[38,39] The high incidence of MTBI due to IED explosions in Iraq soldiers supports this concept. Specific cognitive symptoms seem to be fairly similar and reproducible from patient to patient.

Perhaps the most consistent area of impairment in MTBI is in speed of information processing.[39] Specific impairment in complex reaction time and also in multiple measures of divided attention[40] are usually seen. These impairments are felt to be secondary to typical primary problems with multitasking and complex attention in MTBI. Distractibility, impairment of short-term memory and inability to concentrate are common complaints.[39,41] Distraction due to ambient noise may prevent patients from engaging in conversation. They will forget events, appointments, and things they have said to other people. Frequently they will block on words, names, or items of familiar information, including over-learned material such as phone numbers and names of acquaintances. When carefully analyzed, most of their cognitive symptoms may be attributable to slowing of information processing and impaired divided or distracted attention, replicating symptoms of attention deficit disorder (ADD).

One of the most persistent and debilitating symptoms is that of profound and pervasive fatigue, both cognitive and physical. With ongoing cognitive demands, patients will "shut down," and be unable to continue with high-level or sometimes even routine cognitive activity. Usually this fatigue will begin in mid-afternoon and prevent any further activity for the rest of the day. Physical exhaustion will usually accompany this, even in the absence of physical activity. Fatigue in minor brain injury is generally combined with other diverse elements of the post-concussion syndrome, but is poorly understood.[42]

Neurological Symptoms

Neurological symptoms involving vision, hearing, and sense of balance are also common. Many whiplash patients complain of difficulty focusing their vision, especially with rapid shift of focus, or with close vision. Examination usually reveals that they have abnormal sacchadic (rapid shifts) and slow tracking movements of the eyes. Binocular dysfunction (using both eyes together) and convergence insufficiency (problems bringing the eyes together with close vision)[21] are common problems seen in whiplash. Binocular dysfunction is particularly difficult to treat. Examination reveals a definite physical impairment of bringing the eyes together with close vision. Exercises to correct it often cause nausea, headaches, and dizziness, as does the use of corrective lenses. Fluctuating monocular refractive errors (blurring in one eye) are also common. All of these findings are usually attributed to MTBI and may be associated with substantial reading difficulty.[21]

Dizziness from several possible causes is common. Patients experience light-headedness, or "head rush," when they arise quickly due to orthostatic hypotension (drop in blood pressure with standing). Vertigo with neck extension or even rotational movements of the head is common, although complaints of dizziness are usually more vague and difficult to define. This symptom has most commonly been attributed to "cervical vertigo," due to abnormal proprioceptive (movement-related) nerve input from sensory movement detectors in the cervical spine. Vertigo has also been attributed to autonomic dysfunction, with faulty regulation of blood pressure.[43] Vestibular symptoms of vertigo and balance impairment also are usually attributed to a concussion of the inner ear, a perilymphatic fistula (hole in the inner ear semicircular canal), or a displaced otolith (tiny stone in the inner ear), but also possibly a reflection of MTBI.[20,44] Tinnitus (ringing in the ears) is also common, often one-sided, and usually with normal audiograms. At times tinnitus may be attributable to one-sided TMJ syndrome, presumably related to edema, or swelling, of the joint, which lies directly in front of the balance center of the inner ear, as noted earlier.[18]

Emotional Symptoms

Finally, emotional symptoms appear in most whiplash victims. For several weeks they may feel numb or detached, but usually they eventually will experience the onset of anxiety and irritability. Anxiety often is specific to automobile travel, especially when a passenger. Actual panic attacks may appear, especially when other cars drive too closely, approach rapidly behind them, or when they drive by the scene of their accident. Visual flashbacks of the accident may be experienced. Repeated intrusive thoughts of the accident may interrupt their train of thought. They may feel jittery, tense, and hypervigilant. They may develop exaggerated startle responses to loud noises, usually after a delay of several weeks. Bright lights and loud or unpleasant noises may become intolerable and cause anxiety and "overload." Awakening at night in a state of alertness or anxiety may develop, sometimes with racing pulse and cold sweat. Nightmares of the accident may periodically awaken them. If enough of these symptoms appear, they will be diagnosed as suffering from post-traumatic stress disorder (PTSD), although many patients will have only a few of the symptoms of PTSD.[45]

As all of their symptoms persist, they may eventually develop apathy, intrusive thoughts, loss of interest in eating, decline in libido, and a sense of hopelessness, leading to a diagnosis of depression. The sleep disturbance may become one of repetitive awakening with difficulty falling back to sleep. As emotional symptoms appear, many physicians will begin to attribute most or all of their symptoms, including their persistent pain, to psychological causes.[46]

Conclusion

In this conceptual model of the whiplash injury, pain is usually attributed to injuries to ligaments and muscles, the notorious and controversial concept of "soft tissue injuries." In other types of soft tissue injuries in which muscles and ligaments are torn, the pain is immediate and severe, associated with swelling of muscles and joints and marked local tenderness. In whiplash, the severe pain usually appears after a delay of several hours, and at times the onset may be delayed for days. Rather than being constant, it fluctuates in proportion to emotional stress. Recovery in other types of soft tissue injuries may be slow, but is usually steady and predictable. In sports injuries, symptoms may fluctuate with use of the affected joint, but do not worsen with incidental life stress, as does the spinal myofascial pain of whiplash. The prolonged recovery from myofascial pain after an MVA therefore defies the usual medical explanations for soft tissue injuries that occur in other circumstances.

In this model of the physical whiplash injury, the cognitive and intellectual problems after an MVA are attributed to axonal shearing as part of a velocity-based cerebral concussion, or minor traumatic brain injury (MTBI). The entire concept of "post-concussion syndrome" includes many of the other emotional and neurological symptoms already described. These include dizziness, headache, blurred vision, irritability, and sleep disturbance. All of these symptoms are believed to be due to injury to the brain and the tissues of the head. Post-concussion syndrome, however, tends to follow MTBI much more often than more severe brain injury, in which prolonged loss of consciousness has occurred for more than twenty-four hours, with no memory of the injury, or even brain surgery. Indeed, some studies suggest that the long-term disability after six to twelve months post-accident is greater in mild concussion than in moderate brain injury where the patient does not remember the accident.[47] As with the physical symptoms, the neurological problems following a whiplash often are dramatically out of proportion to the severity of the injury, especially when compared to more severe injuries to the brain.

The broad spectrum of symptoms and disability in whiplash are simply incongruous. I therefore will discard the concept of physical and structural injuries to the spine, jaw, and brain as the model for whiplash-based injury. Instead, I will explore the concept of the whiplash syndrome as a model of trauma, with long-standing and at times permanent neurophysiological and neurochemical changes in the brain that are experience-based, rather than injury-based. In this model, these changes are triggered by a cascade of neural impulses and neurotransmitters precipitated by a continuous state of intense arousal, alternating with recurrence of the freeze response, resulting in turn from an unresolved perceived life threat in a state of relative helplessness. In short, all of the symptoms reflect the sensory experiences and motor responses of the body, stored in procedural memory and replicated over and over in the face of internal and external cues to the traumatic experience. This is a dramatic departure from the long-standing and traditional concept of whiplash as spinal injury. It presents, however, a compelling and logical theory, bringing together the diverse elements of the whiplash syndrome into a cohesive whole. It also provides a means of treating and curing the symptoms as a whole through therapy for trauma that incorporates these intolerable physical complaints in the therapeutic process.

Notes

1. Trimble, M.: *Posttraumatic Neurosis.* Chichester, England: John Wiley & Sons, 1981.
2. Marshall, H.: Neck injuries. *Boston Medical Surgical Journal,* 1919; 180:93–98.
3. Davis, A.: Injuries of the cervical spine. *JAMA,* 1945; 127:149–156.
4. Gay, J., Abbon, K.: Common whiplash injuries of the neck. *JAMA,* 1953; 152:1699.
5. Severy, D., Mathewson. J., Bechtol, C.: Controlled automobile rear-end collisions, and investigation of related engineering and medical phenomena. *Canadian Services Medical Journal,* 1955; 11:728.
6. Allen, M., Weir-Jones, I., Eng, P., Motiuk, D., Flewin, K., Goring, R., Kobetitch, R., Broadhurst, A.: Acceleration perturbations of daily living: A comparison to "whiplash." *Spine,* 1994; 19(11):1285–1290.
7. Bosworth, D.: Editorial. *Journal of Bone and Joint Surgery,* 1959; 41-A:16.
8. Radanov, P., DiStefano, G., Schindrig, A., Ballinall, P.: The role of psychosocial stress in recovery from common whiplash. *Lancet,* 1991; 338:712–715.

9. Balla, J.: Report to the Motor Accidents Board of Victoria on Whiplash Injuries. In Chapter 10, "Headache and Cervical Disorders" in Hopkins, A. (Ed.). *Headache: Problems in Diagnosis and Management* (pp. 256–269). London: Saunders, 1988.

10. Pearce, J.: Whiplash injury: A reappraisal. *Journal of Neurology and Neurosurgery,* 1989; 52:1329–1331.

11. Friedmann, L., Malin, E., Padula. P.: Biomechanics of Cervical Trauma. In Tollison, C. David, Satterthwaite, J. (Eds.). *Painful Cervical Trauma: Diagnosis and Rehabilitative Treatment of Neurosmusculoskeletal Injuries* (pp. 10–19). Baltimore: Lippincott Williams and Wilkins, 1992.

12. Packard, R., Ham, L.: Posttraumatic headache. *Journal of Neurology and Neurosurgery,* 1994; 6:119–136.

13. McNab, I.: The whiplash syndrome. *Orthopedic Clinics of North America,* 1971; 2:389–403.

14. Luo, Z., Goldsmith, W.: Reaction of a human head/neck/torso system to shock. *Journal of Biomechanics,* 1991; 24(7):499–510.

15. McConnell, W., Howark, R., Guzman, B., Bomar, J., Raddian, L., Benedict, V., Smith, H., and Hatsell, C.: Analysis of human test subject kinematic responses to low velocity rear end impacts, 1993; Society of Automotive Engineers 930899.

16. Pettersson, K., Hildingsson, C., Toolanen, S., Fagerlund, M., Bjornebrink, J.: MRI and neurology in acute whiplash trauma. *Acta Orthopedica Scandinavia,* 1994; 65:525–528.

17. Ommaya, A., Faas, F., Yarnell, P.: Whiplash injury and brain damage—an experimental study. *JAMA,* 1968; 204:285–289.

18. Veinherg, S., LaPointe, H.: Cervical extension-flexion injury (whiplash) and internal derangement of the temporomandibularloint. *Journal of Oral and Maxillofacial Surgery,* 1987: 45:653–659.

19. Wickstrom, J., Martinez, J., Rodriguez, T.: Cervical Sprain Syndrome and Experimental Acceleration Injuries of the Head and Neck. In Selzer, M., Gikas, P., Huelke, P. (Eds.). *Proceedings of Prevention of Highway Accidents Symposium* (pp. 182–187). Ann Arbor: University of Michigan, 1967.

20. Oosterveld, W., Kortschol, H., Kingma, G., de Jong, H., Saatsi, M.: Electronystagmographic findings following cervical whiplash injuries. *Acta Otolaryngol* (Stockholm), 1991; 111:201–205.

21. Roy, R.: The role of binocular stress in the post-whiplash syndrome. *American Journal of Optometry and Archives of American Academy of Optometry,* 1961; November:1–11.

22. Simotas, A., Shen, T.: Neck pain in demolition derby drivers. *Archives of Physical Medicine and Rehabilitation,* 2005; 86(4):693–696.

23. Helleday, U.: Om mysitis chronica (rheumatic). Ett bidrag till dess diagnostic och behandling. *Mord Med Ark,* 1876; 8:art 8.

24. Gowers, W.: A lecture on lumbago: Its lessons and analogues. *British Medical Journal,* 1904; 1:117–121.

25. Peritz, G.: *Med Klinik,* 1906; 2:1145.

26. Travell, J., Rinzler, S.: The myofascial genesis of pain. *Postgraduate Medicine,* 1952; 11:425–434.

27. Travell, J., Simons, D. *Myofascial Pain and Dynsfunction: The Trigger Point Manual.* Baltimore: Williams & Wilkins, 1983.

28. Simons, D.: Clinical features of myofascial trigger points. *Journal of Musculoskeletal Pain,* 1996; 4(1.2):95–121.

29. Hubbard, D.: Chronic and recurrent muscle pain: Pathophysiology and treatment and review of pharmacological studies. *Journal of Musculoskeletal Pain,* 1996; 4(1,2):123–143.

30. Hong, C., Simons, S.: Pathophysiologic and electrophysilliogic mechanisms of myofascial trigger points. *Archives of Physical Medicine and Rehabilitation,* 1993; 79:863–871.

31. Donaldson. C., Nelson, D., Schulz, R.: Disinhibition in the gamma motoneuron circuitry: A neglected mechanism for understanding myofascial pain syndrome? *Applied Psychophysiology and Biofeedback,* 1998; 23(1):43–57.

32. Elson, L.: The jolt syndrome: Muscle dysfunction following low-velocity impact. *Pain Management,* 1990; November/December:317–326.

33. Ellison, D., Wood, V.: Trauma-related thoracic outlet syndrome. *Journal of Hand Surgery,* 1994; 19B:424–426.

34. Lader, E.: Cervical trauma as a factor in the development of TMJ dysfunction and facial pain. *Journal of Craniomandibular Practice,* 1983; 1:88–90.

35. Levandoski, R.: Mandibular whiplash. Part I: An extension/flexion injury of the temporomandibular joints. *The Functional Orthodontist,* 1993; January/February:26–33.

36. Mild Traumatic Brain Injury Committee of the Interdisciplinary Special Interest Group of the American Congress of Rehabilitation Medicine. *The Journal of Head Trauma Rehabilitation,* 1993; 8:3:86–88.

37. Jane, J. A., Steward, O., Gennarelli, T.: Axonal degeneration induced by experimental noninvasive minor head injury. *Journal of Neurosurgery,* 1985; 62:96–100.

38. Povlishock, J., Becker. D., Cheng, C., Vaughan, G.: Axonal change in minor head injury. *Journal of Neuropathology and Experimental Neurology,* 1983; 42:225–242.

39. Gronwall, D., Wrightson, P.: Memory and information processing capacity after closed head injury. *Journal of Neurology, Neurosurgery and Psychiatry,* 1981; 44:889–895.

40. Stuss, D., Stethem, L., Hugenholtz, H., Picton, T., Pivik, J., Richard, M.: Reaction time after head injury: Fatigue, divided and focused attention, and consistency of performance. *Journal of Neurology, Neurosurgery and Psychiatry,* 1989; 52:742–748.

41. Gentilini, M., Nichelli, P., Schoenhuber, R., Bartolotti, P., Tonelli, L., Falasca, A., Merli, G.: Assessment of attention in mild head injury. In Levin, H., Eisenberg, H., Benton, A. (Eds.). *Mild Head Injury* (pp. 163–175). New York: Oxford University Press, 1989.

42. Binder, L.: Persisting symptoms after mild head injury: A review of the postconcussive syndrome. *Journal of Clinical and Experimental Neuropsychology,* 1986; 8:323–346.

43. Boquet, J., Moore, N., Boismare, E., Monnier, J.: Vertigo in postconcussional and migrainous patients: Implication of the autonomic nervous system. *Agressologie,* 1983; 24:235–236.

44. Glimm, R., Hemenway, W., Sebray, P., Black, E.: The perilymph fistula syndrome delined in mild head trauma. *Acta Otolaryngol* (Stockholm), 1989; 262(supplement): 1–40.

45. Blanchard, W., Hickling, E.: *After the Crash.* Washington, DC: American Psychological Association Press, 1997.

46. Miller, H.: Accident neurosis. *British Medical Journal,* 1961; 1:919–925; 992–998.

47. Alexander, M.: Neuropsychiatric correlates of persistent postconcussive syndrome. *Journal of Head Trauma Rehabilitation,* 1992; 7(2):60–69.

four
The Whiplash Syndrome II: A Model of the Brain in Trauma

At this point, we will revisit the complex and varied symptoms in whiplash from the standpoint of what happens in the brain specifically related to the sensorimotor experience in an auto accident. How does the brain organize itself in the face of all of the acute and profound messages it is receiving from the body in this situation? How does it organize this information into a conceptual whole, and then make sense of it? And finally, how does it learn and adapt to this novel and overwhelming information?

Memory Mechanisms in Trauma

Memory mechanisms play a critical role in forming the complex neurophysiological fabric of trauma. Highly emotional events are much more likely to be stored in long-term memory.[1] One usually tends to remember important life events with little difficulty. They have specific meaning to us, and are part of our autobiographical memory. Those in my generation tend to remember with vivid clarity what they were doing at the exact moment they learned that President Kennedy had been shot. The same kind of vivid memories now accompany any reminders of the tragic events of 9/11. Although memories linked to high emotional states tend to persist, but the passage of time they may be distorted by subsequent life events and may lose their accuracy. We usually remember with remarkable detail the events of our weddings, the funerals of loved ones, the greatest moments of our children's success, the news that we have a critical illness, or the vivid experience of a serious physical injury. All of these events are associated with heightened emotions, alertness, or arousal. Animal experiments reveal that they also learn certain tasks more quickly if the task is paired with an arousing stimulus instead of a neutral stimulus. A review of the role of memory in trauma would be helpful at this point.

Declarative Versus Nondeclarative Memory

Basically there are two clearly distinguishable and separate memory systems. Declarative, or explicit, memory is concerned with verbal and semantic memory for facts, events, and information—i.e., "knowing that."[2] It is conscious, intentional, and is the part that we use in acquiring information and a formal education. It contains subsystems for episodic memory related to personal experience, and semantic memory for information acquired from someone else, as in education. Reading this book and remembering some of its content involves declarative semantic memory. Damage to the hippocampus, the brain region probably most important in declarative memory, results in the inability to store new conscious information, as well as exaggerated responsiveness to environmental stimuli.[3,4] Posttraumatic amnesia is characterized by the loss of a segment of declarative memory.

Declarative memory is one of the earliest functions lost in Alzheimer's disease and other organic dementias. It is notoriously fragile and subject to decay in the absence of repetition and over-learning. If semantic declarative memory—memorizing facts—isn't used repeatedly, much of it is eventually lost. Doctors like me probably remember only a fraction of all the information they "memorized" in medical school using semantic memory. Declarative memory probably represents only a small fraction of stored memory. It is also affected and sometimes distorted by the emotional content of the associated experience, and may be notoriously inaccurate. So, although declarative memory in trauma becomes relatively permanent, it also may be distorted and inaccurate. This is clearly illustrated by the varying stories told by survivors of the same traumatic natural disaster or life event, and by the occasional change and distortion of old memories through new life experiences. Of course a highly emotional relationship to declarative memory may well distort its accuracy.

Nondeclarative, or implicit memory, is responsible for storing acquired skills, conditioned responses, and emotional associations—i.e., "knowing how."[2,5] It is unconscious, and governs much of that part of our daily activity that is automatic and instinctual, based on past experiences and training. The part of nondeclarative memory that serves skills and habits as well as conditioned sensorimotor responses is called procedural memory—i.e., related to motor procedures. We have used that term a great deal already, and will continue to do so. False procedural memory is the core of all that ails us in trauma and PTSD.

All of the motor skills that we learn and never forget are stored in procedural memory. We learn to walk, run, gain athletic skills, dance, and play musical instruments through this process. Procedural memories are readily acquired without intention, and retained forever without awareness, especially if they are linked to a coincident emotional event.[6] They are acquired and stored without the necessary involvement of conscious memory brain centers serving declarative memory, such as the hippocampus and pre-frontal cortex. Motor skill memories are stored in the motor cortex, brainstem, cerebellum, and midbrain centers such as the basal ganglia that control postural reflexes.

Another type of nondeclarative memory is unconscious conditioned responses. Conditioned responses or memories may involve the sensorimotor or autonomic nervous systems and are by definition unconscious. In Pavlov's classic experiment, the production of consistent salivation in a dog by ringing a bell after pairing the bell with feeding is linked to nondeclarative, conditioned procedural memory mechanisms. Conditioned responses of this type require reinforcement by continued pairing of the external stimuli to maintain the conditioned behavior. If the bell rings enough times without presentation of the food, the salivation response will undergo extinction and will disappear. This type of conditioning, unlike most procedural memory, is only partially permanent because of its possibility of extinction. On the other hand, many years after extinction of salivation had been accomplished in Pavlov's dogs, the conditioned response was re-established with only one or two trials.

Conditioning only occurs when survival is at stake, and therefore is never totally extinguished. If, however, the paired stimuli include a component involving high arousal or emotion, it will take fewer trials of exposure to produce the conditioned behavior, and more trials of unpaired stimuli to extinguish it. In fact, if one of the stimuli represents a life-threatening event, the conditioned response may appear after one trial and never be extinguished. Conditioned responses are therefore clearly critical to the survival of the organism. They are the substance of our survival skills. With these concepts of procedural and conditioned memory linked to arousal we can begin to reexamine the whiplash syndrome in an entirely new light.

Somatic Responses to Stress

At, or even before, the moment of impact of two automobiles, the occupants' brains undergo a predictable series of changes. Anticipation of the impact based on the presence of preceding sensory input may have a bearing on these events and the resulting symptoms. Studies to determine whether symptoms are worse in the presence or absence of a warning have had mixed results. The prevailing opinion is that any anticipation that allows the person to brace for the impact should diminish injuries. At least one study suggests that the element of surprise results in more severe injuries but the ultimate outcomes are probably similar.[7] Sensory input usually involves visual or auditory awareness of the impending crash and may have an effect on the content of subsequent memories related to the trauma. In either case, within milliseconds, the thalamus and the amygdala receive a barrage of messages from sensory organs of the head, neck, and body. The sensory messages of threat, with input from locus ceruleus through the neurotransmitter norepinephrine, will trigger the cycle of arousal through the amygdala and other pathways discussed previously. The hypothalamus and autonomic nervous system will trigger the systemic release of epinephrine (adrenaline) from the adrenal medulla, preparing the body for fight or flight.

The body's responses of the fight/flight response are of course predictable, but worth reviewing in the context of the accident itself. The eyes will widen, the pupils will dilate, and the eyes diverge (move outward) slightly in order to maximize the field of vision. The pulse, systolic blood pressure, and cardiac output will markedly increase to provide oxygen and glucose to the brain, heart, and muscles. Skeletal muscles will contract and exhibit increased tone in preparation for action or self-protection, but at the same time will be subjected to powerful forces involving stretch and torque in a variety of directions.

As the car is moved in one direction from the impact, inertia will cause the body to move in the direction of the impact. If someone shoves you from behind, your head snaps backward. Stretch receptors in muscles on the side opposite the source of impact will be activated, resulting in selective intense reflex contraction of these muscles through the spinal stretch reflex circuitry. This reflex is analogous to the "knee jerk" when you tap the patellar tendon with a hammer. As the rate of acceleration decreases, the body will then rebound forward, again activating stretch receptors on the opposite side of the body, but to a lesser degree. Based on any rotational positions of the body, torque forces will also activate varied muscle groups on both sides of the body. This will cause a complex and diffuse pattern of muscle bracing that is predictably asymmetrical and affecting different regions.

The rapid acceleration/deceleration of the head in varied directions will cause marked stimulation of vestibular (balance) receptors in the semicircular canals of the inner ears. Messages from the inner ear via the spinal cord will be sent to muscles of the body, which will further contribute to bracing patterns based on directions of movement of the head. Proprioceptive, movement-triggered messages from tightened ligaments, tendons, and stretched muscles will amplify reflex defensive holding patterns. Hands on the steering wheel and feet on brake or accelerator pedals will react defensively based on learned driving skills.

At the same time, the marked fight/flight sympathetic tone will inhibit the vegetative functions of the viscera and cardiovascular system. With the MVA victim in an acute state of fight/flight readiness, and subjected to powerful gravitational forces, the next physiological demand calls for high-level physical activity for survival. At this point the meaning of the event and the relative empowerment of the victim to pursue the physical activity of the fight/flight response become critical. The basic concept of transport in a high-speed vehicle actually becomes a profoundly important issue.

The Meaning of Speed

Vehicular Transport and Society

Although human beings have traveled in wheeled vehicles drawn by horses or other animals for centuries, the speed of travel has been generally slow, and the distances short. The advent of mechanized, relatively high-speed travel with the invention of the steam engine in the nineteenth century has had a remarkable effect on human society. Distances have shrunk, the pace of life and the amount "accomplished" in a unit of time have increased, and humans have become accustomed to the unnatural sensations of traveling at high rates of speed. Nevertheless, a person's first experience with the sensations of rapid acceleration and centrifugal force is often arousing and even frightening. Fear of flying in an airplane for the first time is common, and even repeated benign exposure to air travel does not always extinguish the fear. Amusement park rides are often terrifying before they become exhilarating. Nothing in our physiological evolution prepares us for the experience of this degree of acute and sometimes violent vestibular stimulation. Although the peculiar syndrome involving painful emotional and sensory symptoms associated with vehicular accidents has probably been around since the Roman chariots, the first apparent recorded reference to this condition probably relates to "Railroad Spine," referred to earlier.[8] During that period of the nineteenth century, this condition was believed to fall into the nebulous category of the neuroses or hysteria, and as with present-day whiplash, was predominantly observed in women.

As mechanized transport has transformed the twenty-first century world, vehicles have assumed roles and meanings far more varied and complex than simply a means of travel. This is especially true in the case of the automobile. In its century of evolution the auto has progressed from a curiosity to a sign of power and control, to a symbol of wealth and accomplishment, and to a source of thrill and exhilaration. In much of the civilized world, the automobile and its operation are considered a God-given right, and a necessity of life.

On the other hand, those individuals subjected to the forces associated with rapid mechanized transport that suddenly operate outside of the boundaries of control seldom consider the experience exhilarating. They tend to report the experience of panic or arousal in situations involving loss of control of a motor vehicle, even if a crash is averted. If a crash does occur, however, they frequently undergo an experience of numbing or shock for a period of time. As first reported in cases of "Railroad Spine," the effects of sudden high speed and unexpected changes in velocity or direction may produce distressing and long-standing symptoms in certain individuals, especially if this loss of control culminates in a crash.

Whiplash is described all over the developed world. The increasing frequency of soft tissue injuries in MVAs, the relative resistance to treatment in whiplash, and the incredible costs of their medical care suggest that some unique process is taking place when the human body is subjected to these forces in the face of a crash. Yet a paradox exists in cases of an automobile crash when the operation of the vehicle is connected with an environment of aggression, competition, or intentional risk taking, or when the driver is inebriated. As noted earlier, there seems to be no significant incidence of true whiplash syndrome in race car or demolition derby drivers involved in high-impact crashes, despite the occurrence of significant physical injuries, cerebral concussions, and life-threatening experiences. In more than 5,000 cases of whiplash that I have treated, I have never seen the whiplash syndrome in a person who is inebriated at the time of the accident. Rather, the common denominator in cases of MVAs in which whiplash syndrome develops appears to be the occurrence of the accident when the individual is in a state of fully conscious helplessness.

The Automobile as a Threat

Fortunately, most automobile drivers respect the risks associated with the operation of their car, and realize that bodily injury and death occur with distressing
frequency with their use. This appropriate sense of vulnerability admittedly seems
to be uniquely lacking during the teen years, but it does develop in most people
who eventually acquire what we define as maturity. Although automobile manu-
facturers have made admirable progress in improving the handling of cars, there
is always a fine line in their control that can easily result in an immediate state of
complete helplessness. Many drivers have experienced the sensation of loss of control at some point, and having done so, will never again feel the complete sense of
driver confidence that they did before that experience. Even a small collision will
usually be enough to change most drivers' sense of safety in a car. Obviously gender, personality, and past life experiences have a major effect on the evolution of
this sense of vulnerability. Nevertheless, for most drivers, operation of a car takes
place with very little sense of risk and helplessness.

The impact of two cars by definition triggers the fight/flight response. In
a state of helplessness, the inability to fight or flee will inevitably trigger the
freeze response, which I think occurs in a substantial number of MVA victims.
The immediate experiences of the whiplash victim are often remembered in
vague and even surreal terms. During the moments after the impact, many
patients will describe a sense of shock, confusion, and detachment, often
with no describable emotional tone. "Numbness" is the word most often used
to describe the quality of this experience. On rare occasions, the patient will
describe the sensation of being "full of adrenaline," or "shaking all over," but
an immediate feeling of arousal is uncommon. Often the memory for specific
events is vague and unclear, and details of the impact are often remembered
piecemeal or out of sequence.

Occasionally a sense of detached calm is present, and the victims may appear
remarkably rational and in control. More often, however, victims will describe
a feeling of helplessness, of being in shock or overwhelmed. Others may have a
sense of unreality. On occasion, a number of my patients have described frank
"out-of-body" experiences. Witnesses may describe victims as dazed. Attempts by
the accident victim to describe the events of the MVA at a later time will frequently
reflect the fragmented nature of their recall. Many of these experiences fall into the
category of de-realization or depersonalization, symptoms typical of dissociation
(see Chapter 7).

The Neurophysiology of Trauma in Whiplash

How then does trauma occurring in the context of an MVA explain the symptom
complex of the whiplash syndrome, involving many systems of the body? The
experience of trauma primarily involves arousal and memory mechanisms as
outlined earlier. Aberrations of memory in trauma involve both declarative and

nondeclarative memory, and are characterized by both exaggerated and impaired memory functions.[6] In many instances, victims of trauma have no memory for various events associated with the traumatic event.[6] Memory of the event itself is frequently distorted and inaccurate. Many adults who have been abused as children have no specific memory of the childhood trauma itself, and have a vague sense only of being mistreated. When memories themselves are "recovered," they often are remarkably distorted. This distortion or suppression of traumatic memories may be proportional to the severity of the freeze response, or dissociation, at the time of the trauma. Memories of the event may be quite strong, leading to involuntary resurfacing of these memories in the face of environmental triggers. This process may result in the triggering of recurrent and intrusive memories of the trauma with even nonspecific arousal, and the triggering of arousal by nonspecific events or perceptions that relate to cues of the old traumatic experience. The triggering of arousal or of traumatic memories by cues in the environment that even slightly reflect the traumatic experience is based on this conditioned response. An example is a patient of mine whose anxiety was triggered by the therapist to whom I referred her. When we explored that experience, she suddenly remembered that both the therapist and her abusive grandmother wore red nail polish.

Specific procedural memories of sensorimotor experiences arising from both current and past trauma may be blended and incorporated into this newly activated brain circuitry. Subsequent arousal may then trigger recurrence of these procedural body memories in the form of pain, dizziness, and the protective neuromuscular bracing response associated with the old MVA. If multiple similar traumatic events occur, procedural memories will be markedly reinforced as these new experiences and sensations are incorporated into the traumatic arousal/memory circuitry. Patients who have experienced many MVAs may be exquisitely sensitive to the slightest experience reminiscent of rapid, uncontrolled body movement. This process of generalization of conditioned cues that can trigger the controlled response was called irradiation by Pavlov.

Kindling and Trauma

The mechanism that imprints this self-sustaining feedback circuit may well be related to the physiological phenomenon of kindling. This term was developed from the description of spontaneous combustion of materials reaching a certain critical temperature, based on the tiny pieces of wood used to start a fire. The physiological model was developed in rats by applying a repetitive electrical stimulus to an area of the brain with a specific frequency and intensity. Each stimulus was insufficient to trigger a convulsion, but if the stimuli were applied with a critical frequency and intensity, they would summate and trigger a seizure.[9] In addition, if kindled seizures were induced in newborn rats with many repetitions, the rats would exhibit the tendency for spontaneous self-perpetuating seizures that thereafter would occur without any stimulus. In other words, these rats developed a relatively permanent change in the excitability of neuronal networks within the kindled part of their brain, and were in fact epileptic. The brain region most susceptible to kindling is to no surprise, the amygdala.

Other authors have addressed the concept of kindling as a potential physiological model for the development of PTSD.[10,11,12] Many of the clinical features of PTSD suggest the presence of exaggerated reactivity of brain circuitry, or neurosensitization. Delay in onset, change in basic characteristics, and the spontaneous worsening of memory and arousal-related symptoms are all typical of the progress of clinical PTSD. Similarly, the cognitive and somatic symptoms of whiplash often do not appear for a variable period after the MVA, and may evolve and change character over many months. One doesn't see such delays in sports-related injuries. In athletics, a neck strain hurts immediately. In whiplash, symptoms may not appear for hours or even days, the time it takes for neurosensitization/kindling to become established.

How does this basic process of kindling occur in PTSD, or for that matter, in the whiplash syndrome? I propose a model that goes back to the basic premise for the occurrence of trauma, the fight/flight/freeze response, as presented in Chapter 2. As you recall, trauma is caused by the absence or suppression of a stereotyped autonomic/somatic "discharge" after recovery from the state of freeze immobility. This discharge serves to "complete" the truncated act of defense/escape in our unconscious survival brain. It essentially erases/extinguishes the traumatic procedural memories for what the body felt, and tried, and failed, to do in self-protection. If the discharge does not occur, all of the autonomic/somatic motor and sensory experiences of the threat will be stored in procedural memory as if the traumatic event were still present, and not a past memory/experience. This intrinsic confusion of time related to internal procedural memory messages from the trauma may well explain the kindled phenomenon of PTSD, and of whiplash.

In this model, unconscious procedural traumatic memories would routinely activate the amygdala, sometimes spontaneously as in dreams and intrusive thoughts and sometimes externally through ambient environmental traumatic cues that reflect the traumatic experience. The amygdala in turn would interpret the resulting emotion-based memories as new threats, not past events. This dichotomy would trigger arousal based on the perception of a new threat from a past experience. The result would be the spectrum of memory events seen in PTSD: flashbacks, intrusive memories, cue-related memories, and nightmares. Another result would be the arousal symptoms of PTSD: anxiety, panic attacks, phobias of events and places reminiscent of the trauma, memory- and situation-induced arousal, mood changes, irritability, stimulus sensitivity, exaggerated startle, and insomnia. Under these circumstances, internal kindled connections between centers of arousal (locus ceruleus, amygdala) and memory (hippocampus, sensorimotor centers for procedural memory) may be established (see Figure 4.1). These pathways would then be increasingly mobilized by internal as well as external cues, causing worsening of clinical symptoms through irradiation. Trauma is basically a corruption of the perception of time through kindled somatic procedural memories.

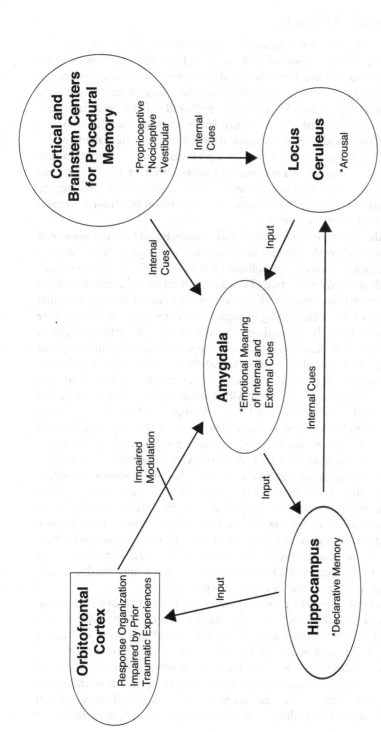

FIGURE 4.1 Theoretical model of arousal/memory kindling in post-traumatic stress disorder. Imprinting of declarative and procedural memories for the traumatic event by lack of completion of the freeze discharge leads to perpetuation of a kindled neuronal loop incorporating locus ceruleus, amygdala, hippocampus, and brainstem, and cortical centers for procedural memory. Internal memory cues, both declarative and procedural, serve to potentiate arousal. The impairment of the modulating influence of a poorly developed right orbitofrontal cortex due to prior life trauma may potentiate this process.

Cognitive Deficits in Trauma

The DSM–IV criteria for the diagnosis of PTSD do not adequately take into account the complex interaction of emotional and somatic experiences in an MVA. Blanchard and Hickling have advocated the designation of a subsyndromal form of PTSD in MVA victims.[13] Their criteria for this subsyndromal form specify inclusion of criteria for Section B (reexperiencing), and either C (avoidance), or D (hyperarousal), to establish the diagnosis. However, a remarkably prolonged freeze response, or period of posttraumatic dissociation, may mask many of the symptoms of arousal and reexperiencing for a prolonged time. This may prevent the criteria-based diagnosis of PTSD, even in a subsyndromal form. Under these circumstances, the predominant symptoms may be those of numbing, distraction, and cognitive symptoms usually attributed to a concussion or minor traumatic brain injury (MTBI) (see Chapter 3).

Even in the absence of any conceivable head trauma, PTSD has been associated with substantial cognitive deficits similar to and severe enough to make the diagnosis of a head injury on neuropsychological test batteries.[14,15] Cognitive deficits attributable only to PTSD in the face of documented traumatic events have been demonstrated in such occurrences as terrorist attacks, imprisonment, vehicular accidents, and combat-related sinking of ships.[16,17,18] These cognitive deficits have a solid theoretical base in the physical and chemical changes in the brain triggered by trauma. Trauma has been shown to interfere with declarative memory, but not nondeclarative or procedural memory. Post traumatic selective impairment of declarative memory appears to be related to the excitatory effect of norepinephrine on the amygdala. High activity within the amygdala inhibits storage and synthesis of declarative memory within the hippocampus while facilitating storage of nondeclarative and procedural memory linked to the norepinephrine-induced arousal.[19] In addition, the release of high levels of endorphins in the brain as part of the response to this arousal further interferes with declarative memory consolidation.[20] Finally, sustained high levels of cortisol have been shown to result in loss of hippocampal neurons, thereby further impairing declarative memory.[21,22,23] Trauma and the freeze response cause impaired declarative memory storage in the face of enhanced storage of trauma-related, nondeclarative procedural memory. Trauma-related memories become intrusive at the expense of conscious declarative memory, and contribute to the documented cognitive and declarative memory deficits in PTSD.[14] Trauma, in other words, impairs cognitive function that is basically indistinguishable from that caused by brain injury.

As noted, endorphins may be involved in memory dysfunction in PTSD. Stress-induced analgesia is a well-known accompaniment of severe trauma. Soldiers with severe wounds have been noted to deny the need for morphine for some time after their injuries.[24] Stress-induced analgesia is consistent with the fact that both norepinephrine and endorphins are released after exposure to severe stress. Animal studies reveal that animals unable to escape a threatening situation and which exhibit withdrawal/despair—i.e., the freeze response—suffer from significant impairment of memory.[20] In these animals, both the freeze response and panic interfered with memory processing, suggesting that both norepinephrine and endorphins contribute to this deficit. Van der Kolk has postulated that the freeze/ numbing response in animals exposed to prolonged severe and inescapable stress may be analogous to dissociation in humans exposed to trauma, and that dissociation may also be mediated by endorphins.

Traumatic memory intrusion may also contribute to the documented deficits in attention, concentration, and multitask thinking in PTSD. In addition, arousal triggered by recurrent and kindled traumatic memories induces release of norepinephrine that once again activates the memory/arousal feedback circuit as well as the hypothalamic/pituitary/adrenal axis (HPA), and sustains the cognitive deficits of PTSD. Memory deficits in whiplash therefore are more likely to be due to freeze/ dissociation than MTBI.

Trauma and Post-Concussion Syndrome

Another matter of concern in the concept of MTBI is the symptom complex commonly referred to as the post-concussion syndrome. This is a vague group of complaints that typically includes atypical headache, visual complaints usually involving blurring of vision, balance disturbance, tinnitus, dizziness and vertigo, orthostatic (going from sit to stand) light-headedness, and mood disturbances. These mood changes have been recognized to contain many of the symptoms of PTSD, and include irritability, stimulus sensitivity to noise and lights, sleep disturbance, fatigue, and depression. Researchers have begun to recognize this association between PTSD and the elements of the post-concussion syndrome.[17,25] In MVA-related concussion, all of the symptoms associated with post-concussion syndrome can be explained by the neurophysiological concept of trauma.

These sources of sensory input to the amygdala include the olfactory system (or sense of smell), the extraocular muscles that move the eyes, the vestibular balance apparatus of the inner ear and brainstem, the hearing apparatus of the inner ear, and the autonomic nervous system and its control of peripheral blood vessels. This concept will also involve procedural memory for the patterns of defensive activity of the muscles that reflexively tried to protect the victim but failed. We shall see that these permanently stored sensorimotor procedural memories will reflect in minute detail all of the perceived sensations and motor patterns of all of these systems for the entire experience. And they will describe all of the symptoms of the post-concussion syndrome.

Binocular Dysfunction

As predators, humans have eyes facing forward in the front of the head thus providing them with the binocular vision that provides precise focus on the prey animal. Prey animals have eyes on the sides of their heads, and sacrifice binocular vision to allow them to scan the environment more effectively for threat.

When involved in an MVA, we human predators revert to the status of prey because of helplessness. As we have noted, under the influence of peripheral epinephrine and brainstem norepinephrine, the eyes will diverge, or move outward, at the moment of trauma or immediate threat in order to scan the environment, and the pupils of the eyes will dilate. These changes take place by reflex activation of the extraocular muscles that move the eyes, and of the circular muscles that make up the iris of the eye and determine the size of the pupil. This response is as automatic as the stretch reflex, and serves to maximize the field of vision in the situation of threat or danger. Predators with their eyes positioned in front to focus on the prey may also face threats, and become prey. Ocular divergence in humans inevitably accompanies any arousal threat when helpless, including that of an MVA. In the event of the freeze response, ocular divergence in response to arousal when helpless is stored in procedural memory, as with all involved muscles. And ocular divergence in the human animal impairs binocular vision, causing blurring. It also causes impairment of convergence, a position required for close vision, such as reading.

If the freeze discharge does not occur, the ocular and pupillary changes triggered by traumatic arousal will be incorporated in the evolving kindled circuit between brain centers for arousal and those for procedural memory, the storehouse for motor skills and habits. Under these conditions, any arousal, whether linked to cues of the accident or even occurring in the stresses of everyday life, will likely trigger ocular divergence and pupillary dilatation, with blurring of vision. In fact, these are basically the clinical findings that have been documented in examinations of patients with post-concussion vision abnormalities. Such patients almost inevitably are found to have impaired binocular movements and convergence insufficiency representing persistent ocular divergence. In this model, however, these changes are not the result of brain injury per se, but rather the incorporation of the eye muscles in the conditioned and kindled circuit of unresolved traumatic procedural memory. I routinely tested ocular mobility in my whiplash patients, and usually noted that, as I brought my finger closer to their face, one or both eyes lost the tracking, and drifted outward, often associated with a feeling of nausea or arousal.

Vestibular and Autonomic Dysfunction

Intense forces of acceleration and deceleration in an MVA will expose the vestibular and proprioceptive sensory apparatus of the inner ears and muscles of the neck to massive sensory input, which will be stored in procedural memory. Vertigo, dizziness, and balance disturbance will thereafter be triggered by conditions of arousal or exposure to traumatic cues of the MVA, including any quick movement of the head.

This has been called "cervical vertigo." Vertigo from both the vestibular and proprioceptive systems in this model therefore represents cue-related survival-based procedural memories.

A labile and unstable autonomic nervous system is known to accompany PTSD. Unstable pulse and blood pressure responses to nonspecific arousal stimuli to sounds, pictures, or smells reminiscent of the trauma, and even to guided imagery of the trauma, have been documented in PTSD victims. Electrodermal skin response (EDR) measures increased electrical conduction in the hands as a measure of sympathetic arousal, which triggers sweat glands in the hands.[26] EDR has also been used with some success in identifying PTSD autonomic overresponders. Conditioned abnormal autonomic responses are common in PTSD and in MVAs.

Victims of PTSD are known to cycle in and out of arousal and dissociation. In the early stages after an MVA, an exaggerated sympathetic response may be prominent. I have documented many MVA patients with systolic blood pressures over 170 with no history of hypertension, and with pulses of 120 to 140 at rest. Most of these patients have been in acute arousal and anxiety, with many symptoms of the adrenaline-driven portion of PTSD. On the other hand, those patients presenting with characteristics of sustained freeze and dissociation will generally present with low systolic blood pressure, occasional bradycardia (slowed pulse), and frequent drop in blood pressure, with dizziness and even fainting. Many of these dissociated patients will also suffer from dramatic alternating constipation and diarrhea, and from symptoms of gastro-esophageal reflux disease (GERD), or irritable bowel syndrome (IBS) indicating parasympathetic, gut-based problems associated with the effect of persistent increased vagal tone related to recurrent freeze.

Autonomic instability is a secondary, conditioned phenomenon linked to the arousal/memory feedback circuit of trauma, with the numbing and the dissociation of the freeze response often associated with cholinergic (parasympathetic) symptoms. The basis for this is found in the role of selected brainstem centers for the vagus nerve, and is discussed in more detail in Chapter 8.

Neuromuscular Dysfunction and Myofascial Pain

Posttraumatic headache, cervical, and lumbosacral spinal pain are the primary symptoms related to whiplash. This pain has been attributed to injuries to muscles, tendons, ligaments, intervertebral discs, spinal facet joints, and nerve roots.[27] I maintain that the prolonged and intractable pain of whiplash is attributable primarily to the condition of myofascial pain. The relationship of myofascial pain in the whiplash syndrome to the arousal/memory link in trauma is quite analogous to the involvement of the other sensory systems that we have discussed.

At the instant of impact, selected muscles are stretched in a coordinated and synchronous pattern depending specifically on the direction of the initial acceleration of the body. This is based on the simple stretch reflex that can be elicited by tapping the knee with a rubber hammer, causing the quadriceps muscle to tighten reflexively, the knee jerk. Muscles contain spindle cell fibers that, when stretched, send signals back to the spinal cord, which then sends back messages that reflexively contract the stretched muscle. This reflex not only allows us to remain standing, but also is the basic reflex for complex patterns of motor function, including those involved in defense/survival.

At the instant of this stretch reflex, proprioceptive (sensory) input from the associated muscle-tendon units also travels to the cerebellum. Cerebellar nuclei then provide neuronal input to the thalamus, brainstem vestibular nuclei, and basal ganglia, the brain centers that coordinate complex movement patterns. These centers in turn provide reflex regulation of complex postural changes by the body in response to the original signals. These unconscious reflex pathways and their messages then create the intricately complex movement patterns of self-defense in response to the messages of the MVA experience.

In addition, input from the thalamus to the amygdala triggers assessment of the emotional content of the experience. The sudden velocity changes accompanying the MVA carry the implication of imminent life threat, and arousal via brainstem norepinephrine pathways, triggering the full-blown fight/flight response. If physiological freezing follows in the face of helplessness, the pattern of the reflexive response of the body to the velocity forces of the accident will be incorporated into procedural memory, just as will any learned motor skill. All of the sensations and movement patterns will be permanently be stored for further use by their association with high arousal and norepinephrine.[28] Finally, these self-protective movement patterns will be incorporated into the kindled arousal/memory circuitry of trauma. In other words, all of the sensory information and complex reflexive movement patterns of all of the muscles involved will be committed to procedural memory as a learned defensive skill. These memories will be for a past life threat that is often perceived as being in the present moment, but in fact is over.

Thereafter, memories of the accident, cues reminiscent of the accident, dreams of the accident, arousal related to those memories, and eventually nonspecific arousal will, like Pavlov's dog, trigger a conditioned motor response. In all these scenarios, procedural memory for regional protective muscular bracing patterns associated with the accident will emerge. Even repetitive use of those muscles that mimics the reflex defensive movements of the accident may trigger arousal and reciprocal muscle spasm. This phenomenon explains the occasional triggering of remote traumatic declarative memories by massage or other types of body therapy. It also explains how we develop certain muscles, usually in the neck or low back that we identify as our "stress" muscles. These "stress points" actually represent procedural memory for use of those muscles in a failed act of self-defense.

Muscles are designed to contract briefly on a reciprocal basis with their opponents. Involuntary sustained contraction of muscle groups sets up a condition of energy failure. This leads to an accumulation of metabolic waste products in muscle fibers, release of kinins (pain chemicals) and other chemical pain generators, and a condition of relative ischemia (impaired circulation) in the involved fibers. Finally, impaired autonomic regulation, intrinsic to trauma, may result in vasospasm (constricted blood vessels), contributing to further impaired circulation to the affected muscles. The result is regional myofascial pain perpetuated by the same kindled feedback circuitry producing the symptoms of PTSD. This theory explains the unusual autonomic and vascular changes documented in muscles involved in myofascial pain.

Those muscles of the body most commonly involved in any intense activity are the so-called core muscles of the spine, especially the low back and neck. They are activated in virtually every skilled motor activity. They also integrate the startle response, a posture of self-defense involving tensing of the spine and flexion of the hips, abdomen, and neck. One cannot operate the arms and legs without precise control of posture. I believe this instinctual pattern of muscular priority for development of myofascial pain selects for the muscles of the startle response, and explains the prominence of neck and low back pain in whiplash, and in fact in any situation associated with stress and trauma.

In one of the most unusual examples of posttraumatic procedural motor memory I have ever encountered, a case of a boy struck by lightning, was presented at a workshop on EMDR, a popular trauma therapy. The child recovered, but thereafter his previously soft hair was noted to stand straight up, especially when he was reminded of his accident. We know that the individual hair fibers each have a tiny muscle that causes them to rise up from the skin (piloerection) with exposure to cold or arousal to protect warmth, hence the appearance of "goose bumps" with cold, and the phrase "It made my hair stand on end!" with arousal. This bizarre phenomenon of piloerection of the boy's scalp hairs disappeared with two sessions of EMDR, as did his symptoms of PTSD. The erection of his scalp hairs with arousal was based on procedural memory for the response of the muscles of piloerection on his scalp that had been triggered by the trauma of the lightning strike. They were conditioned to contract and elevate the hairs on his head with subsequent minimal arousal, and this "purely physical symptom" was cured by therapy for PTSD.

Head and Neck Myofascial Pain

In any MVA, the muscles of the head, neck, and jaw are invariably the most involved in residual long-term regional myofascial pain. Whether the mechanism of the accident involves a rear-end, head-on, or rollover impact, neck pain, headache, and jaw pain usually are inevitable. In the velocity-change, whiplash model of physical injury to these structures, the cause is felt to lie in the pendular effect of the skull on the neck. The relatively heavy skull renders the neck more vulnerable to damaging forces. However, this does not explain the same cluster of painful symptoms in low-velocity accidents, or when the head and neck were not subjected to unusual forces based on the particular dynamics of the accident. It also does not explain the relative absence of permanent myofascial pain in sports and competitive driving pursuits. (Hint: sports participants and competitive drivers are functioning as predators, not prey—they tend not to freeze when injured.)

Another explanation lies in the intimate neuronal connections of the locus ceruleus with sensory end organs and especially joint proprioceptors of the head and cervical spine. These sensory receptors provide the locus ceruleus with information about environmental threat through positional orientation of the head and its sensory apparatus. The orienting reflex is a gradual side-to-side rotation of the head allowing scanning of the environment for information. It utilizes all of the sense organs of the head, and is a basic and universal instinctual motor pattern for gathering sensory information in all species. Muscles of the head and neck are therefore intimately involved in sensory information in all situations, both with regard to feeding and to fight/flight survival.

Because of their intrinsic role in survival, bracing of head and neck muscles in response to threat renders them uniquely vulnerable to the conditioned incorporation of this pattern of muscular holding in survival-based procedural memory, with subsequent persistent cervical myofascial pain. In addition, most of the muscles of the head and neck are derived from branchial arch (gill) muscles of the embryo, and originally were involved in the process of respiration, also explaining their unique role in survival.

The jaw muscles have specific importance in survival. Jaw clenching (bruxing) is a primitive reflex, with its origins based on instinctual patterns involving use of the teeth and jaw in the most basic of survival activities: alimentation (eating), and as both offensive and defensive weapons. Bruxing (jaw clenching) after an MVA is part of the nonspecific protective muscular bracing patterns linked to unresolved arousal, leading to the well-known but perplexing condition of temporomandibular joint (TMJ) syndrome. TMJ, therefore, may have nothing to do with injury in whiplash, but simply may reflect the primitive role of the jaw muscles in basic instinctual survival. This bruxing occurs mainly during sleep, a period of time in which the day's experiences are integrated during dreams with old declarative and procedural memories linked to survival for the purpose of adding to one's storehouse of survival skills. And of course bruxing at night is also a well-known symptom of nonspecific stress.

Conclusion

Clinical experience suggests that many victims involved in MVAs experience dissociation, or freezing, at the moment of the accident. Dissociation is known to be a major predictor of eventual development of PTSD, and is thought to reflect the freeze response seen in animals. The acculturated human species, unlike creatures in the wild, tends not to go through the stereotyped and instinctual neuromuscular discharge of the freeze response in the face of trauma. This instinctual defect may relate to issues of suppressing inappropriate social behavior. The absence of the freeze discharge does not allow "completion" of the thwarted act of escape in procedural memory. The survival brain is "fooled" into thinking the threat is still present. Thereafter, resurrection of these procedural memories in the face of internal and external cues to the trauma eventually result in neurosensitization, or kindling, providing the context for the symptoms of complex PTSD, especially multiple somatic symptoms.

This model provides a unitary hypothesis for the myriad symptoms of whiplash. It also provides a model for the concept of somatization, one of the more prominent co-morbid conditions seen in complex PTSD. In this model, myofascial pain is caused by inhibition of completion of the act of self-preservation through the freeze discharge after a life threatening experience. The specific distribution of the involved muscles is based on the self-protective muscular bracing response to movement patterns of the MVA, which will be stored in motor procedural memory. Those specific muscle groups will thereafter be activated to contract with any internal or external cues to the unresolved trauma. Blood circulation to those muscles will be impaired because of autonomic dysregulation intrinsic to unresolved trauma. Prolonged contraction with diminished circulation will lead to spasm/myofascial pain in the involved muscles. This hypothesis explains whiplash as a problem of altered brain memory circuits and false conditioned procedural memory, rather than injuries to muscles or other soft tissues. It also explains the frequent regional persistence of myofascial pain, and the only temporary benefit of treating the spine with manipulation or the muscles with massage or physical therapy.

Similarly, vestibular, auditory, visual, and autonomic symptoms of the post-concussion syndrome also represent somatic experiences of the MVA that are stored in procedural memory and linked to arousal circuitry within the amygdala. These symptoms will be perpetuated by any head movement reminiscent of the trauma, and also by nonspecific arousal or by declarative memory cues of the accident. For instance, many whiplash victims experience headache and neck tightening whenever they get into a car. The frequently delayed onset of symptoms in low-velocity accidents is consistent with the development of kindling. This supports my premise that all of these symptoms are based on changes in brain physiology, not structural injury.

Although MTBI may be a cause of specific and sometimes persisting cognitive deficits in victims of MVAs, cognitive impairment in the whiplash syndrome is also explainable by the attention deficit, thought intrusions, and short-term memory deficits seen in trauma and dissociation related to the traumatic experience of the accident. In very low-velocity accidents, these alterations in brain function associated with trauma are more than likely to be the primary cause for significant persisting cognitive symptoms and impairment. Whiplash, in other words, is predominantly a syndrome based on experience and the brain, rather than on injury and the tissues.

Notes

1. van der Kolk, B., van der Hart, O.: The intrusive past: The flexibility of memory and the engraving of trauma. *American Imago*, 1991; 48:425–454.

2. Roediger, H.: Implicit memory: Retention without remembering. *American Psychologist*, 1990; 45:1043–1056.

3. Squire, L., Zola-Morgan, S.: The medial temporal lobe memory system. *Science*, 1991; 253:2380–2385.

4. Altman, J., Brunner, R., Baler, S.: The hippocampus and behavioral maturation. *Behavioral Biology*, 1973; 8:557–596.

5. Duffy, C.: Implicit memory: Knowledge without awareness. *Neurology*, 1997; 49:1200–1202.

6. van der Kolk, B.: The body keeps the score: Memory and the evolving psychobiology of posttraumatic stress. *Harvard Review of Psychiatry*, 1994; 1(5):253–265.

7. Sturtzenetter, N., DiStafano, G., Radanov, B., Scilnidrig, A.: Presenting symptoms and signs after whiplash injury: The influence of accident mechanism. *Neurology*, 1994; 44:688–693.

8. Trimble, M.: *Post-traumatic Neurosis*. Chichester, England: John Wiley & Sons, 1981.

9. Goddard, G., McIntyre, D., Leetch, C.: A permanent change in brain functioning resulting from daily electrical stimulation. *Experimental Neurology*, 1969; 25:295–330.

10. Post, R., Weiss, S., Smith, M.: Sensitization and kindling: Implications for the evolving neural substrate of post-traumatic stress disorder. In Friedman, M., Charney, D., Deutch, A. (Eds.). *Neurobiological and Clinical Consequences of Stress: From Normal Adaptation to PTSD* (pp. 203–224). Philadelphia: Lippincott-Raven Publishers, 1995.

11. Miller, L.: Neurosensitization: A pathophysiological model for traumatic disability syndromes. *The Journal of Cognitive Rehabilitation*, 1997; November/December:12–23.

12. Charney, D., Deutsch, A., Krystal, J., Southwick, S., Davis, M.: Psychobiologic mechanisms of post-traumatic stress disorder. *Archives of General Psychiatry*, 1993; 50:294–305.

13. Blanchard, E., Hickling, E.: *After the Crash*. Washington, DC: American Psychological Association Press, 1997.

14. Bremner, D., Scott, T., Delaney, R., Southwick, S., Mason, L., Johnson, D., Innis, L., McCarthy, G., Charney, D.: Deficits in short-term memory in posttraumatic stress disorder. *American Journal of Psychiatry*, 1993; 150(7):1015–1019.

15. Alexander, M.: Neuropsychiatric correlates of persistent postconcussive syndrome. *Journal of Head Trauma Rehabilitation*, 1992; 7(2):60–69.

16. Gill, T., Calev, A., Greenberg, D., Kugelmas, S., Lerer, B.: Cognitive functioning in post-traumatic stress disorder. *Journal of Traumatic Stress*, 1990; 3:29–45.

17. Miller, L.: The "trauma" of head trauma: Clinical neuropsychological and forensic aspects of chemical and electrical injuries. *Journal of Cognitive Rehabilitation*, 1993; 11(4):6–18.

18. Weiner, H.: *Perturbing the Organism: The Biology of the Stressful Experience*. Chicago: University of Chicago Press, 1992.

19. McGaugh, J., Weinberger, N., Lynch, G., Granger, R.: Neural mechanisms of learning and memory: Cells, systems, and computations. *Naval Reserve Review*, 1989; 37:15–29.

20. Siegfried, B., Frischknecht, H., Nunes de Souza, T.: An ethological model for the study of activation and interaction of pain, memory, and defensive systems in the attacked mouse: Role of endogenous opioids. *Neuroscience Biobehavioral Review*, 1990; 14:481–490.

21. Sapolsky, R., Uno, H., Rebert, C., Finch, C., Hippocampal damage with prolonged glucocorticoid exposure in primates. *The Journal of Neuroscience*, 1990; 10(9):2897–2902.

22. Sapolsky, R., Packall, D., Vale, W.: Glucocorticoid toxicity in the hippocampus: In vitro demonstration. *Brain Research*, 1988; 453:367–371.

23. Uno, H., Tarara, R., Else, J., Suleman, M., Sapolsky, R.: Hippocampal damage associated with prolonged and fatal stress in primates. *The Journal of Neuroscience*, 1989; 9(5): 1705–1711.

24. Beecher, H.: Pain in men wounded in battle. *Annals of Surgery*, 1946; 123:95–105.

25. Machuda, M., Bergquist, T., Ito, V., Chew, S.: Relationship between stress, coping, and postconcussion symptoms in a healthy adult population. *Archives of Clinical Neuropsychology*, 1998; 13(5):415–424.

26. Shalev, A. Y., Rogel-Fuchs, Y.: Psychophysiology of the post-traumatic stress disorder: From sulfur fumes to behavioral genetics. *Psychosomatic Medicine*, 1993; 55:413–423.

27. Evans, R.: Some observations on whiplash injuries. *Neurologic Clinics*, 1992; 10(4):975–996.

28. LeDoux, J. E., Romanski, L., Xagoras, A.: Indelibility of subcortical emotional memories. *Journal of Cognitive Neuroscience*, 1989; 1(3):238–243.

five
Bonding, Attunement, and Concepts of Homeostasis

The Neurophysiology of Attunement and the Developing Brain

In my early medical training, I was taught that the infant brain was extremely tolerant and resilient to physical injury and emotional experiences. Because of the relative simplicity of the infant brain, we were taught that it could still develop to its full potential despite oxygen deprivation or even brain hemorrhage at birth. We never even considered that the brain might be vulnerable to impaired development because of emotional or relational deprivation. However, Bowlby in the 1980s developed the concept that attachment between mother and child dramatically shaped the child's emotional development.[1] He documented that disorders of attachment produced predictable dysfunctional behavior patterns in the affected child. Bowlby believed that the earliest bonds formed by children with their caregivers have a tremendous impact on the infant's behavioral development that continued throughout life. According to Bowlby, attachment also served to keep the infant close to the mother by reinforcing her own attachment to the infant, thereby improving the child's chances of survival. The central theme of attachment theory is that mothers who are available and responsive to their infant's needs establish a sense of security in their children. The infant "knows" that the caregiver is dependable, which creates a secure base for the child to then explore the world. Bowlby's student, Mary Ainsworth, expanded on his theories, defining attachment disorders by the reactions of infants to strange situations.[2]

Schore carried that concept further, making the case that attachment/attunement between mother and infant had a profound and measurable effect on physical brain development.[3] He grounded his concept in brain plasticity, providing a neurophysiologic model for infant brain development based on the attachment experience. Shore has assembled a vast portion of this research in both animals and humans, and has integrated it into a compelling theory of the effect of maternal-infant interaction on the structure and function of the developing brain.

Emphasizing neurophysiological aspects of infant development, Schore explored the effects of complex patterns of social interaction between infant and maternal caregiver on the infant's structural brain development. He states that this interaction between mother and infant "indelibly set(s) the stage for every aspect of an organism's internal and external functioning throughout the lifespan" (p. 3). This process takes place through the regulation of brain hormones and arousal-based neurotransmitters in the infant's developing brain through visual and touch-based maternal/infant sensory interaction. Predominance of a specific type of neurotransmitter may affect the specific structural development of areas of the infant's brain. The infant's brain chemistry is regulated by the positive, symbiotic relationship experienced through closely attuned visual interaction between infant and mother. This process stimulates the development of pathways regulating positive emotional states. Face-to-face interaction between mother and infant is actually promoting the development of new neuronal pathways in the infant's brain that are critical for long-term regulation of the emotional brain and the autonomic nervous system.

The most important brain region in this case is the right orbitofrontal cortex (OFC). The right OFC grows rapidly in the early months of life, and its relative increase in size and structure has been documented to be proportional to the effective development of the maternal-infant dyad (two-as-one). This dyadic attunement specifically stimulates the growth and neuronal development of the right OFC. The OFC, as you will recall, is specifically involved in the regulation and modulation of the limbic (emotional) brain and the autonomic nervous system. It serves as the primary regulator of the amygdala.

Schore also postulates that impairment of this maternal-infant interaction during critical periods of growth and development can produce impaired development of the infant's OFC.[3] This deficit can result in abnormal organization of neurons in this critical regulatory brain center, and results in persistent abnormal emotional and autonomic regulation. An abnormally regulated limbic system in turn may contribute to the development of psychopathological behavior patterns in adulthood.

In other words, if this process of attunement and bonding between mother and infant is impaired or disrupted, it can lead to structurally abnormal brain development in those parts of the brain that regulate our basic emotional state as well as the autonomic control of our visceral organ systems. Poor OFC development therefore is also likely to subject the poorly attuned infant to many emotional and physical diseases of adulthood. Schore notes that orphaned children who are denied an adequate experience of this brain shaping, interactive external stimulus in the early months of life fail to develop those modulating brain regions. fMRI studies in well-attuned infants demonstrate rapid growth of the right OFC in the first weeks and months of life, to the extent that it physically overlaps the left OFC. Orphaned infants demonstrate poor development, or even shrinkage of the right OFC.

In animal models, the continued survival of certain brain centers may be dependent on the repetition of appropriate experiences that stimulate those centers. Studies of the structural development of the visual cortex in immature animals suggest that specific visual input and experience may be necessary for proper growth and function. It is likely, therefore, that the developing brain is a fertile template for the growth of neuronal centers and synaptic connections formed by specific sensory input as part of complex early life experiences. We become whom we will be for better or worse during this critical period of brain development. Physicians formerly thought that the infant brain was malleable and resilient. In fact, the infant brain is exquisitely sensitive to experience and can be permanently damaged by impaired maternal attunement, bonding, and attachment. As we'll see, impaired attunement as an infant, and cumulative negative life experiences throughout childhood, may be a potent predictor of emotional and physical health throughout the lifespan.

Emotional and physical health is dependent on a steady state of autonomic regulation called homeostasis. Homeostasis is the body's maintenance of a "steady state" of function of the autonomic nervous system. Within this state, the sympathetic and parasympathetic systems alternate in a smoothly regulated fashion, sympathetic with arousal and fighting/fleeing and parasympathetic with resting and digesting. The process replicates a sine wave, the rhythmic oscillation of systems of the universe and of all of the body's systems, autonomic, hormonal, and immune. As we'll see, trauma, including impairment of attunement in the newborn infant, disrupts homeostasis, creates exaggerated autonomic oscillation, and the heritage of dysregulated emotional and autonomic nervous systems. The capacity to deal with stress and trauma through the optimal development of the OFC in infancy ensures optimal homeostasis over the lifespan unless interrupted by significant traumatic events along the way.

The Development of Character

Grigsby and Hartlaub present another model of neural plasticity in the concept of formation of character as a function of procedural learning.[4] Temperament can be defined as a primarily genetic trait, prone to generalities (inhibited vs. gregarious, sensitive vs. resilient) and persists in basic form, although shaped by experience. "Character" may be defined as the exhibition of characteristic behavior in the face of specific internal and external stimuli, and probably is developed through repeated interpersonal experiences in infancy and childhood. Character is built on the template of temperament, but is stable across the lifespan.

Procedural learning and memory, of course, refer to the processes of skill learning and conditioning—functions of non-declarative, unconscious memory. Information is acquired through this sequence unconsciously, and logically takes place through procedural memory mechanisms. We "learn" who we are through the accumulation of experiences and their positive or negative effects on us. Our subsequent behavioral responses to positive or negative life experiences reflect that learned, procedural memory. Grigsby and Hartlaub maintain that "This automatic, unconscious repeated performance of routine behaviors is the essence of character" (p. 362).

So character can basically be defined as how we consistently and unconsciously behave in response to experiences under any specific circumstance. Since character is acquired through unconscious mechanisms, people are generally not aware of most of their individual character traits. In addition, procedural memories are by nature separable from declarative memories that are by definition largely conscious. As a result, we can't determine the causes of character traits simply by logically analyzing historical events and how they impact the individual. This only provides an explanation for the behavior, not how it was acquired, and does not change the unconscious, conditioned nature of the character trait. Character, therefore, tends to remain very stable throughout life, similar to our reservoir of conditioned procedural memories related to motor and survival skills. It tends to be changeable only through specific procedural learning that is directly related to further unconsciously acquired traits. These types of traits are often acquired through intense negative life experiences.

I have emphasized that many of the clinical characteristics of trauma are associated with conditioned imprinting of sensorimotor experiences/memories through procedural memory circuits. Procedural learning associated with high negative emotional intensity—i.e., potential trauma—has the capacity to produce significant character change, illustrating the plasticity of neuronal circuits that have been relatively "hardwired" in childhood. As a result, it makes sense that treatment approaches for both dysfunctional character traits and for PTSD logically will be limited if one uses techniques involving declarative, conscious memory and verbal interaction. Treating character dysfunction as well as trauma must by definition therefore involve therapeutic techniques that approach unconscious memory through the limbic, autonomic, and somatic nervous systems. Traits acquired through traumatic experiences and basic character structure also are primarily based on classical conditioning. Appropriate therapeutic techniques therefore must include the unconscious mechanisms of extinction, quenching, or desensitization, not the use of declarative memory and words alone. This fact has great importance for therapeutic techniques for trauma, which by this definition require the extinction of somatic conditioned procedural memories.

The Polyvagal Theory

The Dorsal Vagal Complex

Stephen Porges has developed a theory that addresses the role of the vagal nuclei in the brainstem with regard to the dorsal vagal nucleus and the freeze response, but also the mammalian ventral vagal nucleus and autonomic regulation.[5] As we noted in Chapter 2, the freeze response is governed by a brain center in the medulla, or reptilian brain, called the dorsal vagal nucleus ("dorsal" implying the top of the medulla). In reptiles, the influence of the dorsal vagal nucleus allows the animal to dive under water for long periods of time without breathing to escape predators or pursue prey. It allows some reptiles, such as frogs, to hibernate under the mud for long periods, with pulses of 3 to 5 beats per minute. Reptiles are cold-blooded and don't require high oxygen utilization. The freeze response, a deep parasympathetic state governed by the dorsal vagal nucleus, is also associated with profound reduction in pulse rate, blood pressure, and breathing. The freeze response therefore can be very dangerous in mammals with their high oxygen needs.

Cannon provides insight into the role that rituals play in human physiology in his exploration of the phenomenon of voodoo death in what we consider to be primitive cultures.[6] Rituals in indigenous cultures are used both in healing ceremonies, and in protecting the tribe's close-knit bonding, a feature necessary in a dangerous natural environment. In voodoo death, a tribal member who has violated a societal taboo is subjected to a voodoo curse by the tribal shaman, or witch doctor. Taboos reflect behaviors or actions that could be harmful to the welfare of the tribe based on the fairly rigorous limits of behavior demanded by dangers inherent in their environment. Breaking such a taboo by a tribal member, depending on its severity, may lead to "boning" (pointing a sacred bone at the person) by the witch doctor. The tribal member in that circumstance will perceive that they have been cursed. As the curse progresses, the "boned" member will retire to their hut, and progressively lapse into torpor, and will eventually sink into a coma and die. The mode of death strongly suggests a state of profound vagal parasympathetic tone, analogous to the freeze response, and mediated by profound tonic influence of the dorsal vagal nucleus.

Sudden death in more advanced cultures may indeed reflect this state of helplessness, frozen by a profound approach/avoidance conflict, both sides of which are either necessary for survival, or conversely intolerable. In the tribe, this state is induced entirely by the culturally determined meaning of the rituals to which the person is exposed. Conversely, a series of rituals, or counter charm, by the shaman or medicine man may actually reverse the entire process and restore the person afflicted by the curse to health, again apparently through the meaning of the healing rituals. Voodoo death occurs based on a profound dorsal vagal parasympathetic state that basically reflects the freeze response.

Richter demonstrated the dorsal vagal role in sudden death with wild rats.[7] He trimmed their whiskers, a principal source of information from the environment. He then held them in his gloved hand until they froze. Then he placed them in a vat of water and timed how long they would swim. The wild rats with whiskers, and not exposed to the freeze response because of this means of survival-based information, swam for 60 hours, whereas the frozen rats without their whiskers sank to the bottom and drowned. The rats that survived had markedly increased pulse rates from arousal, whereas the frozen rats had markedly low heart rates, reflecting the parasympathetic, dorsal vagal nucleus influences in freeze/helplessness. Once again, the freeze in mammals is a hazardous state.

However, the other autonomic role played by the dorsal vagal nucleus is life-affirming, the role of rest, recuperation and digestion. It is the engine of much of the function of the parasympathetic nervous system—slowing the heart rate, lowering the blood pressure, dilating blood vessels of the intestines, stimulating intestinal contractions and releasing saliva and enzymes from glands for digestion, contracting the colon and bladder for excretion of wastes, and stimulating sexual organs for procreation. This role is one of energy storage and restoration. But, as so often the case, excessive activation of the dorsal vagus even in its restorative role may also produce painful over-activity of the gut and its secretions, producing what I have called diseases of the freeze response.

The dorsal vagal complex also has a sensory component—the nucleus tractus solitarius, or solitary nucleus. All of the visceral organs contain sensory receptors that warn the brain about disease, as in the "stomach ache." The intestines contain vast numbers of neurons, some of whose functions are rather obscure. Some people refer to these neurons as "the brain in the gut." When we say, "I have this gut feeling," we actually are referring to the fact that strong emotional states always are associated with "feelings"—actual sensations within the viscera, as well as the throat, that correlate with the primary emotions—apprehension, fear, terror, shame, guilt, joy, ecstasy—and so on. The brainstem nucleus where the solitary nerve connects with the brainstem not surprisingly has direct connections with the limbic/emotional brain, including all of the centers we have been discussing, and helps us define how we are "feeling" at any given time. Visceral sensations are sent to a limbic area called the insula a patch of cortex deeply embedded beneath the temporal fissure. The anterior insula receives messages from the viscera, and the posterior insula from the somatic body. As we'll see, visceral and somatic awareness is an important function in sustaining emotional well-being. The reptilian dorsal vagal complex (motor and sensory) therefore, even in the mammal, has evolved a role in the limbic functions of emotions, feelings, and memory beyond the physical freeze and the storage of nutrients.

The Ventral Vagal Complex

Mammals have evolved another brain nucleus in the medulla, the ventral vagal nucleus (VVN), which also sends nerve fibers via the vagus nerve to the heart. Its purpose is to regulate the high energy needs of mammals by providing a "brake" on initiating the fight/flight response to threat. If mammals responded with an all-out fight/flight response to every event that looked like there might be danger present, the mammal would literally be exhausted by repetitive fight/flight burn-out. This "vagal brake" serves to slow the heart rate initially in the face of threat to the mammal, releasing this "hold" if the threat is validated, thereby allowing initiation of the fight/flight response. This balancing function in mammals is the basic source of homeostasis, or maintaining optimal stable sympathetic/parasympathetic oscillation in the face of the dangers inherent in life.

Porges notes that this state can be measured in mammals by the difference in heart rate between inhalation and exhalation of breath. The heart rate normally rises with inhalation, and slows with exhalation, a state called "heart rate variability" (HRV).[5] The greater the difference in pulse rates during breathing in and out, the "healthier" the mammal is, and the better their state of homeostasis. Low HRV correlates with most of the causes of death. This ventral vagal function is significantly impaired in trauma. HRV is therefore quite low, homeostasis is disrupted, and the trauma victim is subject to many diseases, as we'll see. Because many of these diseases represent abnormal regulation and not a fixed state of diseased tissue, Western medicine has had a hard time pinning down the state of these kinds of pathologies. Because one can't measure a fixed point of the abnormality through a blood or imaging test, and because strong emotions accompany fight/flight and freeze responses, physicians usually attribute these diseases of regulation to being psychosomatic. This dichotomy will be expanded considerably in Chapter 8.

But the ventral vagal nucleus has other critical functions that intersect with homeostasis and actually interpersonal attunement. Porges calls this the "Social Engagement System."[5] The Polyvagal Theory clearly describes an incredibly complex system of functions, from the primitive reptilian freeze, to the maintenance of homeostasis through vagal brake and maintenance of optimal HRV, and to the complex process of mammalian attunement. The original name given to the ventral vagal nucleus is the nucleus ambiguus (NA). The dorsal and ventral vagal nuclei are respectively located in the top and bottom of the medulla, the reptilian brain. After they exit the skull, they are combined in a common nerve sheath.

When discovered, anatomists could not determine a defined role for the ventral vagal nucleus, thus the name nucleus ambiguus. However, Porges notes that the NA shares its evolutionary origin with many of the brainstem motor and sensory nuclei that control the head and neck. All of these brainstem nuclei, including the NA, have their origins in the developing gill arches that we all still possess as embryos. These nuclei include the origin of motor and sensory fibers that innervate the muscles of the face, jaw, throat, middle ear, larynx, and neck.

In other words, the NA has a role in facial expression, and the intense, unconscious communication that the face provides when two people are "face-to-face," as with the mother and newborn infant, the members of a family, a tribe, and a culture. Humans have far more muscles of facial expression that any other mammal. We read each other's intent, safety, and emotional state all the time through recognition of the facial expression reflecting another person's emotions.

The jaw muscles are critical to many acts of survival—attack by the predator, defense by the prey, and chewing/eating (alimentation) by all species. They are innervated by the fifth cranial nerve, another motor nucleus linked to the VA. These motor fibers, along with the facial nerve (cranial nerve VII), also innervate the tiny muscles of the middle ear that dampen the vibration of the ear drum (tensor tympani), and auditory ossicles (stapedius). But these muscles don't just protect the ear drum and inner ear by dampening loud sounds—they also are attuned to the auditory modulations of human speech, and select for the correct pitch and tone. These nuances of speech patterns are specifically social in their function, and are called "prosody," the emotional meaning attached to verbal speech. Just as with the facial muscles, prosody allows us to connect unconsciously with the emotions and intent of other humans. There is evidence that prosodic auditory dysfunction of this part of the social engagement system is prominent in autism.

Muscles of the neck, especially the sternomastoid muscles, are the generators of the orienting response, the side-to-side head movements that engage the primary senses of vision, smell, and sound. These muscles are also innervated by the pathways linked to the VA. They are the source of sensory localization of the threat in the case of the prey animal, and prey in the case of the predator. The orienting response sets up the survival brain for information from the head's sensory receptors for flight or attack. This most basic of reflexes always ushers in the act of pursuit of survival. The gill-derived muscles of the neck provide this orienting function, orienting the sensory organs of the head and neck to receive messages that promote survival.

The muscles of the pharynx, or throat, and the larynx, or voice box, contribute to swallowing and vocalization. Speech of course is also one of the primary sources of social interaction, and as with all of the other muscles of the NA, is critical to effective social engagement. Coordination of sucking (mouth, tongue), vocalizing (larynx), and swallowing (pharynx) is critical in order to prevent aspiration of food and liquids into the lungs, especially in the infant. This complex multitasking is also handled by the NA. So here we have an array of coordinated functions, derived from the mammalian vagus, not only coordinating the complex act of sucking, swallowing, and breathing critical to the newborn infant, but also the nuances of social communication throughout the lifespan.

The limbic, or emotional brain, evolved because of the need for social attunement and bonding, and conservation of energy in the evolving mammalian species. Reptiles could produce hundreds of progeny at a time, so that a reasonable number could survive and perpetuate the species. They are ready for survival after emerging from the egg, except for rapid winnowing by predators (and by the voracious mother), but require no critical numbers of species members to survive. Reptiles' energy demands are low, and they survive as predators not by pursuit, but by lurking and ambushing.

Mammals are dependent on the social cluster for hunting and self-protection. Infants develop slowly, and require total care for a time. These features demand a means of social organization and special means of communication to meet these critical needs. All of these needs are provided by the evolution of the social engagement system, which interestingly evolved in the reptilian part of the brain, but has bonded to the limbic emotional mammalian brain.

Conclusion

Whatever the climatic conditions that fostered the evolution and development of mammals, the need for contact and coordination of behavior between members of a herd, pride, flock, tribe, or other social grouping has been universal. Social grouping provides nurturing, communication, and devotion to the welfare of other members of that group within the species. Because mammals are born in a state of utter helplessness, the state of social connection is especially critical in the mother/

newborn bond. Social scientists have now recognized that this is not so much a "psychological" need, as it is a neurophysiological necessity. The brain—specifically the right orbitofrontal cortex (OFC)—is dependent on this neonatal experience to develop normally. If optimal, the OFC will modulate emotions and fight/flight arousal throughout the lifespan. We human beings desperately need this optimal brain development to live a life of physical and mental stability, a state called homeostasis. In its impairment or absence, we are condemned to a shortened life, fraught with disease and emotional disorder. The life associated with impaired infant attunement swings wildly between states of exaggerated sympathetic tone—fear, panic, anxiety, paranoia, aggression—and parasympathetic tone—terror, collapse, dissociation, and freeze. Both of these extremes are productive of most of the diseases that create vulnerability to emotional disturbances and shorten the lifespan.

We mammals, especially the human species, have also developed the capacity for achieving homeostasis, or auto-regulation, primarily through the evolution and development of the mammalian ventral vagal nucleus in the reptilian brainstem. This nucleus has developed parallel to the mammalian limbic system, and complements its function of regulating emotions and autonomic function. Because attunement is based on communication afforded by the sensory-motor systems of the head and neck, the ventral vagal nucleus operates in conjunction with these systems to facilitate that communication. These systems depend on facial expression, sound quality (prosody) of speech, visual connection, vocal intonation, and positioning of the head and neck—all products of these sensorimotor systems. At the same time, the ventral vagus modulates the cardiac response to arousal/threat, inhibiting fight/flight physiology until the serious nature of the threat has been identified, thereby providing energy conservation.

So here we have two brain centers, one in the frontal cortex, the other in the reptilian medulla, working in concert to regulate our emotions and our autonomic function. They both operate on the same principal that is dependent on our innate need to connect with other members of our human species. Contribution to homeostasis by the ventral vagal nucleus is always there for us, but is dependent on optimal function of the OFC. And development of a functional OFC is dependent on capacity of the mother/caretaker to enlist the Social Engagement System to facilitate bonding.

It will come as no surprise that most of the diagnoses of mental illness have their roots in the failure of this process. And many of the most common diseases that plague our current civilization clearly have their roots in failure of homeostasis—heart disease, hypertension, obesity, peptic ulcers, immune disorders,, and Type II diabetes. And many of the diseases that plague, but don't kill us, many called "somatization disorders"—are based on exaggerated autonomic cycling—GERDs, IBS, mitral valve prolapse, to name a few. We shall address this in Chapter 8.

Notes

1. Bowlby, J.: *Attachment and Loss, Vol. 3: Loss, Sadness and Depression*. New York: Basic Books, 1981.

2. Ainsworth, M. D. S., Blehar, M. D., Waters, E., Wall, S.: *Patterns of Attachment*. Hillsdale, NJ: Lawrence Erlbaum Associates, 1978.

3. Schore, A.: *Affect Regulation and the Origin of the Self*. Hillsdale, NJ: Lawrence Erlbaum Associates, 1994. pp. 204–209.

4. Grigsby, J., Stevens, D.: *The Neurodynamics of Personality*. New York: Guilford Press, 2001.

5. Porges, S.: *The Polovagal Theory: Neurophysiological Foundations of Emotions, Attachment, Communication and Self-Regulation*. New York: W.W. Norton & Company, Inc., 2011.

6. Cannon, W.: "Voodoo" death. *Psychosomatic Medicine*, 1957; 19:182–190. Reprinted from *American Anthropology*, 1942; 44:169.

7. Richter, C.: On the phenomenon of sudden death in animals and man. *Psychosomatic Medicine*, 1957; 19:191–198.

Negative Neuroplasticity: Does Trauma Damage the Brain?

Sandy had been injured in a rollover accident and had suffered from a long period of cognitive impairment, driving phobias, sleep disturbance, and headaches. She had received several years of treatment, both cognitive therapy for her minor traumatic brain injury, and somatically based trauma therapy, including eye movement desensitization and reprocessing (EMDR) and somatic experiencing (SE). Although she continued to experience problems with memory and speed of information processing, she had managed to complete a master's level degree during her recovery, and went on to train as a skilled SE practitioner. Her phobic and arousal symptoms had largely cleared, except for difficulties with sleep maintenance. Two years after the accident, she lost control of her car on an icy road, and ran head-on into a tree. She totally destroyed her car, and suffered multiple bruises. At the scene she immediately applied her therapeutic skills, and effectively discharged the intense shock of the accident through a period of trembling and shaking. A fellow therapist met her at the emergency room and continued to assist her in discharging the shock of the trauma. Although she experienced a predictable period of pain, anxiety, and fatigue, she never went through the prolonged and painful recovery that she had experienced after the first accident.

* * *

The concept of trauma and its effects on the central nervous system and human behavior has evolved dramatically throughout the history of psychiatry. Theories of causation have fluctuated radically from psychological to physiological, from chemical brain alterations to impairment of willpower, from issues of secondary gain, to malingering. The frequent shifts in bias and emphasis often have reflected the basic societal trends of the time. They have also been influenced by the culture or country represented by the most influential psychiatric theoreticians during that particular period. The recurring theme in this history of trauma has been the systematic denial of the validity of symptoms in trauma victims, especially those associated with warfare. Societies as a whole have had difficulty accepting the concept that their members can be severely and permanently damaged by negative life experiences. A fascinating and comprehensive review of the history of the concept of trauma in psychiatry may be found in van der Kolk, Weisaeth, and van der Hart.[1] A brief review of this history will serve as a background to the exciting and relatively recent reemergence of research into the neurophysiological bases for trauma, and the development of the theory of post-traumatic stress disorder (PTSD) as a permanent change in brain physiology and structure.

The History of Post-Traumatic Stress Disorder in Psychiatry

The fields of neurology and psychiatry evolved from a single discipline in the latter part of the nineteenth century, with the earlier clinicians in these specialties dealing with both physical diseases of the central nervous systems and diseases of the emotions, or neuroses. Although theories of hysteria had emerged in prior decades, much of the important early work in this area took place in the Salpetriere Hospital in Paris. There the neurologist Jean-Martin Charcot and his student, the psychologist Pierre Janet, first recognized that patients with hysteria appeared to have the basis for their symptoms in histories of childhood trauma.

Charcot first identified the association of hysteria with the phenomenon of dissociation, although he approached the concept from a purely neurological point of view, considering it a hereditary degenerative process.[2] Janet expanded the concepts of dissociation in trauma and postulated that intense emotional experience interfered with integration of memory into awareness.[3] He believed that these emotional experiences caused memories associated with them to be split off, or dissociated, from consciousness and to be stored instead as physical sensations of arousal and panic or as visual memories, such as flashbacks or nightmares. He also felt that subsequent efforts to keep these memories out of consciousness led to a gradual disintegration in personal functioning.[4] Thus, he introduced the roles of dissociation and memory into the concept of trauma and addressed the potentially permanent and progressive nature of the disorder.

The Austrian neuropsychiatrist, Sigmund Freud, and his mentor, Joseph Breuer, adopted many of these concepts from the Salpetriere in early papers, and initially acknowledged the association of conversion hysteria with childhood sexual abuse.[5] When Freud presented these findings and opinions to his Viennese colleagues, however, he was met with a storm of criticism, reflecting the cultural rigidity of his

Victorian times and the unwillingness of the psychiatric community to acknowledge the pervasiveness of child abuse in existing middle-class society.[6]

As Freud developed his theory of psychoanalysis around the premise of repressed infantile sexuality, he progressively abandoned the concept of trauma as a physiological disturbance of memory associated with dissociation. Instead, he related hysteria to active repression of the sexual and aggressive fantasies of the Oedipal complex with the mother, and denied the validity of reports of childhood sexual abuse in his hysterical patients.[7] He basically validated the perpetrators, abandoned his incest victims, and turned the blame onto their childhood sexuality. The almost universal acceptance of psychoanalytic theory by the field of psychiatry resulted in the almost total rejection of the effect of child abuse and trauma on personality development, character traits, and psychiatric illness for almost eighty years.

World War I ushered in a new manifestation if hysteria in the form of the unique diagnosis of shell shock. Soldiers in the trenches of France would often be found paralyzed after a shell bombardment, their posture locked and frozen in the position of self-defense they had assumed. Dramatic motor and sensory disorders in shell shock reflected in many ways the behavior of Charcot's patients in the Salpetriere. Ferenczi, a contemporary of Freud, noted that a "tic" represented an "over-strong memory fixation on the attitude of the body at the moment of . . . trauma." He of course was implying that repetitive, stereotyped movement patterns in shell shock—or for that matter, in Freud's patients with conversion hysteria—reflected procedural memories for aborted physical acts of self-defense.

Although the two world wars brought back to reality the fact that overwhelming life trauma resulted in profound emotional dysfunction, sporadic attempts to relate this association in a clinical setting were overwhelmed by the prevailing concepts of psychoanalytic theory. An exception was the work of Abram Kardiner (1891–1981), a psychoanalyst who attempted to restructure his theories of war neurosis based on his observations of the pervasive hypervigilance and sensitivity to environmental stimuli of his patients. He actually introduced the concept of a physioneurosis related to trauma exposure, and commented on the progressive nature of the syndrome in many of his patients.[8] Kardiner documented many of the peculiar maladaptive traits of trauma victims that would later be incorporated into current definitions of PTSD. World War II afforded the opportunity to study trauma in soldiers and concentration camp inmates. These studies in general documented the catastrophic effects of severe trauma on subsequent general health, and on the capacity to tolerate stress in later life.[9,10] Many of the post-war clinical investigators who studied these effects of trauma had themselves been part of wartime or concentration camp experiences.[1] Unfortunately, the members of the "greatest generation" were soon abandoned once again, and left to cope with their nightmares and depression. The incidence of alcoholism and many of the diseases of stress and trauma among this group of soldiers bears witness to their sacrifice.

The Vietnam War resulted in another resurgence of interest in the effects of traumatic stress. This in turn rekindled interest in the work of Kardiner, and in 1980 led to an attempt to compile a list of symptoms related to trauma from the existing literature into a unitary syndrome. The new name for this syndrome was post-traumatic stress disorder, and it was included for the first time in the *Diagnostic and Statistical Manual of Mental Disorders, Third Edition* (DSM–III). At the same time, attention was finally given to the previously ignored and relatively vast population of traumatized women and children.[11,12] Revisions of the definition of PTSD in the DSM (DSM–III–R, 1987; and DSM–IV, 1994) have continued to clarify and focus the epidemiology and clinical features of PTSD, but still have not completely defined the symptom of dissociation as specifically related to traumatic stress (see Chapter 7).

Since 1980, there has been an explosion of interest and research into the effects of trauma on the human brain and psyche, with the establishment of numerous journals and the publication of many books solely devoted to the study of human traumatic stress. Particularly noteworthy has been the increasing emphasis on the chemical, humoral, and physiological changes in the brain produced by the experience of trauma and the resulting breakdown of the separation of psychological and biological processes in mental illness. Physiological and behavioral studies in animals exposed to extreme stress have contributed greatly to the expanding knowledge of the basic science of trauma.[13] Movement of trauma research away from the psychoanalytic model has resulted in an increased awareness of the prevalence of trauma in all societies, and its pervasive effects on dysfunctional social and personal behavior. It has also fostered further research in the growing area of brain plasticity, not only in the face of physical damage from stroke or injury, but also associated with exposure to extreme stress.

Brain Plasticity in Trauma

Numerous studies of autonomic and neuromuscular responses to trauma-related stimuli in PTSD patients suggest that relatively hard-wired changes in brain circuitry and response have occurred. Studies testing exposure of combat veterans to combat-related visual and auditory cues consistently show exaggerated heart rate, blood pressure, skin conductance, electromyography (EMG), and plasma epinephrine responses.[14] Based on these findings, Kolb has postulated that PTSD might be due to "conditioned emotional responses" similar to fear conditioning in animals.[15] The consistency of a conditioned response (autonomic arousal) in combat veterans to a stereotyped conditioned stimulus (trauma-related memory cue) certainly supports this hypothesis.[16] This method of testing specific conditioned responses in trauma, however, is difficult to adapt to other types of trauma, such as child abuse, rape, accidents, and natural disasters. These sources of traumatic stress are often associated with more varied and complex conditioning stimuli, resulting in the procedural memory storage of diverse and often unpredictable traumatic cues.

Mental imagery should be quite adaptable as a conditioned stimulus to general populations of trauma victims. Studies of autonomic responsiveness to trauma-related mental imagery are reviewed again in Shalev and Rogel-Fuchs.[14] As might be expected, combat veterans with PTSD show exaggerated sympathetic autonomic response to combat-related imagery, whereas veterans without PTSD do not. Victims of sexual assault with PTSD show the same abnormal physiological traits, as do patients with motor vehicle accident (MVA)-related PTSD.[17] This enhanced arousal response is dependent not just on exposure to the traumatic conditioning stimulus, but on whether clinical symptoms of PTSD resulted from that exposure. The consistency of an exaggerated autonomic response resulting from mental imagery also suggests a conditioned response to a conditioning stimulus, in this case a memory. Pavlov, in fact, hypothesized the existence of a "secondary system of representation," involving memories, as well as verbal and visual images that were retained in memory. This "system" should be able to enhance learning and even conditioning without external sensory input.[18] This theory would fit with the concept of the kindled procedural memory/arousal/neuromuscular feedback circuit discussed in Chapter 3.

In this model, declarative memory in the form of reminiscence serves as an additional trigger for the conditioned response. The introduction of memories into the self-perpetuating neural circuits of PTSD in a safe therapeutic setting could reduce traumatic arousal and the symptoms of PTSD through the process of extinction.[14,19] As one might expect, however, the contributions of declarative memory to the neural pathways serving trauma appear easier to change through flooding than those served by procedural memory circuits that, in fact, may well be the major type of memory that contributes to traumatic kindling. The measurable conditioned autonomic responses to an arousal stimulus noted in the previous studies tend to be the most permanently imprinted on procedural memory in trauma, and seem to be the most resistant to change with existing forms of therapy. Their persistence and constancy of expression suggest a change in brain structure and physiology as permanent as that of character traits. The persisting conditioned somatic procedural memories related to a traumatic event may hold the key for ultimate healing.

Objective Measures of Brain Change in Trauma

A permanent change in sympathetic autonomic reactivity in patients suffering from chronic PTSD has been well documented in the literature. This change also correlates with documented consistent cognitive changes in these patients, specifically in the area of verbal memory.[20] Further evidence for traumatic experience-based anatomic changes in brain structure have been documented with recent advances in brain imagery. Brain MRI studies suggest a significant reduction in the size of the hippocampus in Vietnam combat veterans suffering from PTSD.[21] Similar reduction in hippocampal volume has been documented in female victims of childhood sexual abuse.[22] The hippocampus, of course, is linked to episodic and verbal declarative memory.

High blood levels of serum cortisol have been implicated in this toxic effect on the hippocampus in both human and animal studies, both in vivo (live subjects) and in vitro (in the laboratory). Activation of the hypothalamic/pituitary/adrenal axis (HPA) as part of the initial adaptive hormonal response to stress results in prolonged elevation of levels of glucocorticoids, including cortisol, in the body. Although glucocorticoids are crucial in modulating the acute response to stress initiated by norepinephrine, prolonged exposure to elevated levels of these hormones results in damage to hippocampal neurons, both in the in vitro rat brain,[23] and in vivo studies in primates.[24] Prolonged exposure to stress in primates also has been shown to cause selective hippocampal damage.[25] These findings of experience-based anatomical changes in brain structure are quite consistent with theories previously cited by Schore.[26]

Another example of dynamic changes in regional brain structure and function has been noted using positron emission tomography of the brain (PET) associated with exposure of traumatized individuals to detailed narratives related to their trauma.[27] Patients read arousing personal narratives, while PET scans were taken of their brains. Localized increased metabolic activity was uniformly documented in the right hemisphere in the specific region in the limbic system associated with the amygdala—the region of the brain serving memory associated with arousal and anxiety. Increased activity in the right visual cortex was consistent with the presence of flashbacks experienced during the study. Interestingly, Broca's area for speech showed reduced activity, consistent with the symptom of alexithymia, the inability of PTSD patients to express emotions in words.[27] One does not need words when one is engaged in intense survival-based behavior. Similar scans of individuals without PTSD did not show this pattern, indicating the existence of a persistent change in regional brain function in PTSD.

The cingulate gyrus, another part of the limbic system, plays an important role in the brain's physiological response to threat, and demonstrates predictable changes in blood flow during fear activation in PTSD. The anterior cingulate serves an inhibitory gating function on fear conditioning by the amygdala, and also plays a role in generation of maternal behavior and social bonding. (This role in bonding will be an important consideration when we address the cingulate's role in the effectiveness of trauma therapy in Chapter 11.) The posterior cingulate helps regulate processing of visual images, a function important in processing of information regarding threatening events, as evidenced by right visual cortical enhancement during traumatic imagery in PTSD.[27] Recall the anterior cingulate gyrus as a brain area that helps to modulate the amygdala. PET scans during exposure to traumatic stimuli show the failure of activation of the right cingulate in PTSD victims, perhaps reflecting a permanent deficit of this process in the trauma victim.[28,29] This deficit may represent a permanent change in brain physiology that might contribute to perpetuation of arousal-based kindling.

The Permanence of Post-Traumatic Stress Disorder

Longitudinal studies of patients with PTSD show evidence not only for prolonged persistence of symptoms, but also for actual decline in standard measures of personal and social functioning.[30] This deterioration would be in keeping with the model of PTSD as self-perpetuated kindling involving brain centers associated with memory and arousal, and closely linked to avoidance and dissociation. It would also be consistent with permanent changes in neuronal interaction that would restrict the behavioral options of the traumatized individual. One would expect this effect to contribute to a sequential decline in functional coping skills in the victim of PTSD based on the verified relationship of prolonged cortisol exposure to permanent changes in hippocampal structure and function. Surprisingly, studies of urinary free-cortisol levels in those patients with late or chronic PTSD show low, stable levels when compared to patients with other types of psychopathology.[31] At the same time, the HPA axis is over-responsive to exposure to cortisol. The basic physiology of trauma obviously changes over time.

In addition, these chronic PTSD patients demonstrate relative elevation of urinary norepinephrine levels, resulting in an unusual elevation of the norepinephrine/cortisol ratio.[32] This finding is in contrast to the well-established elevation of both norepinephrine and cortisol in acute stress. One explanation for this unusual late suppression of serum cortisol in late PTSD might be that adaptive mechanisms to the continuously kindled arousal of PTSD might suppress rather than stimulate the HPA axis without suppressing adrenergic arousal. Several studies have shown that certain psychological defense mechanisms, especially denial, can powerfully suppress urinary cortisol levels, both chronically,[33] and even lower in acute stress.[34] The possibility that adrenal cortical exhaustion explained the suppression of low chronic cortisol levels in PTSD was ruled out in one of these studies by the administration of adrenocorticotrophic hormone (ACTH), and the production of a normal cortisol response.[35] Cortisol, of course inhibits, or "puts a lid on," the immune system. This paradoxical state of suppression of serum cortical levels has important implications for autoimmune states in late or complex trauma. Cortisol, therefore, seems to exhibit a paradoxical role in acute traumatic stress versus late PTSD, suggesting that the evolution of the post-traumatic syndrome is associated with basic changes in the core physiology of the brain and the body.

On a psychodynamic basis, denial and dissociation share many similarities. Dissociation is one of the cardinal features of the late adaptive mechanisms of PTSD. Dissociation at the time of a traumatic experience predicts the later development of PTSD more than any other measured variable.[36] This is quite logical, since dissociation reflects the state of consciousness in the freeze response. Those individuals who dissociate at the time of the trauma will tend to dissociate under later conditions of stress, especially if the initial trauma was in childhood (see Chapter 7). The persistence of dissociation in chronic PTSD may play a role in suppression of the HPA axis, and contribute to the loss of adaptation to the continued cyclical arousal in chronic PTSD. Suppression of serum cortisol in these patients in that model would prevent the modulating effect of cortisol on the acute effects of epinephrine, serving to perpetuate the seemingly permanent neurophysiological changes of this condition. These theoretical considerations, and the role of the parasympathetic nervous system in PTSD are explored in more detail in Chapter 7.

Conclusion

Exposure to stress and trauma have profound effects on the brain and the endocrine system, especially the HPA axis. This effect is crucial for the initial autonomic and neuroendocrine response to a threatening event in order for the person to adapt to the threat. But these responses soon begin to have harmful and ultimately long-standing harmful effects on neuronal structure and function. Imaging studies of the brain, both anatomical and functional, suggest that these effects on the brain are long lasting and in some instances probably permanent. The implications of these data provide a real challenge to the effective treatment of trauma, especially in its chronic stages.

The concept of kindling as a source of development and perpetuation of the neurophysiological basis for PTSD is quite consistent with the permanence of PTSD. Kindling also provides a theoretical basis for the possibility of associated permanent anatomical and physiological neuronal change in traumatic stress. These concepts are also in keeping with emerging theories addressing the hardwired experiential basis for brain development, the development of character, and the vulnerability to psychopathology. Thus far, the elusive changes in brain function seen in imaging studies, as well as the contradictory findings in HPA axis function in victims of trauma, appear to be the faintest of clues to a process that we are only beginning to unravel. These changes, however, appear to support the concept of PTSD as a "physioneurosis," a condition involving multiple systems of the brain and body, and one that may indeed be progressive and self-perpetuating. These findings may also contribute to the healing of trauma through techniques based its neurophysiology, whether behavioral or pharmacological.

Notes

1. van der Kolk, B., Weisaeth, L., van der Hart, O.: The history of trauma in psychiatry. In van der Kolk, B., McFarlane, A., Weisaeth, L. (Eds.)., *Traumatic Stress: The Effects of Overwhelming Experience on Mind, Body, and Society* (pp. 279–302). New York: Guilford Press, 1986.

2. Noyes. A., Kolb, L.: *Modern Clinical Psychiatry*. Philadelphia: W.B. Saunders Company, 1958.

3. Janet, P.: *L'automatisme Psychologique*. Paris: Alcan, 1889.

4. van der Kolk, B., van der Hart, O.: Pierre Janet and the breakdown of adaptation in psychological trauma. *Journal of Psychiatry*, 1989; 146:1520–1540.

5. Freud, S.: The aetiology of hysteria. In Strachey, J. (Ed. and Trans.). *The Standard Edition of the Complete Psychological Works of Sigmund Freud* (Vol. 15. pp. 1–240; Vol. 16, pp. 241–496). London: Hogarth Press. (Original work published 1896).

6. Miller, A.: *Banished Knowledge: Facing Childhood Injuries*. New York: Anchor Books, Doubleday, 1990.

7. Freud, S.: The interpretation of dreams. In Strachey, J. (Ed. and Trans.), *The Standard Edition of the Complete Psychological Works of Sigmund Freud* (Vol. 7. pp. 125–243). London: Hogarth Press. (Original work published 1905).

8. Kardiner, A.: *The Traumatic Neuroses of War*. New York: Hoeber, 1941.

9. Eitinger, L., Strom, A.: *Mortality and Morbidity After Excessive Stress: A Follow-Up Investigation of Norwegian Concentration Camp Survivors.* Oslo, Norway: Universitets-forlaget, 1973.

10. Hocking, F.: Psychiatric aspects of extreme environmental stress. *Diseases of the Nervous System,* 1970; 31:1278–1282.

11. Burgess, A., Holstrom. L.: Rape trauma syndrome. *American Journal of Psychiatry,* 1974; 131:981–986.

12. Kempe, R., Kempe, C.: *Child Abuse.* Cambridge, MA: Harvard University Press, 1978.

13. van der Kolk, B., Greenberg, M., Boyd, H., Krystal, J.: Inescapable shock, neurotransmitters and addiction to trauma: Toward a psychobiology of post-traumatic stress disorder. *Biological Psychiatry,* 1985; 20:314–325.

14. Shalev, A., Rogel-Fuchs, M.: Psychophysiology of the post-traumatic stress disorder: From sulfur fumes to behavioral genetics. *Psychosomatic Medicine,* 1993; 55:413–423.

15. Kolb, L.: A neurophysiological hypothesis explaining the post-traumatic stress disorder. *American Journal of Psychiatry,* 1987; 144:989–995.

16. Grigsby, J.: Combat rush: Phenomenology of central and autonomic arousal among war veterans with PTSD. *Psychotherapy,* 1991; 28:354–363.

17. Blanchard, B., Hickling, E., Taylor, A.: The psychophysiology of motor vehicle accident related post-traumatic stress disorder. *Biofeedback and Self-Regulation,* 1991; 16(4):449–458.

18. Pavlov, J.: *Conditioned Reflexes: An Investigation of the Physiological Activity of the Cerebral Cortex* (1927). Anrep, G. V., ed. and trans. New York: Dover, 1960.

19. Keane, T., Kaloupek, D.: Imaginal flooding in the treatment of a posttraumatic stress disorder. *Journal of Consulting and Clinical Psychology,* 1982; 50:138–140.

20. Bremner, J., Scott, T., Delaney, R., Southwick, S., Mason, J., Johnson, D., Innis, R., McCarthy, G., Charney, D.: Deficits in short-term memory in posttraumatic stress disorder. *American Journal of Psychiatry,* 1993; 150:1015–1019.

21. Bremner, J., Randall, P., Scott, T., Bronen, R., Seibyl, J., Southwick, S., Delaney, R., McCarthy, G., Charney, D., Innis, R.: MRI-based measures of hippocampal volume in patients with PTSD. *American Journal of Psychiatry,* 1995; 152:973–981.

22. Stein, M., Hannah, C., Koverola, C., Yehuda, R., Torchia, M., McClarty, B.: Neuroanatomical and neuroendocrine correlates in adulthood of severe sexual abuse in childhood. Presented at the 33rd annual meeting of the American College of Neuropsychopharmacology. San Juan, PR, 1994.

23. Sapolsky, R., Packan, D., Vale, W.: Glucocorticoid toxicity in the hippocampus: In vitro demonstration. *Brain Research,* 1988; 453:367–371.

24. Sapolsky, R., Uno, H., Rebert, C., Finch, C.: Hippocampal damage associated with prolonged glucocorticoid exposure in primates. *Journal of Neuroscience,* 1990; 10(9): 2897–2902.

25. Uno, H., Tarara, R., Else, J., Suleman, M., Sapolsky, R.: Hippocampal damage associated with prolonged and fatal stress in primates. *Journal of Neuroscience,* 1989; 9(5): 1705–1711.

26. Schore, A.: *Affect Regulation and the Origin of the Self.* Hillsdale, NJ: Lawrence, 1994.

27. Rauch, S., van der Kolk, B., Fisler, R., Alpert, N., Orr, S., Savage, C., Fischman, A., Jenike, M., Pitman, R.: A symptom provocation study of posttraumatic stress disorder using positron emission tomography and script-driven imagery. *Archives of General Psychiatry,* 1996; 53:380–387.

28. Shin, L., McNally, R., Kosslyn, S., Thompson, W., Rauch, S., Alpert, N., Metzger, L., Lasko, N., Orr, S., Pitman, T.: Regional cerebral bloodflow during script-driven

imagery in childhood sexual abuse-related PTSD: A PET investigation. *American Journal of Psychiatry*, 1999; 156(4):575–584.

29. Bremner, J.: Alterations in brain structure and function associated with posttraumatic stress disorder. *Seminars in Clinical Neuropsychiatry*, 1999; 4(4):249–255.

30. Tichener, J.: Post-traumatic decline: A consequence of unresolved destructive drives. In Figley, C (Ed.), *Trauma and Its Wake* (Volume 2, pp. 5–19). New York: Brunner-Mazel, 1986.

31. Mason, J., Giller, E., Kosten, T., Ostroff, R., Podd, L.: Urinary free-cortisol levels in post-traumatic stress disorder patients. *Journal of Nervous and Mental Disease*, 1986; 174(3):145–149.

32. Mason, J., Giller, E., Kosten, T., Harkness, L.: Elevation of urinary norepinephrine/cortisol ratio in post-traumatic stress disorder. *Journal of Nervous and Mental Disease*, 1988; 176(8):498–502.

33. Friedman, S., Mason, L., Hamburg, D.: Urinary 17-hydroxycorticosteroid levels in parents of children with neoplastic disease. *Psychosomatic Medicine*, 1963; 25:364–376.

34. Mason, J.: Clinical psychophysiology: Psychoendocline mechanisms. In Reiser, M. (Ed.). *American Handbook of Psychiatry* (Volume 4. pp. 551–582). New York: Basic Books, 1975.

35. Shalev, A., Peri, T., Caneti, L., Schreiber, S.: Predictors of PTSD in injured trauma survivors: A prospective study. *American Journal of Psychiatry*, 1996; 153:219–225.

36. van der Kolk, B., Greenburg, M., Orr, S., Pitman, R.: Endogenous opioids and stress-induced analgesia in post-traumatic stress disorder. *Psychopharmacology Bulletin*, 1989; 25:108–112.

seven
Somatic Dissociation

Sam had suffered fractures of his right wrist and ankle in a particularly traumatic head-on motor vehicle accident. Thereafter, along with significant PTSD, he developed intractable burning pain associated with variable heat and coolness of the right hand and foot. This condition was eventually diagnosed as reflex sympathetic dystrophy (RSD), a particularly malignant and painful condition that occasionally follows injuries. Despite extensive treatment including multiple sympathetic nerve blocks, treatment in a pain center, and multiple medication trials, Sam was ultimately disabled by his RSD. His physical examination revealed measurably increased warmth along the outside of his right lower leg and foot, and coolness of his right hand, with extreme painful sensitivity to touch of the skin in those areas. I performed visual boundary testing during one of his visits with me. I passed my out-stretched hand around his 180-degree visual field at a distance of about 6 feet. When I entered his right visual field, he flushed and experienced discomfort. When I asked him what he had experienced, he told me that he had felt a flash of anger toward me. He then had a sudden memory of his grandfather striking him on the back of his right leg with a fireplace poker as a child, a preferred form of punishment in his family. His RSD had developed in an injured leg that represented a region of his perceptual field held in procedural memory as a persistent latent threat to his sense of safety. This was the region of his body that had experienced repeated, painful traumatic messages as a child.

* * *

Dissociation is a term coined by Janet in the late nineteenth century to describe mental states characterized by a disruption of conscious awareness.[1] In this state of altered consciousness, the individual may experience distortion of memory, affect, perception, or sense of identity. The dissociated person may experience altered perceptions of somatic sensations and time, periods of amnesia, unreality, and depersonalization. More profound clinical states include symptoms of conversion hysteria, fugue states, and multiple personality disorder (dissociative identity disorder).[2-5] Psychiatrists believed that dissociation occurred when anxiety became so overwhelming that certain aspects of the personality became dissociated or split from one another. They believed that the various manifestations of dissociation served to protect the individual from the conflict producing the anxiety. Dissociation, in other words, served as a psychological escape mechanism from fear.

Examples of Dissociation

In the traumatized person, dissociation occurs in many forms—at many times in the evolution of traumatic stress and post-traumatic stress disorder—and has emotional, perceptual, physical, and memory-related manifestations. In a motor vehicle accident, dissociation presents as the emotional and perceptual confusion and numbness often experienced at the time of the accident. Many people describe it as being in shock. Dissociation is clearly linked to the freeze response, and actually may represent the state of one's perception when in the freeze. The out-of-body, third person perception that people sometimes feel at the moment of traumatic stress is an example of depersonalization, a classic symptom of dissociation. The victim of childhood incest who perceives her disembodied self as looking down from the ceiling of her bedroom feeling sorry for the little girl on the bed who is being abused by her father is experiencing this form of dissociation.

Several of my MVA patients have described this phenomenon vividly. One patient was sitting in the front passenger seat of a car driven by a friend. They stopped at his mountain home after a trip as they completed a conversation. Suddenly, she saw from her left a car traveling erratically down the steep road toward them. As the car lost control and hurtled over an embankment toward their car, she began to perceive events as occurring in slow motion, and then realized that she was looking down on the scene from above the car, in which she could still see herself sitting next to the driver. The oncoming car then descended through the air, landed on the hood of their car, bounced off, and landed on its top ten feet from their car. During this shocking event, the patient remained calm and detached. She then found herself "back in her body," unhurt and apparently unshaken. She calmly exited the car and went to check on the driver's son, who had climbed out of the car before the impact to check the mail. She then checked on the driver of the other car, and went into the house to call the police and ambulance. All of this was done in apparent complete emotional control, although later she would report that she did all of this in a state of "automatic pilot." The next morning she awoke with an agonizing headache and neck pain, and thereafter experienced the full-blown whiplash syndrome that I have described, even though the car in which she was sitting was shaken but not moved by the impact. Her symptoms included intractable headache and neck pain, prominent cognitive impairment, the vertigo and blurred vision of post-concussion syndrome and full-blown acute PTSD.

Another patient involved in a moderate impact, rear-end MVA experienced a profound out-of-body experience similar to the one described previously. When she emerged from her car, she experienced a sudden revelation that the heavens opened up and filled her with an amazing power with the implication that it would forever change her life. She even perceived a bright light in the sky at the time. This is called *derealization*: the sense that immediate perceptions are unreal, or in this case supernatural, and is another example of dissociation. An experience such as the one just described might be considered delusional, and in this case the doctors who evaluated the patient in the emergency room believed that she was probably a psychiatric patient.

Almost all of my patients with clinical PTSD after an MVA say that they have lost their sense of self, that they no longer know who they are, and that they are now living a strange and unrecognizable life. This sense of unreality pervades their life, and is often referred to as a "fog" that exists between them, their sense of awareness and the rest of the world. Although this foglike perception is often described as almost palpable, its main feature seems to be a clouding of consciousness, both cognitive and emotional, with numbing, distraction, and loss of emotional tone. At times in the course of a patient's recovery, this "fog" may lift rather suddenly, and this event is almost always associated with improvement in cognitive impairment. It clearly represented a state of prolonged dissociation. Symptoms of arousal and hypervigilance actually may increase when this state of numbing begins to clear. Dissociative symptoms in general are often bizarre by the usual medical standards and seem to defy rational physical explanation. In my experience, however, the clearing of this sense of clouded perception is frequently a positive result of therapy for the trauma.

Perhaps the most extreme instance of depersonalization in dissociation involves the development of "multiple personalities," or dissociative identity disorder (DID). This rare condition is clearly an example of traumatic dissociation, with the incidence of severe child abuse in these individuals approaching 80 percent.[6] The various personalities exhibited in this disorder may show difference in hand and apparent cerebral hemispheric dominance, different psychophysiological responses to stress, and may even suffer from different diseases as evidence for remarkable physiological and somatic dissociation.

Memory in Dissociation

Distortions of memory in PTSD may also be a manifestation of dissociation. Traumatic amnesia is perhaps the most common example.[7] While many traumatized patients experience recurring and intrusive memories of the trauma, a significant number have partial or complete amnesia for the experience. This form of amnesia is especially common in adult survivors of child abuse, who may have little if any memory for their abuse,[8] or else remember it in grossly distorted terms. Although recovered memories of child abuse may be distorted or inaccurate, they frequently clearly represent dissociative amnesia for actual events.

Many victims of child abuse may have remarkably little memory of any events of their childhood as a result of this process. Several of my MVA victims, suffering from amnesia for an accident presumed to be due to a head injury, have recovered complete memory for details of the accident with trauma therapy alone. Memories for the traumatic event may also be distorted by the perceptual alterations associated with a traumatic experience.[9] The process of derealization leads to remarkable memory alterations, including the clear memory of an out-of-body experience.[4] The memory for the sense of the passage of time is often greatly altered,[10] and usually is experienced as the dramatic slowing of time, "as if my life passed before my eyes." Frequently sounds, smells, and other sensations are greatly amplified in traumatic memory as part of the dissociative experience. In MVAs, the impact is often described as "a bomb going off." The powder released by the air bag is remembered as "suffocating." As the traumatized individual cycles in and out of dissociation, these somatic memories may serve as conditioned cues that may trigger panic, flashbacks, and somatic dissociative symptoms.

The most profound type of dissociative amnesia is called a fugue state. In its most dramatic form, this type of dissociation is probably what the Hollywood movie industry is trying to represent in fictional stories about persons experiencing prolonged periods of amnesia. These persons are depicted as suffering profound emotional trauma, or sometimes a blow to the head. Thereafter, the victims go so far as to begin another life with no memory for prior life events, including their own name or past life history. Although obviously stretching reality in the interests of drama, these stories have a kernel of truth.

A fugue state is often characterized by a prolonged time for which the patients have no memory, but during which they continue to talk and relate in a somewhat normal fashion. During this time, they may not remember their name or personal facts, but otherwise appear normal. In other fugue states, they may appear confused, dramatic or histrionic, socially inappropriate, or bizarre. When such a fugue state clears, as it eventually does, these patients usually have no memory of the events that occurred during that time. This type of reaction occurring in the context of an MVA usually occurs at the time of, or just after, the accident. Once again this may be difficult to distinguish from the occasionally confused behavior that may accompany a closed head injury. During the period of amnesia following a moderate closed head injury, agitated, delusional, or even combative behavior may occur that later may be very difficult to distinguish from similar behavior due to a traumatically induced fugue state.

Another dissociative memory disturbance, also seen in a number of my whiplash patients, is the loss of memory for remote, familiar autobiographical events, some of them containing strong personal emotional content. Although this phenomenon is often attributed to the effects of a minor traumatic brain injury, these patients have accurate recall of the accident itself, and in addition to cognitive complaints, all of them had other dissociative and arousal symptoms of PTSD.

Selective amnesia for autobiographical events in these patients is very likely dissociative in nature, and relates to similar traumatic amnesia for childhood events in victims of child abuse.

Actual flashback memories associated with trauma also represent dissociative events. They are almost always associated with intense emotional arousal, and often panic.[11] The patient's sense of awareness and reality during a flashback memory is usually distorted, with a sense of detachment from one's immediate surroundings. The patient may report the "foglike" sense previously described, and other sensations may be similarly altered. Memory associated with the flashback will almost always relate to the specific trauma and may be quite accurate, but also may be altered, exaggerated, symbolic, or otherwise distorted from the actual event. Flashbacks may last from minutes to hours, or even days. Needless to say, the person is essentially completely disabled during the flashback experience, both from the confusion accompanying the memory and the associated intense arousal. Flashbacks as well as repeated intrusive memories of a traumatic event are representative of the fact that memory in trauma, in addition to being absent for certain events, may also be exaggerated and distorted. Unlike the dissociative nature of flashbacks, intrusive memories tend to be more accurate and representative of the traumatic experience, perhaps even more so than common declarative memories unlinked to emotion or arousal.[12]

Cognitive and Emotional Features

Dissociative symptoms in trauma also affect attention, cognition, and emotional intensity, mainly by constriction, withdrawal, and detachment. All of these behaviors serve to protect traumatized persons from experiencing arousal by literally removing them from the scene of the action. Constriction impairs both the victims' awareness of events around them and the emotions associated with those events. Mood, affect, and range of emotion may be blunted and flattened. Fear and panic may be dulled, but joy, pleasure, and satisfaction may be muted as well. Social isolation may accompany withdrawal, and may become so complete that the trauma victim may literally become a hermit. The image of the traumatized Vietnam veteran retreating to a cabin in the forest as depicted in several motion pictures is not entirely exaggerated.

Dissociation may produce a distorted sense of time. The victims may spend their days in random and disjointed behavior, missing meals, not attending to personal hygiene, and confusing night and day. Neglect and confusion of purpose may be severe and quite disabling. Conversely, trauma victims may rigidly plan every hour of their waking day in order to avoid the intrusion of anxiety that appears whenever they do not have everything in their life scheduled, planned, and organized. Obsessive-compulsive behaviors may result from this aspect of traumatic stress. Such patients will organize and reorganize details of their life, especially as they relate to the MVA after whiplash. They may drive the medical provider to distraction with constant requests and demands to deal with what they perceive to be daily life crises, with many of these demands being perseverative and anxiety driven. These patients are very likely to review the copy of the medical consult that the physician has performed, and to make multiple minute corrections of facts as related to the case history described in that report. All of these obsessive, controlling behaviors serve to protect the person from exposure to ambient traumatic cues and intolerable anxiety.

Other problems of cognitive and mental processing functions may result from dissociation. Constricted attention may affect the person's ability to access information, with distraction leading the person to neglect and ignore the details of the information that is heard, seen, or read. This symptom may often present as forgetfulness, absent-mindedness, or simply as an attention deficit. In fact, in PTSD patients, neuropsychological test batteries reveal a variety of deficits, usually in the areas of short-term memory and attention.[13–19] Adult victims of trauma have more recently been diagnosed as having adult ADD (attention deficit disorder). They may also show impaired higher-level intellectual information processing and executive function. The ability to make judgments based on complex pieces of information and the ability to problem solve based on complex associations may be dulled.[20,21] They may neglect the details in making decisions, instead reaching conclusions based mainly on initially constricted impressions. This process of constriction may limit access to the full range of available information and, as a result, common sense, judgment, and logic may at times be impaired, or stereotyped. Often the victims of trauma, sensing the difficulties associated with cognitive demands, may make every effort to avoid participating in life decisions in order to reduce the complexity of their life to avoid traumatic cues.

The literature cited previously documents significant cognitive impairment in trauma survivors unexplained by coincidental minor brain injury. I have noted in many of my whiplash trauma victims that test scores on neuropsychological test batteries are even worse than one would expect from their apparent level of daily function. Several such patients have completed college and graduate level degrees with neuropsychological test scores that would suggest that this achievement should not be feasible. I believe that the very process of exposure to the demands of this type of testing may accentuate fear and anxiety, trigger distraction and dissociation, and lead to artificially depressed test scores.

Dissociative Physical Symptoms

Perhaps the least appreciated manifestations of dissociation in trauma are in the areas of perceptual alterations and somatic symptoms. As noted, time perception is often altered, especially with the dissociative response related to the initial traumatic freeze episode. The popularly described perception of "time standing still" is indeed a frequent experience of the MVA victim at the moment of impact, as documented in hundreds of my patients. Slowing of time is the most common alteration of time perception. A sense of time alteration may persist for some time after the impact, and its duration often reflects the length of time of the post-MVA freeze episode, or period of dissociation.

Visual perception and acuity are also commonly affected in dissociation. Flashback memories are often characterized by marked distortion of shape and color, usually with vivid and bizarre changes that reflect the accompanying state of enhanced arousal, as noted in prior references to MVA experiences. The MVA victim will often remember the other car in flashbacks and intrusive memories as being enlarged and distorted, and traveling at exaggerated speeds. In earlier chapters, we discussed the frequent association of binocular visual acuity impairment and convergence insufficiency in whiplash patients. These patients often also have less easily explained monocular (one eye) visual alteration, including monocular diplopia (double vision) and blurring of vision.

One such patient was referred to me because of partial vision loss in her right eye following an auto accident two months prior. She had not experienced a blow to her head. The patient had lost control of her car on an icy mountain road, and as the car spun out of control, it slid off of the right side of the road into a shallow ditch. On the other side of the ditch was a cliff. As she watched the edge of the cliff approaching from her right side (perceived in slow motion, of course), her car was stopped by impacting a tree, and came to rest. Thereafter, she developed persistent blurring of vision in her right eye. Ocular refraction showed a consistent refractive error that appeared to be correctable, and she was fitted with a lens that provided clear vision in that eye. Within minutes after putting on the glasses with the new lens, she developed nausea, palpitations, flashback memories of the accident, and panic. Any further attempts to restore or correct the measurable refractive error in her right eye continued to produce attacks of panic and reexperiencing of the traumatic event through flashbacks. Her visual impairment was diagnosed as being hysterical in nature, despite the consistency of the refractive error.

This remarkable patient presents an example of this somatic group of symptoms. The measurable but physically unexplained refractive error in her right eye was clearly a somatic dissociative response driven by the moment of life-threatening danger perceived in that eye at the time of the MVA. Visual images perceived in her right eye activated procedural memory for the terrifying events of the potentially fatal accident and triggered emotionally charged flashbacks and panic. Blurring of vision in that eye became a dissociative phenomenon that protected against anxiety. The unusual feature of this case, of course, is that the refractive error was consistently measurable and reproducible. Dissociation had resulted in a probably temporary but physiologically measurable alteration of function in the dissociated eye. The occurrence of this type of visual distortion in MVAs usually appears related to the association of visual cues accompanying the threat at the moment of the accident. In my patient population, it occurs much less often in rear-end accidents in which the victim did not see the car approaching, and is especially common when direct visual perception of the impending threat occurred from one side or the other.

Distortion of proprioceptive awareness of the victim's body is a common dissociative phenomenon. This is often associated with an injured part or region of the body, especially one of the extremities. The patient will note altered sensation, usually a vague sense of numbness, but the exact sensation is usually very difficult to describe. The extremity may be neglected or ignored, and postural abnormalities may result that can be quite remarkable. Examination of the part of the body involved may reveal sensory changes on a variety of tests that will usually be interpreted as "nonphysiological" in nature by the physician. Stocking or glove patterns of loss of pain, touch, and vibratory sensation are common. Strength testing often shows giveaway weakness. Patients presenting with these atypical neurological findings will frequently be diagnosed as suffering from conversion hysteria.

An exceptional example of somatic dissociation was seen in an MVA victim treated in my chronic pain program. This young lady had been involved in a rollover accident during which her left arm was crushed by the car as it rolled, tearing off almost the entire skin of her forearm. Amazingly, she suffered minimal nerve damage, but required extensive skin grafting of the forearm. The sensation in the grafted skin was obviously deadened and never returned to normal, but as she recovered she developed increasing vague, hard to describe aching pain that was resistant to all treatment, although it did not fulfill criteria for sympathetically maintained pain or RSD. She essentially stopped using the arm and hand for any activity. The pain was actually worse in the shoulder than the forearm, and was associated with some evidence of myofascial pain and spasm in the muscles of the neck and shoulder. The most unusual feature of her physical examination, however, was her posture. In the standing position, her head was side bent and rotated to the right, and her torso was also rotated to the right. Her left shoulder blade was rotated backward and the arm almost held behind her, literally out of her view. She was totally unaware of this position of total rejection and dissociation of her entire left arm, even when looking in a mirror. When shown a face-on, full-body photograph of herself, however, she was surprised and shocked at her unusual appearance. With somatically based trauma therapy and postural education, the pain largely disappeared in a sequential fashion as her posture approached a more normal status.

In our chronic pain program, we invariably noticed that the patient's unconscious posture reflected not only the pain, but also the experience of the traumatic event that produced the pain. The asymmetrical postural patterns, held in procedural memory, almost always reflect the body's attempt to move away from the injury or threat that caused the injury. Many of these patients manifested the "nonphysiological findings" that have branded them as chronic pain patients, or hysterics, by their physicians. With careful exploration of the mechanisms of the source of the pain, however, one will usually find strong evidence for a history of traumatic stress specific to that area of the body. Specific neuromuscular postural patterns that have developed related to their injury are often visible markers for the presence of somatic dissociation, and explain the patterns of "nonphysiological findings."

Conversion Hysteria and Dissociation

Even nonpsychiatric physicians generally place nonphysiological findings in the diagnostic category of a "conversion reaction," or conversion hysteria. This psychiatric condition was described in detail by Janet and Freud.[1,2] As noted earlier, conversion is considered to be an unconscious protection against intolerable levels of anxiety or phobias. The anxiety is "converted" into symptoms in organs or other parts of the body, and usually presents as sensory or motor neurological symptoms. These symptoms tend to represent the mental conflict creating the anxiety, and also meet some need of the patient—provide "secondary gain"—on an unconscious basis. Conversion of an intolerable anxiety to a physical symptom indeed provides great emotional relief, hence the frequently documented indifference to the disabling physical condition (*la belle indifference*). Hysterical paralysis, for example, has been noted regularly in traumatized soldiers suffering from "shell shock" or "battle fatigue." Hysterical paraplegia at the turn of the century was classically attributed in women to sexual ambivalence—i.e., to a confused mixture of erotic feelings and disgust with regard to sexuality.[2] The term "hysteria" derives from the Greek word for the uterus, *hystera*, essentially branding conversion reaction as a feminine condition. These young women were initially suspected, and are now thought to have been, victims of incest, and the secondary gain achieved is now believed to have been a form of protection from further exposure to their source of trauma.

In the DSM–IV, conversion has been assigned to the category of somatoform disorders, and is technically not believed to represent a true dissociative disorder. As part of the thesis of this chapter, however, I believe that all somatoform disorders constitute subsets of the dissociative response, and that they have a measurable physiological basis and origin. Conversion reaction, then, is an example of regional somatic dissociation as a reaction to trauma. The body part that provided the sensory messages of the trauma to conscious awareness or unconscious perception is rejected/dissociated because it now represents a threat as the source of intolerable arousal and fear.

It is apparent that the patient with a conversion reaction will almost always have been a victim of trauma in the past, usually in addition to the new trauma that may have precipitated the conversion symptoms. Often this past trauma will have been severe childhood abuse. Children typically dissociate in the face of traumatic stress, as we have noted. They sustain this tendency to freeze in the face of perceived threat as they grow older, with each episode of dissociation tending to reinforce the susceptibility to freeze in the face of subsequent threat. As a result, adults with a history of child abuse typically experience a greater tendency to freeze at the moment of subsequent trauma and to develop dissociative symptoms. As we have noted, dissociation is the primary predictor for the later development of PTSD.[22] Individuals who actively dissociate at the time of a traumatic event are much more likely to develop subsequent symptoms of PTSD than those who do not.[23,24,25] People with a history of trauma or PTSD also are susceptible to arousal, freezing, and being retraumatized after exposure to arousal stimuli unrelated to prior traumatic life experiences.[26] They also have trouble differentiating relevant from irrelevant stimuli with regard to content and meaning of threat.[27] The tendency to freeze in the face of trauma appears to be a self-fulfilling prophecy, rendering the victim increasingly sensitive to dissociation with ever-decreasing severity and specificity of threat exposure. This phenomenon of sensitization to increasingly minor and apparently irrelevant threat in victims of childhood trauma may well explain the remarkable incidence of dissociative symptoms and PTSD in my patients with a history of childhood trauma injured in relatively trivial MVAs.

Although poorly understood, a number of neurophysiological processes likely contribute to the clinical phenomenon of dissociation. Recently, attention has been drawn to the role of the dorsal medial prefrontal cortex (MPFC), or anterior cingulate, in PTSD.[28] Reference has been made to this region with regard to concepts of brain plasticity in PTSD in Chapter 2. Hamner and colleagues noted that lesions of the anterior cingulate might facilitate the acquisition of fear conditioning, suggesting that this region may provide an inhibiting influence on the amygdala, inhibiting fear conditioning.[29] You will recall that the amygdala receives input from the locus ceruleus in states of potential threat, and evaluates that information for its emotional or arousal-based content. Continued activation of the amygdala by further input from the locus ceruleus may then set up a state of fear conditioning. The gating or control function of the anterior cingulate is believed to occur through inhibition of activation of the amygdala at the time of fear arousal. Lack of this inhibition of fear conditioning by the cingulate may lead to increased sensitivity to internal and external trauma-related cues (see Figure 7.1).

In Hamner's model, inhibition of the anterior cingulate by overwhelming adrenergic input from the locus ceruleus with traumatic arousal may limit this inhibiting function of the cingulate on the amygdala. This in turn, would allow exposure of the amygdala to overwhelming internal and external arousal cues, thereby producing the exaggerated emotional and behavioral symptoms of PTSD. Once established, locus ceruleus/amygdala kindling would continue to suppress anterior cingulate function, and perpetuate the conditioned fear response. In addition, the anterior cingulate appears to play a role in emotionality, selective attention, and certain social functions, including emotional attachments and parenting, as well as generation of the concept of the self in relation to society. Fragmentation of these functions through inhibition of the anterior cingulate in PTSD may explain the inability of its victims to form social bonds, to manifest avoidance and isolation, and to experience fragmentation of the sense of self that typifies dissociation.

Dissociation almost certainly is also mediated at least in part by the effects of endorphins, which may in turn partially explain the dissociative phenomena of numbing, confusion, and cognitive impairment. Certainly the analgesia associated with the freeze, or immobility, response—the precursor and extreme expression of dissociation—is related to effects of endorphins. Current theory also strongly relates endorphins to the phenomenon of trauma reenactment.[30] Increasing sensitization to dissociate in the face of threat may well be based on endorphin reward systems.

Dissociation, or freezing, may represent the perpetuating mechanism that fuels the kindled arousal/memory feedback circuit of sustained PTSD. If so, it may be the reason why victims of prior traumatic stress, especially childhood abuse, are so susceptible to the development of PTSD symptoms in otherwise minor episodes of life stress, including low velocity MVAs, as noted in my patient population. The

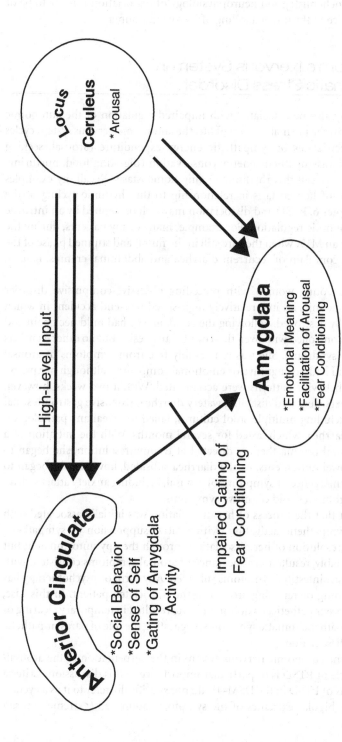

FIGURE 7.1 Theoretical role of the anterior cingulate in post-traumatic stress disorder. The anterior cingulate may exert a braking action on activation of the amygdala, and therefore provide a gating mechanism on the development of fear conditioning in traumatic stress. Excessive or prolonged arousal input from the locus ceruleus in unresolved trauma may impair this gating action through cingulate inhibition, thereby potentiating fear conditioning and traumatic kindling in PTSD.

underlying neurochemistry and neurophysiology of dissociation is likely to be of critical importance to the understanding of its role in trauma.

The Autonomic Nervous System in Post-Traumatic Stress Disorder

Dissociation may also be associated with impaired regulation of the autonomic nervous system. In the normal rhythm of life, the autonomic nervous system cycles smoothly between states of sympathetic energy expenditure (arousal, seeking food, sex) and parasympathetic energy conservation (digesting food, nurturing, social bonding). We call this rhythmic cycling homeostasis. Recall my examples of the sine wave of homeostasis in relationship to the rhythmic cycling of the universe in Chapter 6. PTSD and dissociation may well be defined by an intrinsic disorder of autonomic regulation. For example, many of my patients, during the early stages after an MVA when they are still in the numb and stunned phase of the freeze response, complain of recurrent diarrhea and abdominal cramps, nausea, and indigestion.

A remarkable young woman with preceding obsessive-compulsive disorder suffered soft tissue injuries in a relatively high-speed rear-end accident in which her car was totally destroyed. Following the accident, she had mild neck pain and headache easily controlled with over-the-counter analgesics, but no other elements of the whiplash syndrome. She was remarkably free from symptoms of arousal and of PTSD, and had no cognitive or emotional complaints, although her preexisting reclusive behavior patterns were accentuated. Within two weeks, however, she developed persistent and disabling watery diarrhea. Extensive gastrointestinal investigation, including multiple stool cultures, failed to reveal any pathological cause for the diarrhea, which lasted for several months. With the initiation of a somatic behavioral trauma therapy directed at trauma resolution, she began to have normal bowel movements. As the diarrhea subsided, however, she began to experience the emergence of symptoms of arousal, including anxiety attacks, driving phobias, nightmares, and cognitive symptoms.

It is apparent that the process of her dissociation was initially associated with dramatic parasympathetic activation, with relative suppression of sympathetic arousal. Partial resolution of her dissociation through therapy unfortunately, but probably predictably, resulted in appearance of arousal symptoms consistent with PTSD as her gastrointestinal symptoms subsided. Any form of psychotherapy has the risk of flooding or releasing arousal in the dissociated patient. In this case, return to a more sympathetically dominant state resulted in temporary clearing of severe parasympathetic somatic symptoms, suggesting the role of parasympathetic dominance in dissociation.

This role of the autonomic nervous system in the perpetuation of the arousal/dissociation cycle of PTSD is of particular importance to this discussion. Criteria for the diagnosis of PTSD in the DSM–IV do not specifically refer to it as a cyclical disease, but the bipolar extremes of the symptoms addressed (extreme arousal/

extreme avoidance) certainly suggest abnormal autonomic and limbic cycling. The three criteria categories of PTSD in the DSM–IV (reexperiencing, avoidance, and arousal) reflect dramatic swings of mood, ranging from panic, hypervigilence, and irritability to numbing, detachment, and flattened affect. Physiological markers for PTSD referenced in the DSM–IV include measurements of pulse rate, and electromyographic and electrodermal responses, all primarily measurements of sympathetic autonomic activity. The role of parasympathetic activation or tone in PTSD, however, has been largely neglected.

Oscillatory phenomena in neurophysiological and behavioral systems have been documented in a variety of settings. Antelman and colleagues propose that the exposure of such systems (e.g., endocrine, autonomic, neurohumoral) to chemical or behavioral stressors can induce cyclical patterns of exaggerated increase and decrease in response to each subsequent exposure.[31,32,33] This phenomenon occurs in such a diversity of systems that oscillation in response to chemical or behavioral input may well represent a general principle of biological functioning.[34] Exposure of such systems to stressors sufficient to produce oscillation is entirely analogous to the theories of sensitization and kindling in PTSD (see Chapter 4). A system, such as the autonomic nervous system, sensitized by exposure to stressors without physiological resolution of the resulting response, will be driven to reverberate, or oscillate, within the limits of its physiological capacity. This may well be an innate biological reflex designed to reestablish homeostasis, the rhythmic and balanced subtle fluctuation of all body systems, be they endocrinologic, neurophysiologic, metabolic, or immunologic.[34] If this sensitized system continues to be bombarded by stressors, homeostasis will be prevented, and the exaggerated oscillatory cycles will continue. In the case of PTSD, internal kindled neurophysiological circuits perpetuated by the lack of resolution of a conditioned fight/flight response may provide internal sensitized arousal-based stressors that serve to perpetuate autonomic oscillation. The result is a perpetuated and excessive cyclical dysfunction of autonomic regulation leading to the alternating symptom categories of arousal and avoidance in the traumatized individual (see Figure 7.2). Exaggerated autonomic oscillation also explains the bipolar somatic manifestations of MVA victims with PTSD, ranging from sympathetic activation of neuromuscular protective responses (muscle bracing, bruxism) to vegetative gastrointestinal symptoms (acid reflux, abdominal cramps, diarrhea). Since hyperarousal is also known to be associated with increased release of endogenous opioids, internal reward systems may well contribute to the perpetuation of this exaggerated autonomic cycling.

Depressed levels of serum cortisol have been found in patients with chronic PTSD. This unusual finding is associated with evidence for a sensitized hypothalamic/pituitary/adrenal axis (HPA) in these patients in that they respond to a dexamethasone suppression test with exaggerated suppression of serum cortisol levels. In the normal response to threat, serum cortisol is elevated by stress and arousal through HPA activation and in turn inhibits continued activation of the HPA axis. This feedback inhibition of the HPA modulates the brain's acute response to stress. Continued and repetitive stress exposure would be expected to result in sustained elevation of serum cortisol. In PTSD, however, the "stress" to which

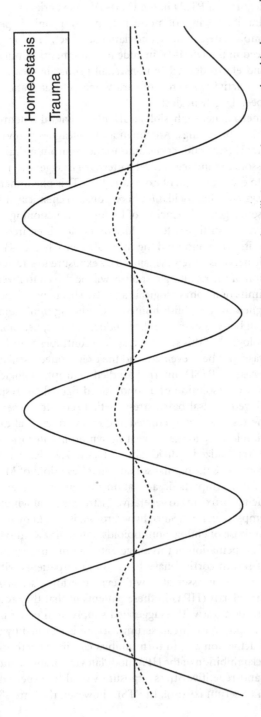

FIGURE 7.2 The autonomic nervous system in trauma. Tonic input into natural oscillatory systems may lead to increasing oscillations to the extremes of physiological tolerance. This phenomenon may in part explain the self-perpetuating exaggerated autonomic cycling between arousal and dissociation in PTSD.

the patient is subjected is through kindled systems that are activated internally by spontaneous recycled memories, and also externally by increasingly nonspecific stress-linked cues. Since there is no possible resistance to or escape from these types of stressors, the victim is essentially helpless. The inevitable response is a cyclical and increasingly recurrent freeze, or dissociative response. Dissociation is primarily a state of parasympathetic activation, one that is associated with reduced muscular and cardiovascular tone. In chronic PTSD, avoidance symptoms become increasingly prominent, as manifested by progressive social isolation, substance abuse, and constricted affect.

Avoidance, denial, and dissociation share many clinical and psychophysiological features, and in general reflect parasympathetic dominance. Depressed serum cortisol in PTSD therefore may well be a reflection of late prominence of parasympathetic influences in its chronic state. On the other hand, evidence supports that the HPA axis in PTSD may be more sensitive and in fact overresponsive to internal biological stimuli. This may reflect neurophysiological sensitization and kindling phenomena also attributed to trauma.[35] An unstable HPA axis is also in keeping with the cyclical model of autonomic fluctuation in PTSD. In late PTSD, however, the cycle is spent increasingly in the parasympathetically dominant states of depression, dissociation, and somatization, as avoidance increasingly isolates the patient from arousal-based cues.

The most compelling model for the evolution of the parasympathetic response to stress lies in the study of infant brain maturation based on early social experience. In his review of the pediatric developmental psychobiological literature, Schore discusses the evolving state of infant brain development on the basis of reactive autonomic oscillation.[36] In the dyadic (two-as-one) emotional interaction between mother and child, a negative maternal response will elicit a state of shame/withdrawal, characterized by a shift from sympathetic "ergotrophic" arousal, to parasympathetic "trophotrophic" arousal, from a hyperaroused to a hypoaroused state. Parasympathetic neurohumoral responses will accompany this shift, including decreased muscle tone, withdrawal from social interaction, vasodilatation (blushing), and loss of facial expression. This phenomenon has been called "conservation withdrawal" in the infant, and clearly represents the early manifestation of the freeze or dissociative response in trauma. Although the development of socialized behavior patterns seems dependent on this process, a pattern of excessive or intense elicitation of this shame response will result in inadequate development of coping strategies by the infant, and contribute to the development of psychiatric and character disturbances, as well as autonomic and emotional dysregulation.[36]

As noted previously, Schore believes that maturational development of the right orbitofrontal cortex (OFC), the primary regulator of autonomic stability, may actually be inhibited by excessive elicitation of shame, rendering these infants more vulnerable to withdrawal. Impaired development of this cortical area through impaired dyadic maternal attunement clearly would render the child and later the adult more vulnerable to the unstable and abnormal oscillatory autonomic state described above. Impaired OFC development would also render the individual more vulnerable to trauma by stressors of relatively less severity, and predispose the individual to freeze/dissociate more readily in the face of subsequent life threat. Impaired physiological and anatomical development of the right OFC may therefore represent the most critical factor in the vulnerability of neglected or traumatized infants or children to later traumatic life events. This process probably explains the frequent past histories of child abuse in my patients who suffered major whiplash disability in minor MVAs.

Further insights regarding the phylogenetic role of the parasympathetic nervous system in PTSD may be drawn from specifics of the Polyvagal Theory of Emotion as presented by Porges.[37] Although we have discussed The Polyvagal Theory in Chapter 6, it is worth reviewing it again in the light of our exploration of homeostasis. The insights in this theory amplify the importance of sustained parasympathetic tone in dissociation and the perpetuation of PTSD. As you will recall, Porges describes the phylogenetic layering of arousal responses in mammals, based on the varied functions of the vagal nuclei. The vagal nuclei are clusters of brain cells deep in the reptilian brainstem, the medulla, and pons. Their purpose is to regulate the viscera, including the heart, lungs, and organs of the abdomen. The dorsal vagal complex (DVC), composed of the dorsal motor nucleus of the vagus and nucleus tractus solitarius (the sensory vagus), is a vestigial and primitive center, primarily useful in reptiles for energy conservation.

The ventral vagal complex (VVC), unique to mammals, is a recent evolutionary adaptation to the high oxygen need of this class of animals, and finely tunes energy utilization by subtle and flexible influences on heart rate. The VVC contributes to the initial relatively muted response to arousal, conserving energy until the degree of threat has been determined. The VVC keeps a brake on excessive arousal for this purpose. This inhibition of arousal by the VVC is reversed if a significant threat is documented, allowing activation of the sympathetic nervous system and mobilization of fight/flight resources. If the mammal is unable to effectively defend or escape through mobilizing sympathetically tuned systems (neuromuscular, cardiovascular), rapid reduction in sympathetic tone may occur. This is then followed by increase in DVC tone, with marked bradycardia, apnea (arrest of breathing), sphincter relaxation, and gastrointestinal activation. The soldier who soils his trousers under assault is experiencing the acute influence of the DVC in a state of helpless terror. DVC activation mimics the freeze/immobility response and is associated with life-threatening cardiac arrhythmias and bradycardia in mammals. This perilous state of autonomic dysregulation has perhaps its extreme expression in humans in the phenomenon of voodoo death, as previously described by Cannon.[38] Profound activation of the DVC, as studied in animals, is associated with death due to cardiac arrest during relaxation or diastole of the heart, which literally stops while flaccid and engorged with blood. Hofer found that, when the freeze response was induced in wild rats by immobilizing them in the gloved hand, a substantial number of those rats died in this state of freeze-induced cardiac arrest, illustrating the dangers of the prolonged freeze in mammals.[39,40] The extremes of dorsal vagal parasympathetic tone therefore is a response to severe emotions, especially those associated with extreme terror and helplessness.

Although the freeze/immobility response may be lifesaving in some cases, recurrent activation of this response as part of the dissociative response in PTSD has clear and serious health and disease implications. As higher levels of adaptation to stress become ineffective, more primitive reflexes no longer useful for survival emerge and exact their toll on the health and survival of the traumatized mammal, and in our case, the human. This phenomenon may well explain the shortened life spans in animals kept in a state of helplessness, such as zoo, domestic, and laboratory animals. As we shall see, it may also explain a host of ailments experienced by the acculturated human animal.

Understanding the role of the polyvagal system as well as endorphins in dissociation may help to define the relationship of dissociation with the basic primitive freeze response in animals, including the human species. As we have noted, the freeze response is probably mediated by the activation of the DVC through failure of autonomic sympathetic arousal to effect escape or defense from a life-threatening event. Although cyclical sympathetic/parasympathetic autonomic and somatic events continue at the onset of the freeze (the brake/accelerator analogy), the victim quickly cycles deep into a state of analgesic immobility mediated by vagal and endorphinergic dominance. This state is characterized by the varying conscious perceptions described at the beginning of this chapter. If trauma occurs, predicated by the absence of "discharge," or completion of the motor sequences involved in flight or defense, the victim may then manifest variations of reemergence of procedural memory for the experiences of the trauma in the form of dissociative perceptions.

These cognitive and somatic perceptions continue to have ongoing meaning to the survival of the victim, because completion of the act of flight has not occurred. Late somatic dissociation, therefore, represents reexperiencing of survival-based messages, and the perception may be cognitive, emotional, autonomic, or sensorimotor. I believe that the entire state and experience of dissociation represents an altered state of cognition and somatic perception, driven by attempts to integrate fragments of unresolved traumatic procedural memories, and shaped by the state of increased endorphinergic and variable autonomic tone of the freeze response.

The Concept of Boundaries

Not only does the concept of autonomic oscillation in PTSD pertain to the physiology of its specific symptoms, but it also relates to the mechanism of somatic nonphysiological symptoms and findings in dissociation. With careful observation, one can find clues to perceptual and physical changes in regions of the body indicating trauma-based somatic and autonomic dysfunction. These body regions and the space around them are altered by dissociation. In this light, let us revisit the concept of boundaries with regard to the perceptual distortions seen in dissociation.

In Chapter 1, we discussed the theoretical concept of perceptual boundaries that guide us in our awareness of our physical sense of self in relation to the outside world. As Joe Kurtz, a psychiatric colleague of mine commented, "The concept of boundaries is to psychology as water is to cooking." The boundaries to which he referred were the intangible areas of sense of self that we perceive in our relationships to others, the regions of subtle behavioral perimeters in personal and social interaction. Although the concept of boundaries to which I refer includes this concept, mine is a much broader use of the term. Boundaries in my context also include our unconscious awareness of a spatial zone around us containing a sense of safety and wholeness, not only as it relates to emotions and relationships but also to the tangible, as well as the intangible, material world. It is, in effect, our personal perceptual surround.

One effect of traumatic stress is to distort or rupture those boundaries, creating a loss of our sense of safety in relation to the world. Boundary rupture occurs not only on a generalized, but also on a regional basis. The resulting sense of perceptual confusion contributes to enhanced arousal, and also to the process of constriction and avoidance seen in PTSD. The other peculiar effect resulting from loss of accurate sense of boundaries is actual physical clumsiness and the tendency to hurt oneself. Many of my MVA-related PTSD patients have experienced repeated minor injuries resulting from what can only be described as clumsiness. When asked about this problem, they invariably excitedly agree that their grace and dexterity have deteriorated. Many such patients experience falls for trivial reasons such as tripping over curbs or objects in their house. They often will bump into objects even in familiar places, especially on the side of the body where somatic dissociation can be documented by "nonphysiological signs." They will slice their fingers preparing food, drop bottles, cups, and pans, break dishes, and drive their spouses to distraction. They seem especially prone to spraining their ankles when stepping off curbs, walking down stairs, or getting out of cars. They seem to be continuously covered with bruises and Band-Aids. I will counsel them with concern about driving, because in addition to injuring themselves during everyday activities, they also are very prone to being involved in further MVAs. This increased risk in traffic probably is related to distraction resulting from dissociation, as well as suppression of attention and visual perception in regions of boundary rupture. These areas of boundary rupture are usually defined and regional, and often are identifiable as developing in the perceptual region where the threat was first identified.

As seen in the patient with a measurable refractive error in one eye due to dissociation, the area of boundary interruption often relates to the region of the perceptual surround where the person first glimpsed or otherwise sensed the threat. The localized area of the body that first experienced an impact or blow, the surrounding area from which the person heard the threatening noise, or the direction in which the body was forcibly thrust might all potentially create an area of impaired boundary continuity. Areas of such changes in perception undoubtedly represent evidence for procedural memory for a threat experienced in that region, leading to a dissociative response in the face of stimuli arising from that area. The generalization of perceived threat from the dissociated region is an example of the tendency for the traumatized individual to become sensitized to increasingly minor and nonspecific sources of arousal.

The presence of localized areas of boundary rupture can also be documented in the clinical treatment setting. As part of our trauma treatment, our therapists prepare patients by seating them in a comfortable chair with their eyes closed. The therapist will ask the patient to report any sensations, both emotional and physical. The therapist then quietly walks slowly around the patient and makes notes of the location if the patient reports distress. As the therapist approaches an area of boundary rupture in the patient's perimeter, the patient may experience a sense of arousal or mild anxiety. Physical symptoms associated with this exercise usually are visceral in nature, including a sensation of tightness in the chest, mild nausea, and "a hollow feeling in the pit of the stomach." These physical sensations undoubtedly represent symptoms related to the early mammalian system of threat awareness involving the ventral vagal complex. These areas of impaired boundary integrity therefore represent regions of potential threat to the patient based on implicit proprioceptive memory for the traumatic event and the region in which it occurred.

I will usually perform a crude test of boundary integrity with my MVA patients. Standing facing the patient, I will slowly move my hand around their visual periphery at a distance of about four to six feet while the patient continues to look at my face. This maneuver will often elicit an arousal response characterized by eye blink, pupillary dilatation, flushing, or even flinching or withdrawal of the body when I reach a specific and reproducible point of visual boundary stimulation. Patients will usually report dizziness, distraction, nausea, or chest constriction at that moment. Frequently the patient will experience pain in the region of the body associated with the boundary rupture. Occasionally the patient may only experience a vague sense of uneasiness, or in some cases, irritability, or anger when vision is stimulated in that region. One can usually relate that area to some meaningful and regional element of the traumatic event, such as being impacted broadside from that direction in an MVA, assaulted from behind in a mugging or rape or receiving a blow to that area of the body in an assault. At times this exercise may be so distressing that arousal is only dissipated if the examiner stands at the door, or even across the hallway.

The area of sensitivity to boundary stimulus usually corresponds to an area of the body associated with nonphysiological symptoms or findings, consistent with their dissociative origin. In cases of a history of severe, multiple traumatic experiences, especially sexual abuse as a child, the patient may have no areas of visual or perceptual stimulation that are not associated with discomfort or arousal, and the whole exercise of visual or perceptual boundary testing may be intolerable. Caution must be applied with this exercise in such cases.

Finally, boundary ruptures also are identifiable by postural changes that reflect unconscious moving of the body away from the dissociated area by assuming bent or twisted static postures, such as in the patient with arm pain after extensive skin grafts. "Nervous tics," or repetitive habitual muscle twitches may be present in this region, since tics reflect procedural memory for a defensive motor act that was suppressed by the traumatic event. At times, however, there may be no associated sensorimotor symptoms to identify the area of impaired boundary. For instance, approaching the rape or incest victim from behind in the office examination room, or requesting that the victim lie prone on the table to examine the back may be enough to trigger a panic attack in the absence of regional symptoms. Even without awareness of an alteration in body sensation, arousal may occur with anticipation of kinesthetic, visual, or auditory sensory input to that region of impaired boundary sense. As a result, the victim of trauma with areas of indefensible boundaries will be repetitively subjected to subliminal arousal stimuli that serve to perpetuate autonomic oscillation. The concept of boundary rupture is a useful tool for understanding somatic dissociation, as well as trauma in general.

The Spectrum of Somatic Dissociation

We have referred to the presence of "nonphysiological signs" in the context of boundary rupture, somatic dissociation, and conversion hysteria. All of these signs of course are neurological in nature, suggesting some arcane impairment of brain function. During my career as a neurologist, I puzzled over the contention by my teachers and peers that conversion hysteria was a psychological phenomenon, and that the disability was in fact imagined. Also as a neurologist, I realized that hysterical patients always ended up in my practice. And they all presented with the same cluster of symptoms, and with the classical nonphysiological signs of stocking-glove anesthesia, give-away muscle weakness, and dramatic, exaggerated balance disturbance. Were they all communicating through some underground system to present with all of the same aberrant "nonphysiological signs"? In fact, Freud himself noted that the areas of paralysis and anesthesia mimicked the areas of the body that experienced the trauma, and the neurological disability therefore protected them from anxiety. In my model of somatic dissociation, the sensorimotor impairment indeed reflects the region of the body that perceived the sensory messages of the threat, and that sensorimotor disability actually reflects the failed motor attempt of defense. In this model, then, all of the common tics, mild postural distortions, asymmetrical facial expressions, limps, and even the slumped posture of depression and aging must reflect the fixed postures of failed survival behavior.

Van der Hart and colleagues explored this phenomenon in shell-shocked soldiers during World War I, describing the sensorimotor impairments in the decidedly dissociative disorder of shell shock as somatoform dissociation. Psychiatrists of that era, including Ferenczi and McDougall, understood that the fixed postures of arms and legs that persisted permanently in their shell-shocked veterans reflected the final postures of self-defense that were "frozen" in place at the moment they were rendered helpless.[41] These soldiers were considered to be hysterics and malingerers, and were institutionalized, sometimes as prisoners. This invaluable heritage of knowledge was lost in the development of trauma theory in psychiatry. Somatic dissociation therefore has its roots in the understanding of conversion hysteria, in the tics and postures of everyday life, and in the strange phenomenon of regional perceptual sensitivity to arousal that reflects boundary rupture, also in the region of an old, unresolved threat.

As we shall see in Chapter 8, that dissociated part of the body bears an additional burden. For one sees disturbances of the autonomic regulation of circulation specifically in the body part and region that provided the warning message to the brain as part of an unresolved life threat. Several psychotherapists have asked me about the appearance of stigmata in their patients. The term, stigmata, was derived from the appearance of the wounds of Christ in devout Christians, occurring in several hundred people sporadically over many centuries. In psychotherapy, many of my colleagues have documented the appearance of change in skin color, usually reddening of a part of the body during a therapy session. Invariably, this area of erythema replicates the area of a blow or injury to that region of the body in a traumatic assault. These stigmata are so precise that in one case a handprint in red appeared on the face of a patient who was describing an assault by her abusive husband during a session of EMDR. These stigmata represent exquisitely specific procedural memory for the sensory experience of a specific trauma, with somatic dissociation of that area, and associated impaired autonomic regulation of circulation in that dissociated region or body part. In Chapter 8 we will explore disease processes that accompany this autonomic, vasomotor manifestation of somatic dissociation.

The Dissociative Capsule

Daniel Stern describes the "present moment" as a variable one-to ten-second "lived story." During this moment, we process sensory information coming from both the internal sensations of the body, and from the external environment. Perception of the present moment is tempered by concepts of time (when?), intentionality (why?) and vitality affects (shifting emotions).[42] Working memory—storage for a limited time—also contributes to our perception of the present moment. This fleeting period of awareness in a sense defines what we perceive as consciousness. The present moment is essential for our ability to process information from our internal and external world, and to act appropriately (intentionality). During the present moment, we continue to develop our constantly evolving sense of self, based on incorporation of the somatosensory components of the moment into the library of our autobiographical memory.[43]

Impairment of perception of the present moment may be caused by intrusion of old body-based procedural memories, as well as declarative memories of past events, especially those linked to old trauma. These traumatic memories are linked to arousal and emotion. In a sense, posttraumatic memories may be considered to be "false," in that they are associated with emotional tone and body sensations that represent a past event as if it were in fact present. The uncorrupted present moment is associated with an appropriate concept of time (when?) based on input from our prefrontal cortex.

This is the dilemma of posttraumatic symptoms: internal and external cues of old traumatic memories continue to trigger emotions and body sensations that do not represent the present moment, but rather past moments when the trauma was experienced. As a result, the present moment may be corrupted by past traumatic autobiographical memories, and the actual experience may be an illusion of time and perception. Because perception of the present moment is relegated to past traumatic experience in the trauma victim, the evolving sense of self will also be "stuck" at that past moment in time. This process is in keeping with the well-known tendency for the trauma victim's sense of self and developmental maturity to be relatively frozen or arrested at the time and age of the sentinel traumatic experience. I would suggest that this unique narrowing, interruption, and corruption of perception of the present moment by past procedural memory in traumatic stress is, in fact, what we define as dissociation.

I have postulated that trauma is due to the storage in procedural and declarative memory of all of the experiences of the traumatic event—autonomic, somatosensory, limbic/emotional, and conscious/explicit—leading to fear conditioning. This storage occurs specifically in the absence of "completion" and extinction because of the absence of the freeze discharge. Each one of these experiences forms a memory "state" or "capsule," the contents of which are precisely specific for the event itself. The content of the capsule may vary based on the unique features of the traumatic experience—it may be predominantly limbic or emotional (grief, emotional shock, shame). It may be profoundly autonomic when little somatosensory input was experienced (terror in warfare, exposure to a mutilated body, shame). Somatosensory memories may predominate (motor vehicle accident, physical assault) where somatosensory input was intense. Finally, declarative memory linked to emotion will usually compose a portion of the capsule, although it may also be absent or distorted. The "size" or intensity of the capsule may be dependent on the relative intensity of the experience itself. It may also be based on the repetitive nature of similar traumatic experiences, as in child and spousal abuse or multiple MVAs. The earlier in life that these traumatic experiences have occurred, the more intense the effects and the greater the relative size of the capsule will be. As such, they would be more likely to obliterate the present moment, and dissociative symptoms and experiences would predominate. I would propose that such procedural memory capsules might be called dissociative capsules, since interruption of the present moment/consciousness by their stereotyped past memory content will be associated with the altered state of perception that we define as dissociation. In such a state, corruption of the concept of time within the present moment will render these memories as being falsely present. The varying nature of the content of the capsules would depend on the varying content of the traumatic experience, explaining myriad manifestations that we attribute to dissociation.

The quantitative impact of many life traumas, especially occurring in childhood, would determine the amount of interference with perception of the present moment that would occur in the trauma victim. In cases of severe, repetitive, and varied childhood trauma, posttraumatic dissociative perceptions would dominate most of their present moment, or consciousness, defining the state and diagnosis of dissociative identity disorder (DID). Because each capsule would have its own unique autonomic procedural memory state, the various "alters" would manifest their own unique autonomic tone, physiology, and even disease states, as has been noted in DID. Poorly understood medical syndromes, such as whiplash, could be viewed as dissociative capsules. The myofascial neck and back pain, vertigo, labile blood pressure, temporomandibular joint syndrome, cognitive impairment, and emotional lability would represent procedural memory for myriad somatosensory, emotional, autonomic, and cognitive experiences of the MVA. They arise repetitively based on internal and external cues, and are perceived as occurring in the present, although they are in fact past procedural memories. Or the dissociative capsule might simply contain emotional and autonomic memories that might be experienced solely as intrusive, distracting ruminative thoughts. In this model, the DSM–IV criteria for PTSD would simply define in generic terms the content of the prototype dissociative capsule. Dissociation would in fact be the altered state of perception produced by a specific capsule, triggered by an internal or external cue related to specific procedural or declarative memory of that capsule and impinging on and corrupting the present moment (see Figure 7.3).

This model is clearly a purely theoretical construct that borrows from a number of thinkers in the field, and ignores a great deal of the vast theoretical literature in the field of dissociation. On the other hand, I believe that it provides a useful platform for the consideration of appropriate therapeutic approaches for traumatic stress and dissociation. It brings together a vast array of clinical symptoms and

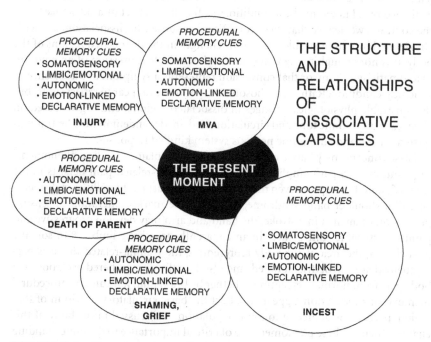

FIGURE 7.3   The dissociative capsule and its interruption of the present moment.

syndromes attributed to trauma into a relatively unitary whole, and it presents a physiological model that lends itself well to the consideration of priorities in trauma therapy. The primary goal of therapy in this model would be the progressive shrinkage and eventual obliteration of each dissociative capsule by extinction of its unique procedural memory cues.

Conclusion

The phenomenon of dissociation may be the most critical element of trauma, and in fact may define it. Dissociation, or freeze, at the moment of trauma is perhaps the main defining event in the development of subsequent PTSD. It may well account for many of the cognitive deficits attributed to a minor physical closed head injury in selected cases. The neurochemical and neurophysiological correlates of dissociation include endorphinergic neural effects, changes in HPA dynamics, and marked autonomic instability in the form of abnormal oscillatory cycling between extremes of sympathetic and parasympathetic tone. These forces may well be the engine driving the kindled brain circuitry of trauma.

The concept of somatic dissociation as a tangible and clinically measurable change in regional somatosensory physiology challenges current concepts of the criteria for somatization and somatoform disorders, conversion disorder, and pain disorder. As defined in the DSM–IV, all of these disorders cannot be fully explained by a known medical condition, or the direct effect of a substance.[44] On the contrary, we believe that these conditions, as subsets of dissociation, are actually defined by demonstrable vasomotor changes in the dissociated regions of the body. It is not enough to say that somatization reflects expression of an emotion in a somatic symptom, or that conversion represents a symptom in the absence of a medical condition. Rather, psychosomatic syndromes appear to reflect subtle but demonstrable physiological changes in dissociated regional end organs based on changes in autonomic tone and circulation, and are dependent in turn on trauma-related central and autonomic nervous system kindled responses.

These concepts may have a correlate in other unexplained medical phenomena. In phantom limb pain, implicit memory for trauma-related pain persists in the form of altered perception even though the injured part has literally been dismembered. In shoulder-hand syndrome, related to the marked alteration in sensory perception of an arm in a stroke, the hand and arm may develop progressive and painful dystrophic contractures in an apparently anesthetic limb.[45,46] In somatic dissociation, the area of the body representing the trauma-related threat is perceptually dissociated, disembodied, and also literally dismembered. Isolation of a body part from normal perception, whether by brain injury, traumatic procedural memory, or dissociation, appears to affect the basic circulatory nutrition of that region, perhaps by altered autonomic regulation as discussed in the body of this chapter. I believe these phenomena are of critical importance to the understanding of many chronic diseases of unknown cause, and may have a major bearing on the progression of any chronic disease.

Finally, I believe that one can provide a model for trauma that incorporates all of the symptoms attributable to it, including the autonomic and somatosensory manifestations, into a unitary whole. By incorporating all of these physiological elements of a traumatic event into a specific state, or capsule, one can explain not only the peculiar and varied manifestations of perception that we consider to be dissociation, but also the entire structure of the posttraumatic syndrome itself.

Notes

1. Janet, P.: *The Major Symptoms of Hysteria.* New York: Macmillan, 1920.
2. Freud, S., Breuer, J.: On the physical mechanism of hysterical phenomena. In Jones, E. (Ed.). *Sigmund Freud, MD, LLD. Collected Papers, Volume I* (pp. 24–41). London: Hogarth Press, 1953.
3. Mayer-Gross, W.: On depersonalization. *British Journal of Medical Psychology,* 1953; 15:103–126.
4. Spiegel, D., Cardena, E.: Disintegrated experience: The dissociative disorders revisited. *Journal of Abnormal Psychology,* 1991; 100:166–178.
5. Bremner, J., Southwick, S., Brett, E., Fontana, A., Rosenheck, R., Charney, D.: Dissociation and post-traumatic stress disorder in Vietnam combat veterans. *American Journal of Psychiatry,* 1992; 149:328–332.
6. Putnam, E., Guroff, J., Silberman, E., Barban, L., Post, R.: The clinical phenomenology of multiple personality disorder: Review of 100 recent cases. *Journal of Clinical Psychiatry,* 1986; 47:285–293.
7. Christianson, S.: The relationship between induced arousal and amnesia. *Scandinavian Journal of Psychology,* 1984; 25:147–160.
8. Briere, L., Conte, J.: Self-reported amnesia for abuse in adults molested in childhood. *Journal of Traumatic Stress,* 1991; 6:21–31.
9. Pynoos, R., Frederick, C., Nader. K., Arroyo, W., Steinberg, A., Eth, S., Nunez, F., Fairbanks, L.: Life threat and post-traumatic stress disorder in school-age children. *Archives of General Psychiatry,* 1987; 44:1057–1063.
10. Terr, L.: Time sense following psychic trauma: A clinical study of ten adults and twenty children. *American Journal of Orthopsychiatry,* 1983; 53:244–261.
11. Mellman, T., Davis, G.: Combat-related flashbacks in post-traumatic stress disorder: Phenomenology and similarity to panic attacks. *Journal of Clinical Psychiatry,* 1985; 46:179–382.
12. van der Kolk, B.: The body keeps the score: Memory and the evolving psychobiology or posttraumatic stress. *Harvard Review of Psychiatry,* 1994; January/February:253–265.
13. Bremner, D., Scott, T., Delaney, R., Southwick, S., Mason, L., Johnson, D., Innis, R., McCarthy, G., Charney, D.: Deficits in short-term memory in posttraumatic stress disorder. *American Journal of Psychiatry,* 1993; 150(7):1015–1019.
14. Goldstein, G., van Kammen, W., Shelly, C., Miller, D., van Kammen, D.: Survivors of imprisonment in the Pacific theater during World War II. *American Journal of Psychiatry,* 1987; 144:1210–1213.
15. Sutker, P., Allain, A., Motsinger, P.: Minnesota Multiphasic Personality Inventory (MMPO-derived psychopathoillgy sub-types among former prisoners of war (POWS): Replication and extension. *Journal of Psychopathology and Behavioral Assessment,* 1988; 10:129–140.

16. Thygesen, P., Hermann, I., Willanger, R.: Concentration camp survivors in Denmark: Persecution, disease, compensation. *Danish Medical Bulletin*, 1970; 17:65–108.

17. Sutker, P., Winstead, D., Galina, Z., Allain, A.: Cognitive deficits and psychopathology among former prisoners of war and combat veterans of the Korean conflict. *American Journal of Psychiatry*, 1991; 148:67–72.

18. Bremner, L., Steinberg, M., Southwick, S., Johnson, D., Charney, D.: Use of the structured clinical interview for DSM–IV dissociative disorders for systematic assessment of dissociative symptoms in post-traumatic stress disorder. *American Journal of Psychiatry*, 1993; 150:1011–1014.

19. Zeitlin, S., McNally, R.: Implicit and explicit memory bias for threat in posttraumatic stress disorder. *Behaviour Research and Therapy*, 1999; 29:451–457.

20. Hilgard, E.: *Divided Consciousness: Multiple Controls in Human Thought and Action.* New York: Wiley, 1977.

21. Krystal, J., Bennett. A., Bremner, J., Southwick, S., Charney, D.: Toward a cognitive neuroscience of dissociation and altered memory functions in post-traumatic stress disorder. In Friedman, M. L., Charney, D. S., Deutch, A. Y. (Eds.). *Neurobiological and Clinical Consequences of Stress* (pp. 244–245). Philadelphia: Lippincott-Raven, 1995.

22. van der Kolk. B., van der Hart, O.: Pierre Janet and the breakdown of adaptation in psychological trauma. *American Journal of Psychiatry*, 1989; 146:1530–1540.

23. Bremner, J., Southwick, S., Brett, E., Fontana, A., Rosenheck, R., Charney, D.: Dissociation and post-traumatic stress disorder in Vietnam combat veterans. *American Journal of Psychiatry*, 1992; 149:328–332.

24. Holen, A.: The North Sea oil rig disaster. In Wilson. L., Raphael, B., (Eds.). *International Handbook of Traumatic Stress Syndromes* (pp. 471–479). New York: Plenum Press, 1993.

25. Cardena, E., Spiegel, D.: Dissociative reactions to the Bay Area earthquake. *American Journal of Psychiatry*, 1993; 150:474–478.

26. Kolb, L.: Neurophysiological hypothesis explaining post-traumatic stress disorder. *American Journal of Psychiatry*, 1987; 144:989–995.

27. McFarlane, A., Weber, D., Clark, C.: Abnormal stimulus processing in PTSD. *Biological Psychiatry*, 1993; 34:311–320.

28. Morgan, M., LeDoux, J.: Differential contributions of dorsal and ventral medial prefrontal cortex to the acquisition and extinction of conditioned fear in rats. *Behavioral Neuroscience*, 1995; 109:681–688.

29. Hamner, M., Loberbaum, L., George, M.: Potential role of the anterior cingulate cortex in PTSD: Review and hypothesis. *Depression and Anxiety*, 1999; 9:1–14.

30. van der Kolk, B.: The compulsion to repeat the trauma: Re-enactment, re-victimization and masochism. *Psychiatric Clinics of North America*, 1989; 12:389–411.

31. Antelman, S., Caggiula, A., Kiss, D., Edwards, D., Kocan, D., Stiller, R.: Neurochemical and physiological effects of cocaine oscillate with sequential drug treatment: Possibly a major factor in drug variability. *Neuropsychopharmacology*, 1995; 12:297–306.

32. Caggiula, A., Antelman, S., Palmer, A., Kiss, S., Edwards, D., Kocan, D.: The effects of ethanol on striatal dopamine and frontal cortical D-[3H] aspartate efflux oscillate with repeated treatment: Relevance to individual differences in responsiveness. *Neuropsychopharmacology*, 1996; 15: 125–132.

33. Antelman, S., Caggiula, A.: Oscillation follows drug implications. *Critical Review of Neurobiology*, 1996; 10:101–117.

34. Antelman, S., Caggiula, A., Gershon, S., Edwards, D., Austin, M., Kiss, S., Kocan, D.: Stressor-induced oscillation: A possible model of the bidirectional symptoms of PTSD. *New York Academy of Sciences*, 1997; 21:296–305.

35. Southwick, S., Yehuda, R., Wang, S.: Neuroendocrine alterations in posttraumatic stress disorder. *Psychiatric Annals*, 1998; 28(8):436–450.

36. Schore, A.: *Affect Regulation and the Origin of the Self.* Hillsdale, NJ: Lawrence Erlbaum Associates, 1994. pp. 204–209.

37. Porges, S.: Orienting in a defensive world: Mammalian modifications of our evolutionary heritage: A polyvagal theory. *Psychophysiology*, 199; 5: 32:301–318.

38. Cannon, W.: "Voodoo" death. *Psychosomatic Medicine*, 1957; 19:182–190, Reprinted from *American Anthropology*, 1942; 44:169.

39. Richter, C.: On the phenomenon of sudden death in animals and man. *Psychosomatic Medicine*, 1957; 19:191–198.

40. Hofer, M.: Cardiac respiratory function during sudden prolonged immobility in wild rodents. *Psychosomatic Medicine*, 1970; 32:633–647.

41. van der Hart, O., van Dijke, A., van Son, M., Steele, K.: Somatiform dissociation in traumatized World War I combat soldiers: A neglected clinical heritage. *Journal of Trauma and Dissocation*, 2000; 1(4):33–66.

42. Stern, D.: *The Present Moment in Psychotherapy and Everyday Life.* New York: W.W. Norton, 2004.

43. Damasio, A.: *Descartes Error: Emotion, Reason and the Human Brain.* New York: Avon Books, 1994.

44. American Psychiatric Association: *Diagnostic and Statistical Manual of Mental Disorders.* Fourth Edition (DSM–IV). Washington, DC: American Psychiatric Association, 1994.

45. Peny, S., Tepperman, N., Greyson, D., Hilbert, L., Jimenez, L., Williams, J.: Reflex sympathetic dystrophy in hemiplegia. *Archives of Physical Medicine and Rehabilitation*, 1984; 65:442–446.

46. Dursun, E., Dursun, N., Ural, C., Cakci, A.: Glenohumeral joint subluxation and reflex sympathetic dystrophy in hemiplegic patients. *Archives of Physical Medicine*, 2000; 81:944–946.

eight
Diseases of Traumatic Stress

Pat had been involved in a relatively minor but particularly terrifying auto accident. While stopped at a light behind a large dump truck, the truck unexpectedly began to back up. Unable to retreat due to the car behind her, and apparently unseen by the truck driver, she watched in horror as the truck slowly bore down on her and crushed the hood and engine compartment of her car. Her car was shaken, but not moved, and the noise of the crushing of metal finally prompted the truck driver to stop. Pat was predictably shocked, stunned, and numb, and took hours to recover her senses and awareness of what had happened to her.

She subsequently developed headaches, neck pain, panic attacks, and full-blown post-traumatic stress disorder, along with significant cognitive problems. Within a week of the accident, she developed influenza, with a severe eruption of herpes sores on her lips. She missed her next menstrual period, and within six weeks, gained twelve pounds, with most of the weight embarrassingly concentrated about her waist. Several bladder infections followed in the ensuing months, and heartburn and symptoms of gastroesophageal reflux prompted a diagnostic workup by a gastroenterologist, with negative results. As her neck pain worsened and spread to her lower back, shoulders, and arms, she noted increasing morning stiffness, and generalized pain and sensitivity to touch. With the development of interrupted, nonrestorative sleep and chronic fatigue, she was ultimately diagnosed by a rheumatologist with fibromyalgia, chronic fatigue syndrome, and irritable bowel syndrome. A physician who performed an independent medical examination for her automobile insurance company, however, concluded that she was probably suffering from conversion and somatization, and that secondary gain issues must be considered, since the accident itself was certainly negligible with regard to the possibility of significant physical injury.

* * *

The Pathophysiology of Stress

The concept that prolonged or excessive exposure to stress could contribute to the development of specific diseases was formulated by Selye in 1936.[1] His original studies are mentioned in Chapter 2, and have led to the conclusion that exposure of an animal or a person to a variety of stressors would result in a complex neuroendocrine response primarily involving the hormones of the pituitary gland and adrenal cortex. These responses were critical to the survival of the organism when subjected to an acute stress, but exposure to prolonged or cumulative stress could result in damage to the organism. Much of this damage was due to prolonged exposure to adrenal cortical hormones, especially cortisol. So Selye's rats subjected to prolonged, inescapable stress were found to develop erosion of the stomach lining, atherosclerosis, and atrophy of the adrenals. Selye's findings have been validated by more than a half-century of research, and support the role of pituitary/adrenal cortical activity in stress modulation and in the development of specific diseases.

We have discussed the role of cortisol and other so-called glucocorticoids in modulating the acute role of the brain neurotransmitter norepinephrine in stress (Chapter 4). Cortisol actually inhibits the acute effects of stress-based arousal by norepinephrine on the limbic system, especially the amygdala. Cortisol also regulates the hypothalamic/pituitary/adrenal axis (HPA) in the ongoing response to stress. It operates via a negative feedback loop that inhibits the hypothalamus and pituitary gland. Elevation of serum cortisol therefore inhibits the release of ACTH, an example of many of the feedback servo-systems in the body that promote homeostasis. The complex effects of gluco- and mineralocorticoids (those that control sodium, potassium, and water) also serve to manage the body's secondary line of defense to stress. These effects include retaining sodium in the body and mobilizing glucose from glycogen in the liver. They increase blood volume and provide increased sources of energy production, both necessary for managing chronic stress. They also include increased insulin secretion, mobilization of calcium from bone stores, increase in fat formation, increase in peptic acid secretion in the stomach, suppression of lymphocyte formation in the bone marrow, and cerebral cortical stimulation. All of these responses prepare the organism to deal with prolonged stress at the expense of long-term health. The resulting immune, metabolic, and neuronal responses are important in the organism's early defenses to abnormal stressors, but if prolonged, may lead to specific organ damage.

The "diseases of stress" that result from prolonged stress adaptation reflect the well-known systemic side effects of prolonged therapeutic glucocorticoid (cortisol) administration. These diseases include diabetes, atherosclerosis, hypertension, peptic ulcer disease, obesity, osteoporosis, and cognitive/emotional impairment, all attributable to the effects described previously. In addition, excess exposure to cortisol in animals has been found to selectively damage neurons primarily in the hippocampus, the brain center for declarative memory (see Chapter 6). All of these diseases appear to accurately reflect the findings in Selye's chronically stressed rats. Clearly, chronic and prolonged exposure to unremitting life stress is associated with a cluster of vascular, hormonal, immunological, neuronal, and degenerative diseases that are largely attributable to exposure to abnormal amounts of glucocorticoids.

Stress Versus Trauma

Prolonged stress and trauma, although they are basically part of the same continuum, differ in a number of ways. Stress may be defined in one sense as any negative stimulus that produces persistent activation of the sympathetic nervous system and related HPA pathways. Trauma may be viewed in this light as an extreme form of stress, one that has assumed life-threatening proportions. Trauma also is usually a sentinel event or events of great threat and magnitude, producing a maximal arousal, fight/flight response. Also, the neurophysiological effects of trauma will often not occur unless there is an element of lack of control or helplessness associated with the stress. When relative helplessness is present, an experience of terror or horror may accompany the traumatic event, an emotional state that is very suggestive of elements of the freeze/immobility response. Once again, the combination of a life threat associated with helplessness is the prerequisite for trauma to occur.

In our previous discussion of the meaning of the freeze response, we noted that the physiology of freezing involves intense vagal parasympathetic tone. If a high-energy, sympathetic fight/flight response has preceded the freeze, the autonomic climate of the freeze may be a rapid and exaggerated sympathetic/parasympathetic cycling, much like the analogy of the simultaneous pressure on the accelerator and brake pedals of a car. However, the freeze response ultimately assumes a state of predominantly dorsal vagal dominance (Chapter 7).

The freeze represents a temporary adaptation to acute stress that is not physiologically sustainable, and one that is certainly not associated with continued arousal associated with adrenaline and elevation of serum cortisol. As we have noted, the freeze response very likely is associated with the perceptual state that we call dissociation, an event that is a powerful predictor of the subsequent development of PTSD in individuals subjected to a traumatic experience. Traumatic stress and the development of PTSD are not inevitable with exposure to stress or trauma, however life threatening. These events very likely depend on the event of the freeze/immobility response occurring in a state of helplessness associated with that threat, and perhaps on the perpetuation of dissociation as a secondary event. By definition, they also depend on the absence of a freeze discharge. As a result, we might expect to see a substantial difference in the pathological changes in the body, and therefore the diseases that occur in chronic stress, trauma, and traumatic stress.

The Hypothalamic/Pituitary/Adrenal Axis

Patients with PTSD exhibit much more complex hormonal changes than those seen in Selye's model of diseases of stress. The changes in PTSD/trauma are primarily suggestive of abnormal function of the hypothalamic/pituitary/adrenal (HPA) axis. Levels of serum cortisol are elevated in acute stress, as in Selye's model of stress-related disease. But studies of serum cortisol in late stage or chronic PTSD show abnormally low levels of serum cortisol and twenty-four-hour urinary cortisol excretion.[2,3,4] It is as if late PTSD has assumed some of the features of the parasympathetic freeze response. In addition, binding sites for cortisol in the brain and on lymphocytes normally tend to increase with low serum levels of cortisol. So it is not surprising in late PTSD, in which serum cortisol is relatively low, that increased numbers of lymphocyte glucocorticoid receptors were also found. This apparent paradox is contradictory to previously noted concepts of the response of the HPA axis to Selye's model of stress. It does suggest, however, that the HPA axis is somehow sensitized in PTSD and trauma.[5]

Further evidence for a sensitized HPA axis in chronic PTSD is found in the Dexamethasone Suppression Test (DST). Dexamethasone mimics the effect of cortisol on inhibiting the HPA axis. So administration of dexamethasone in the normal individual suppresses release of CRH by the hypothalamus as well as adrenocorticotropic hormone (ACTH) by the pituitary.[6] By inhibiting the HPA axis, dexamethasone secondarily inhibits cortisol release by the adrenal cortex by substituting for the patient's own cortisol, thereby "fooling" the HPA axis into shutting down. But chronic PTSD patients actually show an exaggerated suppression of cortisol release with the DST, again suggesting a highly sensitized HPA axis in these patients. In addition, an over-stimulating exposure to hypothalamic CRH causes impairment of the release of ACTH by the pituitary in PTSD patients. This is further evidence for HPA dysfunction in this group of patients. What we may be looking at here is an intrinsic state of autonomic and neurohormonal dysregulation in trauma.

Admittedly these findings are far from conclusive in defining the abnormal stress response in PTSD. They do, however, tend to separate PTSD from other psychiatric conditions with regard to their relationship to the sympathetic nervous system, the HPA axis, and the more traditional model of the stress response developed by Selye.[7] They also may have implications regarding the unique spectrum of diseases that may accompany chronic symptoms of PTSD.

Stress, Post-Traumatic Stress Disorder, and Immune Function

Alteration of the immune system has been one of the more thoroughly studied examples of the health effects of inordinate stress. Studies of the effects of stress on viral immunity have generally shown consistently increased vulnerability to infection. Cold virus inoculations in unstressed subjects and in those exposed to stress have shown increased vulnerability to respiratory infection in the stressed subjects.[8] Antibody levels to Epstein-Barr virus (EBV), hepatitis B virus, herpes simplex virus, and cytomegalovirus have been noted to consistently rise with stress.[9,10,11] Increased viral antibody titers in these cases represent reduced cellular immunity, indicating immune suppression. Immune responses to stress in human immunodeficiency virus (HIV) in limited studies show that stress may induce reduction of total lymphocytes and natural killer cells.[12,13] Clearly, exposure to high levels of chronic stress may increase susceptibility to infectious diseases due to immune suppression.

Natural killer (NK) cells constitute a main line of defense by the immune system against not only infectious agents, but also mutated cancer cells. In acute stress, elevation of epinephrine (E) and norepinephrine (NE) as part of the fight/flight response is associated with increased NK cell activity, or increased immune function. The fact that this increase in immune function is directly due to effects of E and NE on an acute basis is supported by the fact that the increase of NK activity in these cases is blocked by propranolol. Propranalol is a peripheral beta-adrenergic blocker, and therefore an inhibitor of peripheral effects of epinephrine on organs of the body.[14] It has also long been known that high levels of cortisol associated with early responses to trauma and stress actually impair immune function. That is the basis for the long-standing use of synthetic forms of cortisol in organ transplants in order to inhibit immune rejection of the organ, and in autoimmune diseases such as rheumatoid arthritis. So in acute stress, there are somewhat contradictory effects of E and NE versus cortisol on immune function, reflecting the modulating effect of cortisol on the arousal systems of the brain.

By contrast, chronic exposure to stress results in reduction in NK cell activity despite continued increase in E and NE levels.[15] In addition, exposure to chronic stress actually inhibits the increased NK activity response to acute stress.[16] Exposure to chronic stress therefore appears to inhibit one of the body's frontline immune defenses, and to inhibit the natural increase in immune defenses in the face of new and acute stress. The clinical effects of chronic stress on viral infections would certainly suggest that stress-induced immune suppression is clinically significant with regard to general health. Therefore, one would expect relative immune suppression and vulnerability to infectious disease in acute PTSD, where serum cortisol is also elevated. Cortisol function in acute PTSD basically appears to be somewhat analogous to that in chronic stress.

In chronic PTSD victims, however, serum cortisol levels tend to be low, a state in which the inhibitory effect of cortisol on the immune system is decreased. Under these circumstances, the biological effects of late PTSD might stimulate immune activity, and contribute to vulnerability to autoimmune diseases. There is considerable speculation about the role of life trauma in the autoimmune diseases based on these findings of potential immune suppression. Scientific evidence for the increased risk of autoimmune disease with lower serum cortisol levels in chronic PTSD is unfortunately not available at this time. A clue to this possible relationship, however, can be found in epidemiological studies of the incidence of chronic disease in populations of patients who have been exposed to prolonged and severe traumatic stress.

The Diseases of Trauma

Chronic Pain

One of the most thoroughly studied symptoms associated with prior histories of severe trauma is chronic pain. Many of these studies address the effects of childhood abuse on chronic pain complaints, especially in women sexually abused in childhood. The baseline incidence of childhood sexual abuse in women has been estimated at anywhere from 12 to 64 percent of the general female population in various studies.[17-22] An average incidence probably falls somewhere around 30 percent. In males, the incidence is predictably less than half of that figure. Many studies document the association between childhood physical and sexual abuse and chronic pain. Perhaps the most thoroughly studied association is found between female childhood sexual abuse and chronic pelvic pain.[23-29] In general, these studies show a significantly higher incidence of childhood sexual abuse in women with medically unexplained pelvic pain than controls or comparison groups, such as women seeking tubal ligation. Other studies, however, show that childhood physical abuse predicted all adult pain syndromes as well or better than sexual abuse.[30] Taken together, childhood sexual, physical, and psychological abuse are powerful predictors of chronic pelvic, abdominal, low back, orofacial, and myofascial pain.[31-35]

Epidemiological events that occur together do not prove a cause-and-effect association. We need a solid theoretical basis, combined with the weight of controlled scientific studies, to arrive at a justified etiological conclusion. Obviously, this goal is not within the scope of this book. I believe, however, that the core concept of the neurophysiology of PTSD and its relationship to the basic features of the whiplash syndrome allow us to expand concepts of perpetuation of symptoms of many chronic diseases, especially chronic pain.

Classical conditioning is the primary process in the brain that we use in developing our storehouse of survival-based procedural memory. Conditioning is not a laboratory phenomenon, but is the key system of accessing information responsible for individual and species survival. Conditioned responses to an identifiable life threat must take place in one or two trials, or else the specific gene matrix of the unfortunate prey animal is discarded, probably for the betterment of the species. Natural selection is meant to cull the genetically weaker members of the herd. Sensory information for all of the experiences associated with any life threat is incorporated immediately, and hopefully forever, into the implicit memory of the surviving animal for future reference and application in a similar threatening situation. We unconsciously learn to survive only through repeated exposure to threat and the lessons it teaches.

In the example of myofascial pain after an MVA, I believe that the proprioceptive memory of the specific protective movement patterns of the body in the accident generated by stretch receptors are immediately and indelibly stored in motor centers as part of survival-based procedural memory. Thereafter, they will be resurrected time and again in situations of perceived life threat or exposure to cues of the accident experience. This process will lead to recurrent regional patterns of muscle tightening and myofascial pain in those muscles that unsuccessfully tried to protect us. In this scenario, that chronic pain at the base of the left side of your neck is actually based on unconscious reflex self-protective tightening of muscles previously used in an old failed attempt at defense from a threat. This event by definition assumes that a truncated freeze discharge has contributed to the late phenomenon of kindled arousal/procedural memory brain circuitry. In other words, the reflexive bracing pattern of those specific muscle groups has a meaning in terms of survival to those centers of the brain responsible for this function. Pain associated with structural somatic injury, occurring in the context of a life threat without freeze resolution, will continue to be incorporated within implicit memory in situations of threat in order to facilitate the "survival brain" in its instinctual goals. Until that pain no longer represents a message about the unresolved threat, it will continue to be recycled into conscious awareness to protect the traumatized creature/individual in situations of cue-related, or eventually nonspecific arousal. The survival brain has been "fooled into thinking" that the unresolved threat is still imminent.

The dramatic incidence of prior life trauma, and the traumatic origins of pain in those patients treated in chronic pain programs is a well-known association. This fact is also in keeping with the previous concept: the incorporation of meaningful pain messages into procedural and implicit sensorimotor memory in the process of traumatic kindling is a contributing cause of persisting pain in the apparent absence of tissue pathology. This concept also explains frequently seen but poorly understood phenomena of chronic pain such as phantom limb pain. Chronic pain in the trauma population is basically procedural memory for the sensorimotor experiences of the trauma, preserved as a dysfunctional survival skill in the absence of resolution of the trauma through the freeze discharge.

The specificity of this procedural pain memory often determines its location, hence the frequency of pelvic and low back pain in adult survivors of childhood sexual abuse. But certain muscles of the body play an intrinsic role in almost all threatening life events. These are primarily the muscles that participate in the startle response, and those that participate in the maintenance of posture, and that are activated in almost all complex movement patterns. The startle reflex is a complex, stereotyped movement pattern that is characterized by opening of the jaw, extension of the upper neck and head, forward flexion of the lower neck, forward rotation of the shoulder girdle, contraction and flexion of the abdomen, extension of the lumbar spine and flexion of the hip girdle. The startle reflex is primarily defined as a defensive maneuver involving flexion of the trunk and neck to protect the vital organs of the neck and abdominal viscera. Muscles involved include the masseters of the jaw, sternomastoids, pectorals, levator scapulae, rectus abdominus, and iliopsoas. The resulting posture mimics the slumped, folded posture that is often attributed to old age, depression, grief, and also defensive arousal. Many of my chronic pain and whiplash patients eventually fell into this posture. Tonic contraction of these muscles would predictably lead to myofascial pain, explaining chronic headache, TMJ syndrome, neck and low back pain, the primary complaints for which patients seek medical attention. Posttraumatic chronic pain therefore may be the most common of all medical complaints.

Somatic Dissociation and Disease

Victims of trauma likely manifest dissociation, or literally suppression of normal perception, of these painful regions of the body as a protection from the arousal triggered by any sensory input from them. Those body parts represent a reservoir of old traumatic memories that trigger arousal, and are therefore selectively dissociated. A more mysterious and remarkable feature of these areas of somatic dissociation is the presence of subtle signs of autonomic dysfunction affecting the dissociated body part, a physical finding that I have documented with increasing frequency as I have explored this phenomenon with my traumatized patients. Among a number of interesting but unexplained findings in myofascial pain is the occasional presence of dermographia over the area of pain. Dermographia is the appearance of erythema, or reddening of the skin associated with lightly scratching it. One can actually draw a number on the skin that appears in red when scratched, suggesting extreme autonomic sensitivity of the circulation in that region. (Recall the references to stigmata in Chapter 7.) Further investigation may also reveal a pattern of alternating flushing and pallor, often associated with cyclical swelling of skin in the involved dissociated body part.

To my great surprise, one patient told me, that, according to her hairdresser, her hair grew half an inch less per month on the right side. This patient had dramatic sensorimotor symptoms affecting the entire right side of her body associated with nonphysiological physical findings that could only be defined as conversion hysteria. She also had coolness of the right hand, with loss of hair and cracking of the fingernails. She had been involved in a broadside MVA on the right side of her car, the boundary region where she had perceived the threat, and she also had a history of childhood abuse. Subsequent histories from numerous patients have revealed a frequent, often asymmetrical pattern of hair loss and delayed hair growth in skin areas that were not necessarily physically injured in the accident, but which presented with unexplainable sensory symptoms or pain. I have observed abnormally excessive hair growth, erythema (skin redness), warmth, and edema in similar areas of the head, face, or extremities in similar individuals. Many of these patients in retrospect demonstrated stigmata in the area of injury or perception of threat, as discussed in Chapter 7. A few such patients with these types of atypical symptoms in their extremities have experienced progression of signs and symptoms to the point of fulfilling criteria for the diagnosis of sympathetically maintained pain syndromes (complex regional pain syndrome or CRPS, Types I and II) or in its old description, reflex sympathetic dystrophy (RSD).

Reflex Sympathetic Dystrophy

Concepts of chronic regional myofascial and somatic pain may well apply to the development of many chronic regional pain syndromes through similar mechanisms. Obviously, sympathetically maintained pain presents an intriguing possibility as an example of traumatically facilitated chronic regional pain associated with autonomic dysfunction. Reflex sympathetic dystrophy (RSD) was first described in the context of wounds suffered on the battlefield.[36] Although RSD has been associated with a bewildering variety of conditions, the majority of precipitating events are associated with a traumatic event, including fractures, dislocations, wounds, traumatic neuropathies, soft tissue injuries, strokes, and acute radiculopathies (spinal nerve root injuries).[37,38]

Sympathetically maintained pain, complex regional pain, and RSD are relatively common, unexplained painful syndromes characterized by severe pain associated with regional vasomotor symptoms and signs, both parasympathetic and sympathetic in nature. They constitute a spectrum of pain syndromes associated with vasomotor signs of which RSD is the extreme expression. RSD is associated with unusual burning, intolerable pain that often follows traumatic physical injuries, but may also follow trivial physical trauma. The use of the term "sympathetic" in reference to this diagnosis relates to the predominance of vasoconstrictive and dystrophic symptoms and signs implying impaired circulation that characterize the later stages of the syndrome. In fact, trophic or parasympathetic signs with vasodilatation, including hair growth and erythema, may accompany the early phases of the syndrome. In its worst forms, the affected region of the body may eventually develop hair loss, dystonic flexor contractures, and atrophy of skin, muscles, bone, and connective tissue. In rare cases, the symptoms of intolerable burning pain may spread to contiguous or remote areas of the body. In some cases, actual cyclical vascular autonomic changes are apparent.

Personality characteristics have been studied in victims of RSD, and early reports have described RSD patients as "hypersympathetic reactors," with behavioral traits of insecurity, lability, and anxiety. Specific studies, however, have failed to document premorbid psychological disturbances in RSD patients, but also have failed to investigate childhood abuse or prior trauma history in these patients.[39,40]

Certainly the typical vasomotor circulatory signs primarily suggest a role for increased peripheral sympathetic activity in the pathology of RSD. Also, the positive therapeutic response to sympathetic ganglia blockade through infusion of the alpha-adrenergic blocker, phentolamine, or through sympathetic ganglia blockade by direct injection, have implicated excessive activity of the sympathetic nervous system as the cause. Specific sympathetic dysfunction in the head and eyes in the form of bilateral postganglionic Horner's syndrome (dilated pupil, drooping eyelid) and supraorbital anhydrosis (loss of sweat) has been documented in cases of posttraumatic headache.[41] Trauma as the source of a symptom would by definition imply a state of sympathetic dominance.

The cause of this perplexing condition has defied explanation, and both central and peripheral neurogenic causes have been proposed. An intriguing study of the H-reflex (a primitive spinal reflex) in dystonia related to end-stage RSD suggests the influence of supra-spinal, or central brain mechanisms, as a cause of this posture. The authors actually state, "In causalgia-dystonia, central motor control may be altered by a trauma in such a way that the affected limb is dissociated from normal regulatory mechanisms"[42] (p. 2198). I would propose the theory that RSD is a continuum, ranging from the most subtle of autonomic symptoms in a dissociated body region, such as stigmata, to the full-blown intractable pain syndrome that has been classically described in RSD. As such, RSD is a remarkably common phenomenon.

We do know that RSD occurs most commonly after a particularly traumatic physical injury, and patients who develop RSD may have a higher incidence of prior life trauma. The pattern of pain and sensory loss in RSD is occasionally dermatomal, corresponding to the segmental sensory distribution of the spinal cord nerves, but more often is in a linear "nonphysiological stocking and glove" distribution in the extremities, much like that seen in conversion or dissociation. The autonomic nervous system is distributed in a linear fashion in many parts of the body, along the pathways of the peripheral vascular system, rather than in the layered, dermatomal pattern of the somatic spinal nerves. This more linear pattern of distribution of autonomic nerves may at least partially explain the linear "nonphysiological" pattern of sensory loss in both conversion and RSD.

I believe that the phenomenon of regional somatic dissociation is directly linked to the freeze, or dissociative response, occurring at the moment of a traumatic event in a state of helplessness. Just as in myofascial pain, the implicit and procedural memory for both motor and proprioceptive messages accessed at the moment of trauma is stored, in this case powerfully so, under the influence of input from amygdala, brainstem motor nuclei, and sensorimotor cortical centers. Unless the experience related to the traumatic event is dissipated through completion of the physiological cycle of trauma by the intense motor activity of the freeze discharge, the sensorimotor experiences of that traumatic stress will be imprinted in implicit memory through basic classical conditioning, to be accessed in the future for the purpose of survival.

Pain perception will be especially powerfully imprinted. In unresolved traumatic stress, dissociation will cause fragmentation and distortion of the traumatic memories accompanying the event, including any pain associated with it. Therefore, the "objective" manifestations of that injury will likewise be distorted and nonphysiological. Abnormally severe pain perception in trauma not only reflects the injury, but also the threat associated with it, with the pain becoming part of the sensory input from the original threat. Thus, one often notes apparent pain exaggeration related to limited objective pathology in traumatized patients and specifically in those with unexplained chronic pain. The linkage of that pain to implicit memory in trauma associated with dissociation may well explain many of the instances of chronic pain that are no longer explainable by imaging techniques or physical findings. As in many unexplainable symptoms, the meaning of the pain with regard to survival in the face of life-threatening traumatic stress may hold the key to understanding its persistence after the apparent physical cause has been "cured" by current medical standards. The root of chronic pain in this model lies in conditioned implicit pain memory as a reflection of traumatic imprinting.

Pain "memory" may be viewed as a defensive survival tool in the face of an unresolved threat, a conditioned survival response and perception rendered ineffectual because the physiological response of freeze/dissociation has literally blocked the survival brain from instinctively "realizing" that the threat is over. In RSD that pain is also associated with variable, but consistent regional autonomic symptoms and signs. I believe that RSD represents the extreme of traumatic pain memory based on the severity of the dissociative response accompanying the traumatic stress. The region of the body experiencing the pain and now representing a perceived threat has been dissociated in much the same way that a threatening memory may be dissociated in posttraumatic amnesia. Exposure of this dissociated region of the body to the abnormal oscillation of autonomic tone that is intrinsic to trauma results in regional autonomic dysregulation. This results in fluctuating signs of abnormal parasympathetic and sympathetic tone, and the variable syndromes of complex regional pain and RSD. Of interest, the one clinical syndrome mimicking dissociation may be the ignoral of the left side of the body in right-sided brain damage with a stroke. In this situation, there is an inordinately common occurrence of RSD in the ignored/dissociated left upper extremity.[43,44] Ultimately, the mechanism of tissue injury and disease in somatic dissociation is sustained vasoconstriction with diminished blood supply to the point of ischemic damage to the tissues of the dissociated body region.

Fibromyalgia/Chronic Fatigue Syndrome

Another common chronic pain syndrome that may have its roots in trauma physiology is fibromyalgia. First described by Gowers in 1904,[45] it has been exhaustively investigated in numerous, generally flawed studies. It has remained as controversial as one might expect of a syndrome with remarkably uniform and reproducible symptoms, but with few if any objective physical or laboratory findings. Clinical criteria for the diagnosis are generally based on consistency of symptoms and the presence of at least seven "tender points" in specific areas over the surface of the body. Typical symptoms include multiple regional or diffuse sites of soft tissue pain, poor and nonrestorative sleep, chronic fatigue, stiffness, headaches, irritable bowel syndrome, anxiety, cognitive dysfunction, and variable neurological symptoms, especially numbness and paresthesias. These symptoms typically are aggravated by stress, weather changes, and physical activity.

Chronic fatigue syndrome (CFS) is another syndrome closely linked to fibromyalgia, with similar symptoms except for the absence of soft tissue pain. In addition to many other similar symptoms, fibromyalgia and CFS share similar sleep disturbances. The electroencephalography (EEG) pattern during sleep in fibromyalgia and CFS is characterized by abnormal presence of alpha (7.5 to 11 Hz) wave activity seen during deeper non-REM cycles of sleep. This EEG pattern is consistent with a recurrent nonphysiological arousal disturbance, and coincides with the repeated nocturnal awakening characteristic of fibromyalgia and CFS. Interestingly, this unusual EEG pattern is also typical of the arousal disturbance seen in myofascial pain, PTSD, ambient nocturnal noise, and painful joint disease in rheumatoid arthritis.[46]

The clinical syndromes of fibromyalgia and CFS have remarkable similarities to those symptoms affecting whiplash victims with delayed recovery, and the later symptom complex of chronic PTSD (see Chapter 3). I have followed several whiplash patients who over several years have eventually progressed from regional myofascial pain to clinically consistent criteria-specific generalized fibromyalgia. All members of this group of patients had experienced childhood trauma except for one rape victim. Posttraumatic fibromyalgia has been reported in numerous studies, and generally follows soft tissue injuries. One study of 176 cases of posttraumatic fibromyalgia documented that 60.7 percent occurred after MVAs, 12.5 percent after work-related injuries, 7.1 percent after surgery, 5.4 percent after sports-related injury, and 14.3 percent after miscellaneous traumatic events.[47] The majority of these events represent substantial trauma in the face of helplessness.

Neuroendocrine changes in fibromyalgia also suggest a traumatic link. Studies of the HPA axis in fibromyalgia and CFS show remarkably similar aberrations to those seen in late PTSD. These changes include low basal twenty-four-hour urine cortisol excretion, blunted cortisol circadian rhythms, exaggerated ACTH response to CRH, and a blunted cortisol response to increased ACTH.[48] The HPA axis in CFS also reveals lowered basal cortisol levels, and an attenuated ACTH response to CRH, as seen in late PTSD.[46] Depressed pituitary insulin-like growth factor (IGF-I) has been documented in those patients with fibromyalgia, and gives further evidence for HPA dysfunction.[49,50] Finally, hypervigilance to a variety of external and internal noxious sensations, including pain, has been documented in fibromyalgia.[51,52] Hypervigilance and nonspecific stimulus sensitivity, of course, are intrinsic to the diagnosis of PTSD. This association, not surprisingly, has attracted a great deal of scientific attention, leading to scores of articles studying the related incidence of childhood physical and sexual abuse in cases of fibromyalgia. Typical reports of the incidence of incest in fibromyalgia patients reveal figures varying from 37 to 65 percent, compared to control group incidence varying from 42 to 52 percent.[53,54] (Perhaps the most shocking figure in these studies is the incidence of childhood sexual abuse in the control groups!) Retrospective studies such as these, of course, are vulnerable to bias on the part of the respondents, as well as to the problems associated with attributing a causative relationship to consistently co-existent life events.

Nevertheless, many clinical and physiological clues appear to link fibromyalgia/CFS to a traumatic etiology. The predominance of fibromyalgia and CFS in women (>75 percent), the gender prevalence of sexual and physical abuse in women, and the tendency for women to dissociate with trauma and to develop typical PTSD place them at greater risk for both conditions. Similar hormonal markers, arousal sensitivity, and symptom complexes of fibromyalgia/CFS and PTSD demand consideration for an etiological relationship between trauma and the fibromyalgia/CFS syndrome.

Somatization Disorders

Symptoms defined as somatization disorders are not surprisingly extremely common in child abuse survivors. Adults who have suffered physical and sexual abuse as children have a substantially higher incidence than control groups of functional gastrointestinal disorders, genitourinary symptoms and lifetime surgical procedures, most of which did not cure the symptom, or in which no pathology was found.[32,55,56] Somatization in psychiatric terms actually refers to a tendency to express painful emotions as physical symptoms in traumatized patients, possibly related to the inability of such patients to remember traumatic memory in a verbal context. Abuse histories for patients in these studies also correlated with greater symptom complaints in general, and greater utilization of health care services. This fact would certainly be consistent with the tendency for somatization to occur in traumatized individuals. A predominance of visceral complaints in these victims would certainly be consistent with their vulnerability to recurrent arousal, autonomic dysregulation, and dissociation. I believe that somatization and conversion represent more than an aberration of pain memory based on trauma. Regional and systemic somatization symptoms and signs of conversion may well represent measurable pathophysiological changes that are associated with objective disease processes in the symptomatic end organs. Because these conditions reflect the cyclical nature of the underlying autonomic dysregulation, it is difficult to establish fixed objective abnormalities on laboratory testing or imaging studies that would document a consistent abnormality or cause. It is hard to identify a point of fixed pathology in a cyclical disease.

This pathophysiology of dissociation, autonomic dysregulation, and vasoconstriction provides a compelling rationale as the cause of many of the diseases of unknown etiology that are linked epidemiologically to traumatic stress. Syndromes of smooth muscle spasm and/or ulceration in the gastrointestinal system are associated with chronic stress exposure in most cases. These include esophageal cardiospasm, gastroesophageal reflux disease (GERD), peptic ulcer disease, ulcerative colitis, regional ileitis, and irritable bowel syndrome. Interstitial cystitis is associated with painful bladder ulcers and symptoms of problems with coordinated bladder muscle and sphincter control, also of unknown cause. All of these diseases have in common the combination of extremes of sympathetic/parasympathetic oscillation, abnormal regulation of sphincter control and contractility of visceral smooth muscle, and in some cases dystrophic ulceration. Classic migraine, of course, is a prototypical example of vascular manifestations of autonomic cyclical dysregulation, and has been linked to prior trauma in a number of recent studies.[57,58] Many of these conditions have been linked to features of character and personality development suggesting a common behavioral and developmental basis, in keeping with Schore's theories of neonatal brain development and susceptibility to later psychopathology and physical disease.[37] Using this conceptual paradigm, I believe that one must consider diseases that fall under the umbrella of somatization disorder to be pathological and measurable disorders of regulation that in fact represent physical diseases, and not the substitution of physical symptoms for emotional ones.

Abuse victims frequently do not report their abuse history to their treating physician. Probably 20 to 50 percent of abuse episodes are unreported, both at the time they occur and later in life, suggesting that the incidence of child abuse in somatization syndromes may be much higher than current estimates.[59] In addition, I believe that the definition of what specifically constitutes a "traumatic life event" is based to a significant degree on cultural bias, gender-specific definitions, and a general lack of understanding of the physiological tolerance to stress of the developing infant. Added to this dilemma is the well-documented tendency for a society to deny its social ills, as exemplified by Freud's recanting of his theories of incest and conversion hysteria under pressure from his peers (see Chapter 6).

The incidence and cost of diagnostic and therapeutic surgical procedures, including laparoscopies, cystoscopies, colonoscopies, and hysterectomies related to these trauma-based functional complaints has not been accurately documented. Walker and colleagues, however, have estimated that the annual medical cost per childhood abuse survivor for symptoms related to somatization averages $4,700. Upon completion of the expensive, essentially normal diagnostic evaluation for a somatization-based complaint, the physician will be reassuring, but will often justifiably address the possible "psychological" basis for the complaint. The somatization patients, unable to express emotion other than by physical symptoms, will be further devalued and traumatized by the denial of the physical validity of their very real pain, and not surprisingly, will continue to pursue the elusive symptom to the frustration of their medical providers.

Morbidity and Mortality

In addition to increased reporting of symptoms and increased use of medical services, victims of trauma also experience increased morbidity and mortality rates.[55] Studies have tended to focus on war-related trauma, with many of them addressing health status of former prisoners of war (POWs).[60,61] Many of these former POWs experienced increased gastrointestinal and cardiovascular complaints and illnesses, especially peptic ulcer disease, hypertension, and myocardial infarction. In addition, increased mortality was noted in these POWs, especially in the areas of accidents, suicide, and cirrhosis of the liver.[62] These mortality statistics, of course, are likely related to the emotional consequences of war trauma, and the associated increased incidence of alcohol abuse. Cardiovascular morbidity and mortality, however, appear to be more specific complications of wartime stress as documented in the previous studies, and in studies of residents of Lebanon and Croatia during civil wars in those countries.[63,64] In cases of childhood abuse, however, the literature is less clear regarding increased incidence of disease processes in adulthood. Most of the problems experienced in adult survivors of child abuse seem to fall into the classification of functional diseases rather than objective organic disease.[65] Felitti and colleagues in their landmark ACE (Adverse Childhood Experiences) study, however, have documented a strong graded relationship between the degree and severity of exposure to abuse or dysfunctional family behavior patterns during childhood and a number of the leading causes of death during adulthood.[66] This study provides convincing evidence for the dangers of unresolved traumatic stress to one's health and life, especially trauma experienced during childhood.

When the clinical diagnosis of PTSD is added to the stress equation, however, the incidence and significance of adverse health effects of trauma increases significantly.[60,67] The greatest area of vulnerability probably involves the cardiovascular system,[68,69] a predictable association considering the cardiovascular effects of the stress and fight/flight responses. Specific studies of the cardiovascular effects of sympathetic autonomic dysregulation in primates certainly support the concept of the role of stress in the development of atherosclerotic cardiovascular disease.[70]

In their review of the relationship between stress, PTSD, and health, Friedman and Schnurr hypothesize that the widespread changes induced by the neurochemical substrate of PTSD have significant adverse health effects.[60] Hypertension and atherosclerotic cardiovascular disease are likely among the most common and obvious effects of autonomic dysregulation. Endocrinological abnormalities, especially HPA dysregulation and altered thyroid and cortisol function, not only may lead to specific endocrine disturbances, but also to immune disorders. Suppression of the immune system by initial HPA activation and elevated serum cortisol might increase susceptibility to infection, as noted earlier in this chapter. Conversely, lowered serum cortisol levels documented in chronic, late stage PTSD might be expected to produce increased immune activation, since cortisol in effect keeps the lid on basic immune function. Alteration in the genetic phenotypes of blood lymphocytes in PTSD indeed suggests the possibility of increased immune activation.[71] Other authors have postulated that resulting immune dysregulation and heightened activity might also predispose PTSD victims to autoimmune disorders.[55]

Conclusion

Although much of the scientific data associating traumatic stress with adverse health effects is circumstantial and subject to debate and interpretation, many studies show physiological alterations in PTSD that correlate with predictable diseases seen in its victims. There also appears to be a small cluster of poorly understood syndromes that have a compelling link to the physiology and incidence of trauma, including irritable bowel syndrome, gastroesophageal reflux disease, interstitial cystitis, chronic pain syndromes, fibromyalgia/CFS, and RSD.

All of these diseases are compatible with a dysregulated autonomic nervous system, especially with parasympathetic dominance. Other so-called diseases of stress, including hypertension, peptic ulcer disease, ulcerative colitis, and atherosclerotic coronary artery disease probably also can be added to the list of diseases of trauma, although they primarily reflect the high cortisol-based diseases of stress. Idiopathic autoimmune syndromes need to be considered as well, specific to the low cortisol levels of late trauma. Because the physiological events associated with stress and trauma are by nature fluctuating and dynamic, consistent measurement of these events in relationship to clinical symptoms or signs remains a challenge. Proof of a direct relationship between trauma and these syndromes therefore is likely to be extremely difficult. The evidence at hand also suggests that stress or traumatic experiences alone are often not sufficient to cause these diseases. The physiological events of traumatic stress combined with freeze/dissociation appear to be important elements in triggering the required pathological events. Since the autonomic nervous system in PTSD may well be associated with the self-perpetuating central nervous system phenomenon of kindling, it is likely that the resulting continuous perturbation of autonomic, vascular, endocrinological, and immune systems is required to contribute to the development of these diseases of trauma. As diseases of kindling, they may be perpetuated by internal brain processes. They may be expected to progress in severity in the apparent absence of an ongoing identifiable pathogenic event. The remarkable prevalence of trauma in modern society is amply demonstrated in the PTSD literature. In this model, therefore, the pathophysiological effects of trauma might well provide the major impetus to development and perpetuation of many chronic diseases of unknown cause.

Finally, the distinction between the "psychological" and physical pathological manifestations of traumatic stress, as suggested in the term "psychosomatic," needs to be discarded. The pathophysiological, neurobiological, endocrinological, and immunological changes induced by trauma form a continuum with the subsequent pathological somatic manifestations of disease. Based on Weiner's[72,73] and Grotstein's[74] observations, Schore[75] states: "Weiner's fundamental understanding that all physical disease represents a disturbance of regulation and Grotstein's penetrating insight that all psychopathology represents disordered self-regulation clearly indicate that a differentiation between physical and psychosomatic disease is meaningless and misleading." The trauma therefore changes the brain, which therefore changes the body.

Unless one closely examines the traumatized patient for these objective physical findings, the somatic manifestations of dissociation may confuse and frustrate the medical professional attempting to treat the patient's physical complaints. Close inspection of regions of somatic dissociation may allow the clinician to gain insight into the sometimes subtle, but meaningful, objective autonomic changes in the involved areas of the body. Only by understanding the mechanism and somatic manifestations of dissociation in each individual can one begin to develop an effective mode of treatment. Unless one is able to break through, extinguish, or quench the somatic elements of the trauma experience and the dissociation capsule, effective treatment may be frustrated for the emotional components of PTSD and the unexplained chronic pain, somatic syndromes, and chronic diseases that often accompany traumatic stress.

Notes

1. Selye, H.: Thymus and adrenals in the response of the organism to injuries and intoxications. *British Journal of Experimental Pathology*, 1936; 17:234–246.

2. Mason, J., Giller, E., Kosten, T., Ostroff, R., Podd, L.: Urinary-free cortisol levels in post-traumatic stress disorder patients. *Journal of Nervous and Mental Disease*, 1986; 174(3):145–159.

3. Yehuda, R., Boisoneau, D., Mason, L., Giller, E.: Relationship between lymphocyte glucocorticoid receptor number and urinary-free cortisol excretion in mood, anxiety, and psychotic disorders. *Biological Psychiatry*, 1993; 34:18–25.

4. Yehuda, R., Southwick, S., Nussbaum, G., Giller, E., Mason, J.: Low urinary cortisol excretion in PTSD. *Journal of Nervous and Mental Disease*, 1991; 178:366–369.

5. Yehuda, R., Giller, E., Southwick, S., Lowy, M., Mason, J.: Hypothalamic-pituitary-adrenal dysfunction in post-traumatic stress disorder. *Biological Psychiatry*, 1993; 30:1031–1048.

6. Breslau, N., Davis, G., Andreski, P., Peterson, E.: Traumatic events and posttraumatic stress disorder in an urban population of young adults. *Archives of General Psychiatry*, 1991; 48:216–222.

7. Yehuda, R., Giller, W., Levengood, R., Southwick, S., Siever, L.: Hypothalamic-pituitary-adrenal functioning in post-traumatic stress disorder. In Friedman, M., Charney, D, Deutch, A. (Eds.). *Neurobiologic and Clinical Consequences of Stress: From Normal to PTSD* (pp. 351–365). Philadelphia: Lippincott-Raven Publishers, 1995.

8. Cohen, S., Tyrell, D., Smith, S.: Psychological stress and susceptibility to the common cold. *New England Journal of Medicine*, 1991; 325:606–612.

9. Petry, L., Weems, L., Livingstone, J.: Relationship of stress, distress, and the immunologic response to a recombinant Hepatitis B vaccine. *Journal of Family Practice*, 1991; 32:481–486.

10. Keicolt-Glaser, L., Fisher, L., Ogrocki, P., Stout, J., Speicher, C., Glaser, R.: Marital quality, marital disruption, and immune function. *Psychosomatic Medicine*, 1987; 49:13–34.

11. McKinnon, W., Weisse, C., Reynolds, C., Bowles, C., Baum, A.: Chronic stress, leukocyte subpopulations, and humoral response to latent viruses. *Health Psychology*, 1989; 8:389–401.

12. Goodkin, K., Fuchs, L., Feaster, D., Leeka, J., Rishel, D.: Life stressors and coping style are associated with immune measures in HIV-1 infection—a preliminary report. *International Journal of Psychiatry and Medicine*, 1992; 22:155–172.

13. Ironside, G., LaPerriere, A., Antoni, M., O'Hearn, J., Schneiderman, N., Klimas, N., Fletcher, M.: Changes in immune and psychological measures as a function of anticipation and reaction to news of HIV-1 antibody status. *Psychosomatic Medicine*, 1990; 52:247–270.

14. Benschop, R., Niewenhuis, E., Trump, E., Godaert, G., Ballieux, R., Vandoornen, L.: Effects of beta-adrenergic blockade on immunologic and cardiovascular changes induced by mental stress. *Circulation*, 1994; 89:762–769.

15. Knudsen, L., Kjaersgaard, E., Jensen, E., Christensen, N.: Percentage of NK-cells in peripheral blood in resting normal subjects is negatively correlated to plasma

adrenaline. *Scandinavian Journal of Clinical Laboratory Investigation,* 1994; 154: 221–225.

16. Benschop, R., Broschot, J., Godaert, G., DeSmet, M., Geenen, R., Olff, M., Heijnen, C., Ballieux, R.: Chronic stress affects immunologic but not cardiovascular responsiveness to acute psychological stress in humans. *American Journal of Physiology,* 1994; 266:R75-R80.

17. Finkelhor, D.: *Sexually Victimized Children.* New York: Free Press, 1979.

18. Kirkpatrick, D., Edmunds, C.: *Rape in America: A Report to the Nation.* Arlington, VA: National Victim Center. Charleston, SC: Clime Victims Research and Treatment Center, April 1992.

19. Rowan, A., Foy, D.: Post-traumatic stress disorder in child sexual abuse survivors: A literature review. *Journal of Traumatic Stress,* 1993; 6:3.

20. Springs, F., Friedrich, W.: Health risk behaviors and medical sequelae of childhood sexual abuse. *Mayo Clinic Proceedings,* 1992; 67:527.

21. Fromuth, M., Burkhart, B.: Long-term psychological correlates of childhood sexual abuse in two samples of college men. *Child Abuse and Neglect,* 1989; 13:533.

22. Courtois, C.: Adult survivors of sexual abuse. *Primary Care,* 1993; 20:433.

23. Bolen, J.: The impact of sexual abuse on women's health. *Psychiatric Annals,* 1993; 23:446.

24. Walker, E., Katon, W., Harrop-Griffiths, J., Holm, L., Russo, J., Hickock, L.: Relationship of chronic pelvic pain to psychiatric diagnosis and childhood sexual abuse. *American Journal of Psychiatry,* 1988; 145:75–80.

25. Reiter, D.: The incidence and prevalence of women with chronic pelvic pain. *Clinical Obstetrics and Gynecology,* 1990; 33:130–136.

26. Toomey, T., Hernandez, J., Gittelman, K., Hulka, J.: Relationship of sexual and physical abuse to pain and psychological assessment variables in chronic pelvic pain patients. *Pain,* 1993; 53:105–109.

27. Walling, M., Reiter, R., O'Hara, M., Milburn, A., Lilly, G., Vincent, S.: Abuse history and chronic pain in women: I. Prevalence of sexual abuse and physical abuse. *Obstetrics and Gynecology,* 1994; 84:193–199.

28. Walker, E., Katon, W., Hansom, J., Harrops-Griffiths, J., Holm, L., Jones, M., Hickock, L., Jemelka, R.: Medical and psychiatric symptoms in women with childhood sexual abuse. *Psychosomatic Medicine,* 1992; 54:638–664.

29. Rapkin, A., Kames, L., Darke, L., Stampler, F., Nabilol, T.B.: History of physical and sexual abuse in women with chronic pelvic pain. *Obstetrics and Gynecology,* 1990; 76:92–96.

30. Walling, M., O'Hara, M., Reiter, R., Milburn, A., Lilly, G., Vincent, S.: Abuse history and chronic pain in women: II. A multivariate analysis of abuse and psychological morbidity. *Obstetrics and Gynecology,* 1994; 84(2):200–206.

31. Curran, S., Sherman, J., Cunningham, L., Okeson, J., Reid, K., Carlson, S.: Physical and sexual abuse among orofacial pain patients: Linkages with pain and psychologic distress. *Journal of Orofacial Pain,* 1995; 9(4):340–344.

32. Woods, D.: Sexual abuse during childhood and adolescence and its effects on the physical and emotional quality of life of the survivor: A review of the literature. *Military Medicine,* 1996; 161:582–587.

33. Wurtele, S., Kaplan, G., Keaimes, M.: Childhood sexual abuse among chronic pain patients. *The Clinical Journal of Pain,* 1990; 6:110–113.

34. Schofferman, J., Anderson, D., Hines, R., Smith, G., Keane, G.: Childhood psychological trauma and chronic refractory low-back pain. *The Clinical Journal of Pain,* 1993; 9:260–329.

35. Goldberg, R.: Childhood abuse, depression, and chronic pain. *The Clinical Journal of Pain*, 1994; 10:277–281.

36. Mitchell, S., Morehouse, G., Keen, W.: *Gunshot Wounds and Other Injuries*. Philadelphia: J.B. Lippincott Co., 1864.

37. Escobar, P.: Reflex sympathetic dystrophy. *Orthopedic Review*, 1986; 15:646.

38. Schwartzman, R., McLellan, T.: Reflex sympathetic dystrophy: A review. *Archives of Neurology*, 1987; 44:555.

39. Steinbroker, O.: The shoulder-hand syndrome. *American Journal of Medicine*, 1947; 3:403

40. Lankford, L.: Reflex sympathetic dystrophy. In Omer, G., Spinner, M. (Eds.). *Management of Peripheral Nerve Problems* (pp. 216–244). Philadelphia: Saunders, 1980.

41. Khurana, R., Nirankari, V.: Bilateral sympathetic dysfunction in post-traumatic headaches. *Headache*, 1986; April:183–188.

42. Koelman, J., Hilgevoord, A., Bour, L., Speelman, J., Ongerboer, B.: Soleus H-reflex tests in causalgia-dystonia compared with dystonia and mimicked dystonic posture. *Neurology*, 1999; 53:2196–2198.

43. Perry, S., Tepperman, N., Greyson, D., Hilbert, L., Jimenez, J., Williams, J.: Reflex sympathetic dystrophy in hemiplegia. *Archives of Physical Medicine and Rehabilitation*, 1984; 65:442–446.

44. Dursun, E., Dursun, N., Ural, C., Cakci, A.: Glenohumeral joint subluxation and reflex sympathetic dystrophy in hemiplegic patients. *Archives of Physical Medicine and Rehabilitation*, 2000; 81:944–946.

45. Gowers, W.: Lumbago: Its lessons and analogues. *British Medical Journal*, 1904; 1:117–121.

46. Moldofsky, H.: Sleep and musculoskeletal pain. *American Journal of Medicine*, 1986; 81 (Supplement 3A):85–89.

47. Waylonis, G., Perkins, R.: Post-traumatic fibromyalgia: A long-term follow up. *American Journal of Physical Medicine and Rehabilitation*, 1994; 73(6):403–412.

48. Crofford, L.: The hypothalamic-pituitary-adrenal stress axis in the fibromyalgia syndrome. *Journal of Musculoskeletal Pain*, 1996; 4(1/2):181–200.

49. Demitrack, M., Dale, J., Strauss, S., Laue, L., Listwak, S., Kruesl, M. Chrousos, G., Gold, P.: Evidence for impaired activation of the hypothalamic-pituitary-adrenal axis in patients with chronic fatigue syndrome. *Journal of Clinical Endocrine Metabolism*, 1991; 73:1224–1234.

50. Bennett, R., Cook, D., Clark, S., Burckhardt, C., Campbell, S.: Hypothalamic-pituitary-insulin-like growth factor-I axis dysfunction in patients with fibromyalgia. *Journal of Rheumatology*, 1997; 24(7):1384–1388.

51. Rollman, G., Lautenbaacher, S.: Hypervigilance effects in fibromyalgia: Pain experience and pain perception. In Vaeroy, H., Merskey, H. (Eds.). *Progress in Fibromyalgia and Myofascial Pain* (pp. 149–159). Amsterdam: Elsevier, 1993.

52. McDennid, A., Rollman, G., McCain, G.: Generalized hypervigilance in fibromyalgia: Evidence of perceptual amplification. *Pain*, 1996; 66:133–144.

53. Taylor, M., Troller, D., Csuka, M.: The prevalence of sexual abuse in women with fibromyalgia. *Arthritis and Rheumatism*, 1995; 38(2):229–234.

54. Boisset-Pioro, M., Esdaile, J., Fitzcharles, M.: Sexual and physical abuse in women with fibromyalgia syndrome. *Arthritis and Rheumatism*, 1995; 38(2):235–241.

55. Rimsla, M., Berg, R.: Sexual abuse: Somatic and emotional reactions. *Child Abuse and Neglect*, 1988; 12:201–208.

56. Drossman, D., Lesermun, J., Nachman, G., Li, X., Gluck, H., Toomey, T., Mitchell, M.: Sexual and physical abuse in women with functional or organic gastrointestinal disorders. *Annals of Internal Medicine*, 1990; 113(11):828–833.

57. Shuper, A., Zehariu, A., Mimounl, M.: Migraine headaches induced by sexual abuse. *Headache*, 1994; 34(4):237.

58. Gill, J., Stein, H.: More on sexual abuse and headaches. *Headache*, 1988; 28(2):138.

59. Bachman, G., Moeller, T., Bennett, J.: Childhood sexual abuse and the consequence in adult women. *Obstetrics and Gynecology*, 1088; 71:631–642.

60. Friedman, M., Schnurr, P.: The relationship between trauma, post-traumatic stress disorder, and physical health. In Friedman, M., Charney, D., Deutch, A. (Eds.). *Neurobiological and Clinical Consequences of Stress: From Normal Adaptation to PTSD* (pp. 518–524). Philadelphia: Lippincott-Raven Publishers, 1995.

61. Beehe, G.: Follow-up studies of World War II and Korean War prisoners: II. Morbidity, disability and maladjustments. *American Journal of Epidemiology*, 1975; 101:400–422.

62. Page, W.: *The Health of Former Prisoners of War*. Washington, DC: National Academy Press, 1992.

63. Cohen, B., Cooper, M.: *A Follow Up Study of World War II Prisoners of War* (Veterans Administration Medical Monograph). Washington, DC: Government Printing Office, 1955.

64. Sibi, A., Armenian, H., Alam, S.: Wartime determinants of arteriographically confirmed coronary artery disease in Beirut. *American Journal of Epidemiology*, 1989; 130:623–631.

65. Bergovec, M., Mihatov, S., Prpic, H., Rogan, S., Batarelo, V., Sjerobabskl, V.: Acute myocardial infarction among civilians in Zagreb city area. *Lancet*, 1992; 339:303.

66. Felitti, V., Anda, L., Nordenberg, D., Williamson, D., Spitz, A., Edwards, V., Koss, M., Marks, J.: Relationship or childhood abuse and household dysfunction to many of the leading causes of death in adults: The adverse childhood experiences (ACE) study. *American Journal of Preventive Medicine*, 1998; 14(4):245–257.

67. Wolff, J., Schnurr, P., Brown, P., Furey, J.: PTSD and war-zone exposure as correlates of perceived health in female Vietnam veterans. *Journal of Consulting Clinical Psychology*, 1994; 62:1215–1240.

68. Falger, P., Opden Velde, W., Hovens, L., Schouten, E., DeGroen, L., Van Kuijn, J.: Current post-traumatic stress disorder and cardiovascular disease risk factors in Dutch Resistance veterans from World War II. *Psychotherapy Psychosomatics*, 1992; 57:164–171.

69. Litz, B., Fisher, L., Keane, T.: Physical health problems in post-traumatic stress disorder: A risk factor analysis. In Keane, T., Wolfe, J. (Co-Chairs). *Components of Health Risk in Veterans With Post Traumatic Stress Disorder*. Symposium presented at the annual American Psychological Association Meeting. San Francisco, CA, August 1991.

70. Kaplan, J., Manuck, S., Williams, L., Strawn, W.: Psychosocial influences on atherosclerosis: Evidence for effects and mechanisms in nonhuman primates, In Blascovich, L., Katkin, E. (Eds.). *Cardiovascular Reactivity to Psychological Stress and Disease* (pp. 49–82), Washington, DC: American Psychological Association, 1993.

71. Wilson, S. van der Kolk, B., Burbridge, J., Fisler, R., Kradin, R.: Phenotype of blood lymphocytes in PTSD suggests chronic immune activation. *Psychosomatics*, 1999; 40:222–225.

72. Weiner, H.: *Psychobiology and Human Disease*. New York: Elsevier, 1977.

73. Weiner, H.: The dynamics of the organism: Implications of recent biological thought for psychosomatic theory and research. *Psychosomatic Medicine*, 1989; 51:608–635.

74. Grotstein, J.: The psychology of powerlessness: Disorders of self-regulation and interactional regulation as a newer paradigm for psychopathology. *Psychoanalytic Inquiry*, 1986; 6:93–118.

75. Schore, A: *Affect Regulation and the Origin of the Self: The Neurobiology of Emotional Development.* Hillsdale, NJ: Lawrence Erlbaum Associates, 1994. p. 440.

nine
Trauma
Reenactment

Tracey was injured when she was knocked off of her bike in a crosswalk by a car that was making a right turn. When I evaluated her two weeks later, she appeared to have suffered only soft tissue injuries, but also she was experiencing a great deal of arousal, irritability, stimulus sensitivity, and sleep disturbance. I prescribed some physical therapy as well as a course of eye movement desensitization and reprocessing (EMDR) to deal with her residual PTSD.

The accident occurred on January 26. On March 26, she lost control of her car on a mountain road and narrowly escaped going over the edge. On May 26, while bending over to pick something up, her roommate's dog leaped up, hit her in her left eye, and blackened the eye. On June 26, she severely sprained her right ankle. At that point, she realized that something strange was happening, and came back to see me. She told me that toward the end of each month, she had developed a sense of depression and foreboding without her actually recalling the accident. Upon looking at her calendar, she was astonished to note that each subsequent accident had occurred on the same day of the month as her original bicycle mishap.

* * *

Introduction

Victims of trauma live in a perpetually altered state of response to stress and arousal. Vietnam veterans suffering from PTSD continue to produce dramatically elevated levels of adrenaline when exposed to a stimulus related to their past traumatic memories, such as the noise of a helicopter flying overhead or the smell of certain oriental foods.[1] When exposed to scenes of warfare in a video, their brains not only produce more norepinephrine, but also release increased amounts of endorphins, the pain-modulating neurotransmitters, or messengers. Testing their pain thresholds at that time showed reduced pain perception even as they were experiencing significant arousal. As far back as World War II, researchers documented that acutely wounded soldiers seemed to require less morphine for pain relief than one would expect from the severity of their injuries.[2] There are many anecdotes of soldiers with painful injuries continuing to fight in the heat of battle, seemingly ignoring their pain. We suspect that endorphins released at times of great stress and threat to life, as well as in situations of great physical exertion, serve to dampen pain perception in order to allow maximal survival effort.[3] Attention to one's wounds in an acute survival emergency could well impede survival behavior. It makes sense that endorphins appear to play a pivotal role in the early as well as the late behavioral characteristics of traumatized individuals. Pain modulation by endorphins in stress may contribute to one of the more bizarre and at times confusing behaviors of victims of trauma: the seemingly subconscious need to reexperience the traumatic event.

I have treated numerous patients who have been involved in a succession of multiple motor vehicle accidents, in one case as many as eight MVAs over a twelve-year period. Sometimes these accidents seem to occur with increasing frequency as symptoms of traumatic stress worsen. Some may be the result of distractibility due to the effects of trauma and dissociation. Others may be related to low-grade arousal, and resulting overreaction to events in traffic. Repeatedly hitting the brakes as a defensive reaction by the hypervigilant driver could well lead to further rear-end collisions. Sometimes the accident is no fault of the victim, and basically makes no sense. One such patient of mine had six rear-end collisions in eighteen months. Often, however, traumatic reenactment seems to be driven by more deep-seated unconscious conditioned behavior, and may even be linked to the endorphin-based reward systems we have been talking about.

The Roots of Reenactment

The psychological literature is filled with reports of self-destructive behavior in children and adults with a history of child abuse or with histories of multiple childhood surgeries. Examples include self-mutilation (usually by cutting), self-starvation, and anorexia.[4,5,6] Female victims of childhood physical or sexual abuse are more prone to entering subsequent abusive male relationships and marriages.[7] Victims of childhood rape or incest are more likely to be raped, and victims of childhood sexual abuse are at higher risk of becoming prostitutes.[8] Some might call such behavioral tendencies self-destructive or masochistic. It is profoundly inappropriate, however, to pass value judgments on this remarkable association. As you will see, trauma reenactment is rooted in unconscious biochemical systems of the brain, and is probably a deep-seated and conditioned neurophysiological response.

Just like most of the features and behaviors that make up what we call our personality, or sense of self, the roots of trauma reenactment go back to our earliest contacts as an infant with our primary caregiver. Schore explores this maternal/infant interaction in detail.[9] He believes that the earliest verbal, tactile, and auditory interactions between the mother and the infant actually help determine the growth and chemical structure of the brain, leading to the development of personality characteristics and ultimately the person's sense of self. Our basic concepts of the maturation of the individual are dependent on these factors. A healthy, reciprocal maternal interaction stabilizes the arousal systems of the infant brain, and inhibits him or her from excessive over- or underresponsiveness to threat.[10] The infant deprived of a safe haven in response to his or her caregiver is in an untenable situation. When that caregiver is also a threat, all of the rules are broken, and the child must create a safe reality for himself or herself. Under these circumstances, the child will turn to the only resource available—the abusive caregiver. This is one of the first examples of behavioral constriction, and what we might call inappropriate bonding. The child, however, really has no choice, and will use self-blame to justify reattaching to the abuser, since some sort of attachment or bonding is the child's greatest unconscious need at this age.[11] Sometimes the child will also resort to provocative behavior, ensuring repetition of the abuse/attachment cycle. This profound, instinctual need for attachment is common to all primate species.[12] Strong evidence supports the fact that this bonding is correlated with heightened levels of endorphins.[13,14] So even when the child bonds to a threat—the abusive caregiver—the experience will be powerfully rewarding.

Clinical Features

Similar to other neurotransmitters, endorphins clearly serve different functions in different situations. In infants and children they serve to modulate the influence of the traumatic experience, and also to reward the continued bonding that provides them with the resiliency they need to deal with threat and loss. So children physically abused by their caregiver will experience increased levels of endorphins as part of the threat and resulting freeze response. They will also be rewarded by the increased endorphin levels associated with social reattachment and bonding to the abuser, even in the face of ongoing threat. A similar pattern of subjugation, abuse, and passionate reattachment is also typical in many cases of female spousal abuse. It is a fairly accurate reenactment of the similar original child/abusive caregiver bonding. As the conflict leading up to an abusive episode escalates, the abused spouse experiences heightened levels of norepinephrine-based arousal, associated with emotions of fear and apprehension. At the same time, release of endorphins provides a subtle sense of familiar pleasure, and even reward.[15] A period of passionate reconciliation often occurs after an episode of abuse, accompanied by a further dramatic release of endorphins. This pattern of endorphin release both with threat and reconciliation provides a powerful reward system for reenactment of the abuse cycle.[16] Analysis of the interaction between couples in an abusive relationship often reveals that the abused member will sometimes trigger abuse with predictable provocative behavior. It is critical in the treatment of spousal abuse to recognize there are endorphin-based rewards in the relationship to achieve any degree of success. It is also absolutely critical to recognize that this behavior is a conditioned response, and not conscious or "addictive."

This complex dual role of brain biochemistry in trauma also probably explains the remarkable phenomenon of the bonding of hostages, kidnap victims, or cult members with their captors.[17] The common feature in these and other abusive relationships is the condition of helplessness. The constricting effect of this help-lessness cuts the victim off from other sources of support, and like the abused child, the threatened and isolated captive seeks the only source of attachment available, the captor/authority figure.

A fascinating social example of this behavior, one that made the national head-lines in the 1970s, is the case of the kidnapping of newspaper heiress Patty Hearst by members of the radical Symbionese Liberation Army. Within weeks Ms. Hearst was videotaped by a bank camera with her former captors, dressed in black combat attire, wielding an automatic rifle while taking part in a bank robbery. Over time she had developed a sexual/romantic bond with one of the men in the group, and apparently had assumed the group's social identity. The roots of this remarkable and seem-ingly inexplicable behavior by Ms. Hearst are clearly derived from the same primitive endorphin reward systems of the brain described in abused children and spouses.

Animals show the same stereotyped behavior in the face of threat associated with a state of helplessness. Rats placed in a maze, and given a shock in certain sec-tions of the maze, will typically return compulsively to the threatening area rather than explore safer escape routes. They behave as if the shock and trauma lim-its their ability to seek out new or different escape options, leading to reenactment of the shock.[18,19] The familiar is more rewarding to the rats than the unknown even in the face of threat, as in the case of the abused child.

This model of trauma reenactment unfortunately creates a scenario of trauma as a self-fulfilling prophecy. Every time the Vietnam veteran experiences the epi-nephrine/endorphin arousal/reward response of the combat-related stimulus, that response is reinforced. Every time the abused spouse completes the abuse/reconciliation cycle, it ensures that this cycle will inevitably be repeated between the couple. The brain/ biochemistry link in this behavior is quite analogous to the brain biochemistry of narcotic addiction that simply substitutes synthetic morphine derivatives for the brain's natural endorphins.[20] Reenactment therefore constitutes a powerful system of reward and reinforcement, and one that basically is conditioning and self-perpetuating.

A dramatic example of reenactment reward is contained in an anonymous report entered on the Web-based blog *Fight to Survive* for OEF/OIF combat sol-diers, titled "The Drug of War," by "Hellblazer," a veteran of the war in Iraq:

> If one constantly exposes themselves to extreme situations, then all sensations thereafter of equal or lesser intensity offer no stimulation. A heroin addict must constantly increase the dose because the mind has grown tolerant to a lower dosage. A cocaine addict must snort more and more to obtain the same rush of endorphins that was felt the first time. This constant increase to obtain a desired

effect is met with graduation to a more intense medium or fatality. However, a higher dosage or different medium does not always exist to take the addict to the next level, and even if he were to continue to utilize his current choices, the supply is not always infinite. When the supply diminishes, one is left numb to all sensation, and hence follows an increasingly desperate situation. For the soldier, war is his drug. His mind grows an addiction to its ravenous stimuli from abnormally stressful situations. His time within this medium is finite, and when it comes to an end, he will find it hard to deal with his unwanted addiction. This is the tragedy of all those who have fallen to the drug of war, myself included.

Gender Differences

Based on what we have said, it is not surprising that persons with childhood trauma, especially when inflicted by their caregiver, are especially vulnerable to being traumatized again. Studies of trauma victims, however, show remarkable differences between males and females in trauma-related behavior. Males, in general, tend to reenact past trauma by assuming the role of the abusive aggressor rather than that of the victim. So the son of an abusive parent will usually become the abusive spouse or parent as an adult.[21,22] Studies of male criminals convicted of violent aggressive crimes show that a majority of these criminals have suffered severe physical and/or sexual abuse as children.[23,24] These men also appear to have a significantly distorted pain perception consistent with their abnormal brain endorphin systems, and are remarkably prone to various forms of self-mutilation.[6]

Perry studied the posttraumatic behavior patterns of the children released from the Branch Davidian complex in Waco, Texas, after the assault on the complex by agents of the Drug Enforcement Administration where a number of people were killed.[25] He documented that the male children tended to exhibit anger, aggression, and antisocial behavior. The young girls, however, exhibited anxiety, panic attacks, and sleep disturbance typical of the PTSD symptoms of victimization. He hypothesized that males tend to have an "external locus of control," displacing symptoms of trauma on other members of society, blaming them, and acting out aggressively as a result. But females possess an "internal locus of control," blaming themselves for traumatizing events and manifesting guilt behavior.

This and other examples suggest that female victims of childhood trauma tend to assume the more familiar role of helplessness, and to become attached to and dominated by abusive men. They seem much more sensitive to developing forms of revictimization rather than aggression. Aggressive self-abuse such as self-mutilation is much less common in women than in men. Female victims of abuse or even adult trauma tend to pursue nonviolent, self-destructive activities such as self-starvation. Anorexia nervosa and bulimia are often self-destructive manifestations of trauma reenactment in traumatized young women. The incidence of abuse, especially sexual in nature, is common in women suffering from these conditions.[6]

Gender differences may also cause markedly different responses in males and females in natural disaster and accident-related trauma. Women seem much more likely to experience a more profound freeze, or immobility response in these situations, and to sustain that response for a prolonged period. The vast majority of my whiplash patients experiencing prolonged symptoms and delayed recovery have been women. As noted, most of my female patients who experienced severe symptoms from trivial auto accidents have a history of significant childhood abuse or medical trauma. The physical and mental symptoms of whiplash can hardly be considered self-rewarding. But the psychic numbing associated with the freeze response and linked to dissociation is clearly a mechanism for pain modulation by endorphins, and is therefore rewarding. Adult victims of child abuse have a higher incidence of dissociation in the face of adult trauma. I suggest in fact that dissociation in the adult exposed to trauma is basically related to inadequate maternal attunement and bonding or of early trauma as an infant or child. We know that dissociation, or freezing, at the moment of trauma is associated with a high risk of later development of PTSD. These factors probably predispose women to the development of PTSD in traumatic events.

Men exposed to social trauma, natural disasters, or accidents predictably will respond frequently with rage and aggressive behavior (the fight/flight response), as exemplified by increasingly common "road rage" in this country. The degree of violence and aggression seen in men under these circumstances appears to correlate with whether they had experienced abuse and deprivation as children. Of course the victimization/freeze response may also occur in men under these circumstances. This may well relate to whether early abuse in the male related to neglect and abandonment or to physical abuse. Although probably related in part to these theories, the roots of gender differences in response to trauma still are not proven. Perhaps the contribution of genetic influences, relative levels of estrogen and testosterone, or differences in interaction with the maternal caregiver based on gender expectations from the moment of birth could contribute to gender-specific vulnerability. Another disturbing possibility, of course, is that females, both in childhood and as adults, are selectively more exposed to trauma and abuse. Unfortunately a great deal of evidence supports that this indeed is true across all cultures.

Perry and colleagues, however, provide a much more logical and compelling rationale for differences in gender responses to trauma and threat.[25] They base this rationale on the intrinsic role of all brain-related functions, which is survival of the species. Their rationale uses an anthropological and Darwinian model for the behavioral response to threat in males, females, and children. They specifically address the adaptive advantages of fight, flight, or freeze when facing a life threat in both genders in members of the primitive tribe or clan. Anthropological literature reflects the tendency in primitive hominid tribes engaged in battle for the victorious tribe to slaughter the adult males of the defeated tribe, and to take the females and children into bondage as property. When a tribe is attacked by another tribe, attempts by children to flee or fight would guarantee death. But freezing might allow their survival, and incorporation into the new tribe if their tribe was defeated. The same analogy applies to the tribal female members, whose value in contributing to the victor's gene pool as slaves would likely ensure their survival if they also froze. In both cases, this freeze/dissociation adaptation to threat by women and children has evolutionary implications for species survival. On the other hand, if the male members of a threatened tribe were to freeze in the face of this threat, defeat and death would be certain. Sustained arousal and aggression in the male tribal members facing threat therefore has greater benefit to the survival of the species. Perry and colleagues once again relate this behavioral response to the tendency for males to develop externalized oppositional emotional disorders, and females to develop internalizing disorders such as depression, anxiety, and dissociative disorders.[25]

The Anniversary Syndrome

The "anniversary syndrome" is another rarely reported but well-documented example of trauma reenactment. Van der Kolk describes a patient who struck a match to light a cigarette while on night patrol in Vietnam in 1968.[26] That brief moment of illumination allowed a Viet Cong sniper to fire at the patrol, and in a moment of terrible tragedy, his bullet killed the patient's friend. After discharge from the army, the patient found himself apparently unwittingly attempting to rob a store each year, from 1969 to 1986, on the exact day, hour, and minute of the anniversary of the death of his friend. On each occasion, he used his finger in his coat pocket as the "weapon," and waited for the police to arrive, presumably to complete the traumatic experience through his own death.

The similarities between this case history and the actual case from my files at the beginning of this chapter are quite remarkable. How can we explain these seemingly bizarre anniversary-related events in traumatized individuals? We need to remember that all animals, the human species included, possess innate neurophysiologic mechanisms sensitive to the passage of time based on seasonal light variations and even the phases of the moon. The monthly female menstrual cycle may be affected by many subtle outside influences, including the cycles of other females in the household. Subtle seasonal light and temperature characteristics, phases of the moon, or hormonal influences associated with the menstrual cycle at the time of the trauma are very likely stored in implicit memory. Periodic recurrence of these phenomena could result in unconscious activation of arousal on a monthly or even annual basis. Dogs are extremely sensitive to mood changes in their owners. The strange injury described by my patient inflicted by her roommate's pet could be due to secondary arousal of the dog based on subtle biochemical mood changes in my patient related to her past traumatic experience, precipitated by time-contingent internal events. Once again, endorphin-based reward systems associated with this cyclical arousal could well provide further impetus to the repetitive reenactment on the anniversary of the trauma.

Reenactment Through Risk Taking

This strange dance between traumatic arousal and reward also exists in one of our most valued cultural pursuits, high-level athletic competition, especially when involving risk. Although the recent development of the field of extreme sports may be a specific example of this, it exists at many levels, and systems of reward are probably proportionate to the level of intrinsic effort or risk of the particular activity. The release of epinephrine in the face of a survival threat may be associated not only with feelings of anxiety and fear, but also with excitement and exhilaration. It is entirely possible that this arousal/reward link is related to the relative balance of epinephrine and endorphin release with the specific experience.

A person's first skydiving parachute jump is typically associated with stomach-churning panic. But eventually the exhilaration and "high" tends to replace fear and trepidation with eager anticipation. That high is so great in extreme sports that participants will often pursue the event with a degree of intensity consistent with addictive behavior. Examples of this kind of extreme sport include free jumping (off of buildings, towers, or cliffs), extreme skiing, boating or driving to set speed records, technical rock climbing without ropes, and high altitude mountaineering. All of these sports involve a potentially life-threatening pursuit with superficially intangible rewards. All are associated with initial fear, followed by exhilaration and reward, followed by compulsive pursuit of the activity. Often this risk-taking behavior is accompanied by "upping the ante," by increasing the difficulty and danger of the pursuit in order to increase the reward.

All such dangerous pursuits are connected with a powerful fear-based arousal, without which the process would not be initiated. Once established, the fear response no longer seems necessary to perpetuate the habitual thrill response. In every sense of the definition, this thrill-seeking behavior is analogous to more destructive traumatic reenactment. It is governed by the same adrenaline/endorphin threat/reward systems that characterize the behavior of the abused spouse. Although clearly less dramatic, the endorphin withdrawal between episodes of exhilaration has many of the characteristics of morphine withdrawal: restlessness, anxiety, disturbance of sleep, and preoccupation with reproducing the activity.[17]

Those sports that involve maximal sustained physical exertion and effort and that are associated with the most severe anaerobic pain probably are also closely linked to the cycle of traumatic arousal and reward characteristics of reenactment. The "runner's high" has been described at length since the boom in recreational running began in the 1970s. This high has been linked to the release of endorphins triggered by extreme exertion, and this relationship between exertion and endorphin release has been reasonably well validated. Marathons, ultramarathons, triathlons, and competitive cycling are all associated with intense aerobic and anaerobic pain and are probably rewarded and facilitated by endorphin release. In these instances, the stimulus appears to be pain rather than fear. Without this pain, the ultimate reward is substantially lessened.

The necessary practice of intense training to reach sufficient fitness levels to achieve a reasonable level of competition in these sports is by definition painful, at times agonizingly so. Athletes in these circumstances comment on the pain, but often refer to the experience as being "in the zone," a condition of distraction that almost certainly has its roots in the endorphin-based condition of dissociation. The time commitment involved often precludes a meaningful social or even family life outside of the training and competition.

This feature of endurance training is probably true to a much greater extent than in typical seasonal game-based sports. In addition, the financial rewards outside of the core of elite athletes in endurance sports are negligible. Yet even those athletes at the fringe of competition, with no hope of victory, wealth, or recognition, continue to pursue the same painful, self-sacrificing lifestyle, driven presumably by the same mechanisms of endorphin reward that characterize trauma reenactment.

In conversations with trainers and physicians who treat elite endurance athletes, I find a kernel of evidence that this pursuit of fear or pain-based arousal and reward is often related to a history of childhood trauma or abuse. This presumption is admittedly speculative at best, but it makes sense and is consistent with the basic principles of trauma reenactment, that victims of childhood trauma would find the endorphin-based rewards of endurance and extreme sports very powerful. If this association is valid, intense athletic pursuit represents a relatively healthy and stable means of managing the powerful forces driving the victim of trauma toward reenactment. In fact, these unique rewards provided by intense athletic pursuits may actually selectively attract people who have endured childhood trauma. Unfortunately, the serious injury and fatality rate in some of the extreme and risky sports raises questions about implications for species survival.

The same reward system certainly exists in less extreme risk-taking game-based sports. The thrill of competition and victory is a powerful narcotic, as any athlete will agree. Clearly it is not the financial reward that makes players compete well beyond their prime, even when permanent physical impairment may result. The boxer who returns to the ring in his forties and the football quarterback who continues to play despite painful, damaged knees are spurred on by the endorphin-based rewards of "the game." Endorphins serve an important phylogenetic role in allowing wounded prey animals to escape the predator by inhibiting the need to minister to their wounds. The same phenomenon may also drive the human creature to continue to pursue the same endorphinergic reward at the risk of health and survival.

Conclusion

In a sense, our species' survival may be dependent on these conditioned responses in which we push on beyond fear and pain to achieve a goal. Endorphin-based reward systems have evolved as a means of facilitating behavior that is specific to survival, not as a means of perpetuating reenactment. If the neurochemical changes of traumatic stress have resulted from dissociation and a truncated freeze response, however, the result may be endorphinergic reward for reenactment rather than survival. Once again the phenomenon of dissociation may serve as the fuel for another of the features of trauma. Within this context, however, other neurochemical forces may exist that drive gender-based behavioral responses to traumatic stress. Just as changes in brain chemistry and function associated with the experience of trauma may lead to specific diseases of the body, they may also lead to inexplicable behaviors such as trauma reenactment. These late effects of traumatic stress reflect the complexity of the process, and suggest that there may be many pathways to behavioral dysfunction resulting from trauma that we need to study well beyond the defined concept of PTSD.

Notes

1. Blanchard, E., Kolb, L., Prins, A., Gates, M., McCoy, G.: Changes in plasma norepinephrine to combat-related stimuli among Vietnam veterans with post-traumatic stress disorder. *Journal of Nervous and Mental Disease*, 1991; 179:6:371–373.

2. Beecher, H.: Pain in men wounded in battle. *Annals of Surgery*, 1946; 123:96–105.

3. van der Kolk, B., Greenberg, M., Orr, S., Pitman, R.: Endogenous opioids and stress-induced analgesia in post-traumatic stress disorder. *Psychopharmacological Bulletin*, 1989; 25:108–112.

4. Pattison, E., Kahan, J.: The deliberate self-harm syndrome. *American Journal of Psychiatry*, 1983; 140:867–872.

5. Rosenthal, R., Rinzler, C., Wallsh, T., Klausner, E.: Wrist-cutting syndrome: The meaning of a gesture. *American Journal of Psychiatry*, 1972; 128:47–52.

6. Simpson, C., Porter, G.: Self-mutilation in children and adolescents. *Bulletin of the Menninger Clinic*, 1981; 45:428–438.

7. Russell, D.: *The Secret Trauma*. New York: Basic Books, 1986.

8. Silbert, M., Pines, A.: Sexual abuse as an antecedent to prostitution. *Child Abuse Neglect*, 1981; 5:407–411.

9. Schore, A.: *Affect Development and the Origin of the Self*. Hillsdale, NJ: Lawrence Erlbaum Associates, 1994.

10. Weiss, J., Glazer, H., Pohorecky, L., Brick, J., Miller, N.: Effects of chronic exposure to stressors on subsequent avoidance-escape behavior and on brain norepinephrine. *Psychosomatic Medicine*, 1975; 37:522–524.

11. Cicchelli, D.: The emergence of developmental psychopathology. *Child Development*, 1984; 55:1–7.

12. Harlow, H., Zimmerman, R.: Affectional responses in infant monkeys. *Science*, 1959; 130:421–432.

13. Kling, A., Steklis, H.: A neural substrate for affiliative behavior in non-human primates. *Brain Behavioral Evolution*, 1976; 13:216–238.

14. Panksepp, J.: Toward a general psychobiological theory of emotions. *Behavioral Brain Science*, 1982; 5:407–468.

15. Amir, S., Brown, Z., Amit, Z.: The role of endorphins in stress: Evidence and speculations. *Neuroscience Biobehavioral Review*, 1980; 4:77–86.

16. Solomon, R.: The opponent-process theory of acquired motivation: The costs of pleasure and the benefits of pain. *American Psychology*, 1980; 35:691–712.

17. Walker, L.: *The Battered Woman*. New York: Harper and Row, 1979.

18. Mitchell, D., Osborne, E., O'Boyle, M.: Habituation under stress: Shocked mice show nonassociative learning in a T-maze. *Behavioral Neural Biology*, 1985; 43:212–217.

19. Sheldon, A.: Preference for familiar vs. novel stimuli as a function of the familiarity of the environment. *Journal of Comparative Physiological Psychology*, 1969; 67:517–521.

20. Erschak, G.: The escalation and maintenance of spouse abuse: A cybernetic model. *Victimology*, 1984; 9:247–253.

21. Carmen, E., Reiker, P., Mills, T.: Victims of violence and psychiatric illness. *American Journal of Psychiatry*, 1984; 141:378–379.

22. Jaffe, P., Wolfe, D., Wilson, S., Zelko, L.: Family violence and child adjustment: A comparative analysis of girls' and boys' behavioral symptoms. *American Journal of Psychiatry*, 1986; 143:74–77.

23. Groth, A.: Sexual trauma in the life histories of sex offenders. *Victimology*, 1979; 4:6–10.

24. Segholl, T., Prentky, R., Boucher, R.: Childhood sexual abuse in the lives of sexually aggressive offenders. *Journal of the American Academy of Child and Adolescent Psychiatry*, 1987; 36:263–267.

25. Perry, B., Pollard, R., Blakley, T., Baker, W., Vigilante, D.: Childhood trauma, the neurobiology of adaptation, and "use-dependent" development of the brain: How "states" become "traits." *Infant Mental Health Journal*, 1995; 16(4):271–291.

26. van der Kolk, B.: The compulsion to repeat the trauma: Re-enactment, revictimization, and masochism. *Psychiatric Clinics of North America*, 1989; 12(2):389–410.

ten
Sources of Trauma

Joan was referred to me by her physical therapist, who thought that Joan might be suffering from PTSD. As she walked into my office, I noted that her posture was quite dramatic, with a position of defensive flexion of the left arm, head, and shoulder, as if protecting her left chest area from assault. Her eyes squinted in the fluorescent lighting, and she spoke slowly with a stutter. Her thoughts were scattered, and it took her almost ten minutes to state that her symptoms had begun two months before, following postmastectomy breast reconstruction surgery. During that procedure, she had awakened shortly after having been anesthetized to find that she was helpless, paralyzed, blindfolded, intubated, and fully conscious while the surgeon made his first incision. She then remained fully awake throughout the surgery while she listened to conversations of the operating room staff, and felt every painful detail of the opening and manipulation of her body by knives and forceps. She made every effort of will to alert the staff to her conscious state, but EEGs, cardiac monitors, and her blood gas levels gave no clue to her being awake. She began to hallucinate toward the end of the ninety-minute operation, and really felt little pain, although she still recalls the content of conversation in the room during the procedure and the coldness of the water used to irrigate her wound. As drugs and tubes were removed at the end, and the paralysis cleared, her muscles involuntarily went into such violent contractions against the restraints used in the surgery that she had massive bruises for weeks on her arms and legs.

In the ensuing weeks, she predictably developed acute PTSD, with flashbacks, nightmares of knives and wounds, panic, intrusive thoughts, confusion, and severe cognitive problems. Remarkably, she also developed all of the physical symptoms of whiplash, with vertigo, loss of balance, sound and light sensitivity, severe nocturnal bruxism, cervical myofascial pain, headaches, and ocular convergence insufficiency. Her surgeon suggested that the experience might have been a dream, and believed that her symptoms would go away with time.

* * *

Introduction

Studies addressing the epidemiology of trauma and post-traumatic stress disorder have been substantially influenced by the definitions of these terms in the *Diagnostic and Statistical Manual of Mental Disorders,* or DSM–III, the DSM–III–R, and the DSM–IV. Standardization of terms is necessary if one is to arrive at any statistical consistency when attempting to determine the frequency of an event or condition. Revision of the definitions of trauma and PTSD through the sequential editions of the DSM over the past fifteen years undoubtedly has affected the ability of researchers to compare the incidence of these conditions.[1,2,3] When the criteria change, you literally have to start from scratch when doing research on a specific disease. An early study of PTSD in 1987 estimated an incidence in the general population of 1 percent.[4] The incidence of PTSD has predictably increased as the clinical syndrome seen in response to a traumatic event became clearer, and the definition of that event became more inclusive of a wider range of societal experiences. Based on current definitions of trauma and PTSD, estimates of PTSD in the general population range from 3 to 6 percent.[5] It is becoming increasingly clear, however, that the true incidence of trauma and the late syndromes of PTSD are vastly underestimated by these statistics.

Early recognition of trauma in individuals was based almost exclusively on war-related experiences. Such terms as "shell shock" and "battle fatigue" reflected this association. Eventually it became apparent that a relatively broad spectrum of experiences could lead to a group of symptoms that basically were the same as those experienced in combat. When psychiatrists recognized this similarity, it led to such diagnoses as "situational maladjustment," "gross stress reactions," and "adjustment disorders" in the International Statistical Classification of Diseases, Injuries and Causes of Death (ICD, revisions 6, 8, and 9), and the DSM–I–II.[6,7] It was not until 1980 that the term PTSD was introduced in the DSM–III.

Differentiating between stress and a traumatic event has also evolved along with the interpretation of the individual's response to such events. Stress has long been known to exert a marked, and, at times, injurious effect on the body and to produce a pattern of predictable emotional responses. However, we recognize that a stressful event alone is unlikely to produce the relatively stereotyped and long-lasting symptoms of PTSD in a healthy individual. The DSM–IV clearly implies that only a relatively catastrophic event will predictably lead to the syndrome of PTSD. Such an event, based on Criterion A, would require that the individual "experienced, witnessed, or was confronted with an event or events that involved actual death or serious injury, or a threat to the physical integrity of self or others"[3] (p. 427).* In addition, the person's response to that event should involve "intense fear, helplessness, or horror"[3] (p. 428).* As I proposed in Chapter 1, however, the meaning of the event to the person exposed to it might well create an environment sufficiently threatening to constitute an adequate criterion for the previous definition, even though another person might not experience a similar event as traumatic. The female victim of incest or rape predictably might develop acute PTSD after an experience of transient fondling on a crowded bus, whereas a female with no similar previous life trauma might respond with anger and fear, but probably wouldn't freeze/dissociate and go on to develop PTSD.

As noted, in my experiences with relatively trivial low velocity MVAs, victims of substantial prior life trauma may respond with a full-blown whiplash syndrome, including PTSD, even though the definition of this type of trauma did not approach the DSM–IV criteria. The somatic expressions of the whiplash syndrome, in fact, may represent a universal constellation of symptoms attributable to recurrent activation of procedural memory for the instinctive physical defensive response to any unresolved life-threatening experience. In the case history at the beginning of this chapter, I initially thought that the patient had suffered a whiplash based on her symptoms until she told me about the surgery. This dichotomy is extremely important in the assessment of what constitutes types and sources of trauma in our society. We must be wary of the inclination to interpret an experience that has been followed by symptoms of trauma to be too trivial to be the cause. The special meaning of the threat to the victim based on his or her past experience must be considered before dismissing the threat as not sufficient to be traumatizing.

Criteria for specific symptoms sufficient to make the diagnosis of PTSD require one or more patterns of reexperiencing, three or more of avoidance, and two or more of arousal. This type of threshold requirement for establishing the diagnosis of PTSD is probably necessary for standardization in order to promote research studies, but creates an artificial barrier to the diagnosis of trauma. The expression of symptoms of trauma is not rigidly set, but composes a continuum based on the type and severity of the trauma, the past experience of the victim, the prevalence of dissociation, the age at which trauma occurred, gender, and many other factors. Like any other natural phenomenon, the symptoms of trauma form a typical "bell curve." Incomplete criteria for symptoms based on the DSM–IV must not imply that victims have not been traumatized by an experience, and that the basis for their expressed symptoms therefore is not PTSD. In the area of PTSD associated with MVAs, Blanchard and Hickling have proposed a "subsyndromal" form of PTSD in an attempt to address this dilemma.[8] The obvious risk of arbitrarily

---

*Reprinted with permission from the *Diagnostic and Statistical Manual of Mental Disorders, Fourth Edition (DSM–IV)* (Copyright 1994). American Psychiatric Association.

broadening the clinical definition of symptoms of trauma is loss of the standardization required for developing a legitimate statistical epidemiological base, and therefore for doing research. That is the dilemma of both ends of the bell curve. On the other hand, ignoring the somatic symptoms of trauma based on dissociation, and of the many subsyndromal expressions of trauma, creates an inappropriately limited appreciation of the potentially disastrous effects of life trauma on the individual victim and on our societal health.

Van der Kolk and colleagues have explored the significance of dissociation, affect dysregulation, and somatization as "associated features" of PTSD.[9] They studied three groups of patients: those currently fulfilling diagnostic criteria for PTSD, those with lifelong PTSD but not currently meeting criteria, and those with no PTSD. Among other findings, they specifically noted that the "associated features" often persisted for many years, even after full-blown PTSD symptoms have subsided. Does this mean that they had recovered from the effects of the trauma, and the "associated features" simply represented neurotic characterological traits? An important implication of their study is that subsidence of acute PTSD symptoms so the specific diagnosis cannot be made ignores the long-term, pervasive, and often somatic consequences of exposure to traumatic stress. These "associated disorders," and indeed many of the diseases of trauma (Chapter 8), must be considered to be part of the continuum of the diffuse physiological changes triggered by the trauma and associated initially with the syndrome of PTSD. For this reason, although I will review statistical data regarding the relative incidence of various sources of life trauma, I will also explore the theoretical basis for other predictable but relatively unexplored traumatic societal events and experiences.

The Definition of Traumatic Stress

Any consideration of the relative incidence of PTSD after specific types of traumatic events obviously depends directly on the accepted criteria for such an experience. Levine would define trauma as any event that produced the requisite physiological event—in his model, an unresolved freeze response, or dissociation.[10] Several other investigators have taken a similar theoretical direction based on the response of the individual to trauma. Krystal has suggested that psychic surrender, or "freezing of the affect," may represent a typical response to extreme stress.[11] Hobfoll also suggests that the response of resource conservation, or "playing dead," may imply exposure to a severe stress sufficient to qualify as traumatic stress.[12] Note that they all have defined trauma by the response to it rather than by its intrinsic nature.

The American Psychiatric Association, in the DSM–III–R, defined a traumatic event as one "that is outside the range of usual human experience and that would be markedly distressing to almost anyone"[2] (p. 250).* This definition does not imply that a specific behavioral or physiological response to the experience is

---

*Reprinted with permission from the *Diagnostic and Statistical Manual of Mental Disorders*, Fourth Edition (DSM–IV) (Copyright 1994). American Psychiatric Association.

essential, other than marked distress. In the DSM–IV, a traumatic event is defined as "The person experienced, witnessed, or was confronted with an event or events that involved actual or threatened death or serious injury"[3] (p. 427).** In addition, the experience of helplessness or horror is added to the definition, thereby incorporating the response of the individual to the event. Breslau and Davis, and Solomon and Canino would agree with the need to define traumatic stress more by the response elicited by it than by a conceptual definition of the event itself.[13,14] By their definition, any stressor sufficient to produce the traumatic symptoms of reexperiencing, arousal, and avoidance should qualify as a traumatic event. Norris, on the other hand, has introduced the concept of violence, involving sudden extreme force from an external agent as a reasonable source of traumatic stress. Designed primarily for research, Norris' concept would include events related to nature, technology, and human behavior as sources of trauma. Like Blanchard and Hickling,[8] she also notes that the limiting constraints of the DSM–IV criteria results in a definition of PTSD that "represents only the tip of the iceberg in terms of experienced distress"[15] (p. 416). She further states, "In reporting rates of disorder that are constrained to be low, one should be cautious not to give the mistaken impression that few people become distressed following traumatic events"[15] (p. 416).

I would question the conclusion that traumatic stress had occurred even without a sufficient behavioral and physiological response to an event. The spectrum of such responses clearly varies widely between individuals: People are primed to respond to a variety of stressful events based on myriad predisposing factors. What may produce surprise and perhaps cause consternation in one individual may induce shock and dissociation in another. Many of my whiplash victims reported no emotional distress at the time of the accident, but on questioning, admitted to symptoms of confusion, shock, numbing, and even out of-body experiences: clear evidence of dissociation. As we have stated, the potential for an event to be traumatizing depends in part on the meaning of the event to the person experiencing it. This assumption, however, has not been entirely supported by researchers in PTSD. The DSM–III concluded that PTSD is a normal response caused by an abnormal incident, and would be expected to occur in the majority of people experiencing that incident.[1] Much of the PTSD literature does not allow for the concept that a full-blown and prolonged traumatic physiological response may occur after a relatively minor stressful event if the victim has a past history of severe trauma, especially as a child. It also does not take into consideration that a threatening experience that replicates similar past trauma is far more likely to be traumatizing.

Childhood trauma may produce a state of sensitization, vulnerability, or diminished reserve capacity to stress that may result in an overwhelming physiological stress response and full-blown clinical PTSD in response to a nonspecific societal

---

** Reprinted with permission from the *Diagnostic and Statistical Manual of Mental Disorders*, Third Edition (DSM–III) (Copyright 1987). American Psychiatric Association.

stress such as a trivial MVA. I strongly support those authors who feel that the response of the victim to a traumatically stressful event is the defining factor for experiencing trauma, taking into careful account that individual's life burden of traumatic stress. I also maintain that the definition of a recognized response to traumatic stress must include not only those symptoms related to reexperiencing, arousal, and avoidance defined in the DSM–IV, but also must address such comorbid and associated symptoms as dissociation, depression, affect dysregulation, and somatic complaints. Such symptoms may be of the type known to be related to past exposure to trauma, but also must include symptoms of somatic procedural memory related to the experience, such as with the whiplash syndrome.

Exposure to Combat

As we have noted, most of the early studies in trauma arose from experiences with victims of traumatic stress related to wartime combat experiences. From "soldier's heart" in the Civil War, to shell shock in World War I, and to battle fatigue in World War II, researchers in trauma derived many of their observations and theories from the study of wartime veterans experiencing emotional distress based on their combat exposure. The term "combat stress reaction" (CSR) eventually was applied to the acute behavioral, emotional, and physical symptoms experienced by some soldiers exposed to combat.[16] These symptoms constitute a complex and variable mix that reflect the linking of psychological and somatic complaints observed in late PTSD, some of which are ignored in the DSM–IV. Agitation, increased startle, stimulus sensitivity, and irritability reflect increased arousal. Apathy, depression, and psychomotor retardation may alternate with increased arousal. Somatic and primarily autonomic symptoms may include nausea, diarrhea and constipation, and abdominal cramping.[17]

Exposure to combat-related traumatic stress in the Vietnam War was probably comparable to previous great wars. The controversial nature of the Vietnam conflict and the difficulties with societal assimilation of many returning veterans, however, may have sensitized the scientific community to the distress seen in many members of the military who experienced combat there. It is also likely that the societal rejection of returning veterans may have contributed to the severity and incidence of post-combat emotional symptoms. Increased awareness of the emotional burden carried by these soldiers has led to extensive follow-up studies of their postwar symptoms.

These studies have yielded a great deal of data regarding PTSD, have led to the term PTSD itself, and have helped to define the syndrome as we now know it. Much of the early data came from the National Vietnam Veterans Readjustment Study (NVVRS), from which the study Trauma and the Vietnam War Generation was published.[18] At the time of the latter study, using DSM–III–R criteria, 15.2 percent of then-current male Vietnam War veterans suffered from PTSD, and 11 percent from partial PTSD. The number of veterans who had a lifetime prevalence that included prior experience of criteria-based symptoms was 30.9 percent. Lifetime prevalence implies the presence of symptoms sufficient to diagnose PTSD at any time in their lives. A National Comorbidity Survey (NCS) by Kessler and colleagues estimated that the risk of developing PTSD after exposure to combat is 38.8 percent.[19] Epidemiological studies of the occurrence of PTSD in the Vietnam War clearly reflect a substantial incidence of combat-related PTSD in wartime, based on relatively strict DSM–III–R criteria. This high incidence of criteria-based PTSD after exposure to the experience of war-related combat is certainly predictable based on the emergence of this diagnosis from the theater of war.

These findings, however, do not necessarily reflect the breadth of varied and long-term symptoms that may occur long after criteria-based PTSD or CSR has subsided. Later problems in combat veterans experiencing CSR include impaired performance in work-related, family-related, sexual, and social functioning that does not appear to improve with time.[16] Increased somatic complaints, poorer indices of both health and attempts at health maintenance have been reported in veterans who have experienced CSR.[20,21,22] Some Persian Gulf War veterans (PGV) returned from combat with a somatic syndrome consisting of muscle and joint pains, headache, weakness, pathological fatigue, memory loss, sleep disorders, skin rashes, hair loss, shortness of breath, and gastrointestinal complaints.[23,24,25] In the majority of these cases, physical diagnostic explanations have included asthma, migraines, and inflammatory bowel symptoms of unknown cause.[25] Psychiatric explanations have included PTSD, anxiety disorder, and depression.[25] Approximately 15 percent have remained unexplained.[23,24,25] The syndrome has since been called Gulf War syndrome.

Amato and colleagues studied neuromuscular symptoms in PGVs and found no objective evidence of neuromuscular disease.[26] They commented on the unusual similarity of symptoms in these PGVs to fibromyalgia and chronic fatigue syndrome, noting that many of their patients also suffered from anxiety, headaches, depression, sleep disturbance, and bowel disorders. We are once again presented with the dilemma of an unexplained somatic/psychological symptom complex clearly following exposure to traumatic stress. When one is locked into the confining definitions of the DSM–IV and adherence to Cartesian dualism, such syndromes defy explanation. When viewed outside of these constraints, however, they fall into the logical niche of trauma-based psychophysiological pathology analogous to the whiplash syndrome and to many syndromes discussed in Chapter 8.

Within the group of soldiers who develop PTSD, a number of factors seemed to contribute to their vulnerability. Bremner and colleagues found that a history of childhood physical abuse appeared to be a significant contributory factor to the development of PTSD in Vietnam veterans.[27] They concluded that exposure to prior trauma was not protective in dealing with a new traumatic event, but might even increase vulnerability to being traumatized. This conclusion is quite in keeping with my observations concerning increased vulnerability to traumatic stress in MVAs when a person has a prior history of trauma, especially when it has occurred in childhood. A number of studies have documented that Vietnam veterans suffering from PTSD differed from their non-PTSD cohorts in their lack of support from postwar social systems, including those from spouses, family members, and fellow veterans.[28-31] These studies, however, were unable to differentiate whether the development and perpetuation of PTSD were enhanced by the lack of social support, or whether avoidance as a symptomatic component of PTSD led to social isolation, and therefore lack of support. Intensity of combat exposure is a predictable factor in the development of PTSD, and this conclusion is supported by many studies.[28-32] Although these studies provide only a few clues to the sources of vulnerability to CSR and PTSD, they support the presence of diminished reserve capacity and resiliency in trauma associated with a history of prior traumatic stress. They also emphasize the importance of the availability of adequate support systems after trauma.

Child Abuse

The well-documented association of childhood psychological, physical, and sexual abuse with a remarkable constellation of physical and emotional symptoms, and mental illness in adulthood, also strongly supports the link between a traumatic emotional experience and subsequent somatic dysfunction. Child abuse has been linked to a wide variety of chronic and often unexplained pain syndromes, including pelvic, low back, orofacial, and bladder pain, as well as fibromyalgia. Irritable bowel syndrome, interstitial cystitis, anorexia, and bulimia have all been linked to child abuse, especially sexual abuse (see Chapter 8).

The vulnerability of the developing brain to positive and negative emotional experiences has been thoroughly explored in recent years, and provides a solid neurophysiological substrate for the development of adaptive and maladaptive changes in brain morphology and function.[33,34] These changes in turn will likely affect not only autonomic adaptations to further stressors, but also tend to cause somatic physiological changes that will predispose the adult survivor of childhood trauma to predictable physical disease and behavioral dysfunction. Exposure to traumatic stress in childhood is particularly likely to result in long-lasting and varied late symptoms of trauma. Traumatic stress at any age produces persistent, and at times, permanent changes in brain structure and chemistry. Exposure to trauma will predictably have a far more profound effect on the developing brain of the infant or very young child, producing permanent patterns of neuronal development that may result in specific disturbances in personality and behavior.[34,35]

Infants and young children, especially females, are especially susceptible to dissociate, or freeze in the face of trauma (see Chapter 9). Males are much more likely to become activated, and enter the fight/flight continuum. This is clearly reflected in the predominance of aggressive, hyperactive, and acting-out behavior in disturbed boys, and the converse tendency for traumatized girls to exhibit depression, anxiety, dissociative, or borderline personality traits. The benefit of aggression in males and freeze/dissociation in females in the face of threat for species survival is obvious.[34] Dissociation in male members of the tribe in the face of danger would inhibit the aggressive defensive behavior on which the survival of the tribe is dependent. Aggressive behavior on the part of physically weaker children or females, however, would jeopardize their survival. This dichotomy is illustrated by the remarkable incidence of a past history of child abuse in prison populations, especially among males, where violent behavior has led to incarceration.[36] Among fourteen male juvenile murderers condemned to death in 1987, Lewis and colleagues noted that twelve had been severely physically abused and five had suffered sodomy at the hands of their relatives.[37]

Even male children traumatized when very young, however, are more likely to manifest symptoms of avoidance, constriction, withdrawal, and further dissociation in the future, especially in the face of episodes of traumatic stress (see Chapter 9). Symptoms and behaviors reflecting the categories of arousal and reexperiencing are less likely to present themselves in these children, and therefore the criteria-based diagnosis of PTSD may be more difficult to make in this subpopulation.

In one study of severely traumatized children with symptoms of hyperarousal, only 70 percent met DSM–IV criteria for PTSD.[38] Part of the explanation for this discrepancy may be that many of the late symptoms of trauma in children are secondary to dissociation, and present as comorbid disorders (depression, obsessive compulsive, adjustment, attention deficit disorders) that may not reflect their origin in traumatic stress. Symptoms of *hypoarousal*, in fact, may predominate in traumatized children.[9] The diagnostic category Disorders of Extreme Stress, Not Otherwise Specified (DESNOS), reflects symptoms associated with self-regulation, impulse control, self-esteem, relationships with others, and dissociative tendencies. Although DESNOS is not recognized as a diagnostic entity by the American Psychiatric Association, one study found that DESNOS as a diagnostic criteria in adult survivors of child abuse correlated more accurately with a poor treatment outcome than did the diagnosis of PTSD based on the DSM–IV.[39] The constraints presented by this dilemma make any attempts at documenting the incidence of traumatic stress and PTSD in children who have experienced abuse extremely difficult if conclusions and diagnostic categorizations are based on DSM–IV criteria.

It is difficult to estimate the actual incidence of societal child abuse because of the intrinsic effect of dissociation on traumatic memory. By definition, dissociation may result in fugue-related amnesia for the traumatic event, and although the validity of recovered memories for remote or childhood trauma has been challenged, ample evidence suggests that traumatic amnesia is common in childhood.[40] When patients say that they really cannot recall much detail from their childhood, it is a red flag for child abuse. In addition, most adults traumatized as children will not voluntarily divulge this information to their physician.[41] When I started taking detailed trauma histories on my whiplash patients, it was like turning over a societal rock, with all manner of ugly stories beneath it. The phenomenon of "effort after meaning," on the other hand, may contribute to amplification of the statistical frequency of child abuse.[42] "Effort after meaning" refers to the tendency for patients who exhibit somatization to search for a specific physical reason for their symptoms, especially when confronted with a skeptical medical profession. Effort after meaning may in fact be a product of skepticism and emotional dismissal of patients perceived as somaticizing by the physician.

Controlling for ethnic, geographic, economic, and cultural variables in studied populations is extremely difficult. Based on these and other factors, it is not surprising that estimates of the societal incidence of child abuse vary widely. In a review of the literature, Wood notes an incidence of childhood sexual abuse in females of between 12 and 64 percent, and in males, between 3 and 13 percent.[43] A study from the National Victim Center reported 2,936,000 children in the United States to have been abused or neglected that year.[44] These statistics undoubtedly reflect the varied populations studied, as well as other factors noted previously. Taking all of these factors into consideration, however, the prevalence of child abuse in our society is remarkable and shocking. Many of the late diseases of trauma reflect the sustained autonomic dysregulation linked specifically to dissociation. Adult survivors of child abuse bear a legacy of altered physiological responsiveness and resulting susceptibility to a wide spectrum of chronic diseases (see Chapters 6 and 8). The emotional, physical, social, and economic toll on our society from the shattered lives of our abused children is far more widespread and overwhelming than we currently seem to realize or admit.

Victims of prior child abuse present one of the most challenging populations to treat for the injuries suffered in a MVA. Since dissociation characterizes the basic response to trauma in these individuals, they usually will relate significant symptoms of dissociation at the time of the accident. These symptoms will often persist for weeks, and the associated confusion and numbing will frequently be interpreted as a brain injury. As dissociation subsides, cyclical arousal in the form of emotional instability and anxiety will appear, along with symptoms of full-blown PTSD. These patients usually develop dissociative somatic symptoms that present in a nonphysiological and bizarre fashion. Such symptoms often are linked to arousal and panic, enhancing their perceived severity. Attempts to link dissociative somatic symptoms to spinal injury or other physical causes are usually fruitless. Efforts to treat these symptoms with physical therapeutic measures often are ineffective, or may aggravate them. Intrinsic autonomic instability and other neurochemical and neurophysiological changes intrinsic to dissociation and PTSD often are associated with intolerance to medications. These patients are extremely sensitive to side effects of drugs. Headache and myofascial pain are often intractable, and may respond only to narcotics, which present a problem because narcotics, with their similarities to endorphins, may enhance dissociation (see Chapter 7). Exposure and other highly interactive forms of psychotherapy must be used with great care because of the risk of flooding and resultant dissociation in these individuals. Clearly, the most dramatic examples of severe morbidity and delayed recovery in whiplash fall into the category of those patients with a prior history of child abuse.

Societal Trauma

The risks of exposure to catastrophic and traumatic events occurring in any urban society are predictably high. Victimization by crime in any form can be traumatizing. Even being subjected to personal or financial loss through nonviolent means may prove threatening to one's future through loss of financial security, and the resulting threat to one's physical well being. The death of a loved one, close friend, or an otherwise important figure in one's life may be threatening enough to induce helplessness. Such personal losses through nonviolent means are generally accepted in our society as part of normal life stress, and therefore not felt to fall into the category of trauma. As part of our basically Calvinistic upbringing in the United States, we are encouraged to "suck it up," get over it, and move on in life in the face of pain and loss. Yet, numerous studies support the concern that prior life traumatic events and psychiatric morbidity are associated with a higher risk of developing PTSD after a new trauma, and that this vulnerability may result in an enhanced traumatic reaction even with less intense traumatic exposure.[45,46,47] As a result, even minor, nonviolent societal trauma should not be dismissed as a source of significant trauma in selected populations, especially if it occurs in a climate of relative helplessness and is out of one's control.

In general, however, the degree of exposure and intensity of the trauma tend to correlate directly with the incidence and severity of resulting depression and PTSD.[48,49] The literature clearly reveals that there is no shortage of social and natural exposure to extreme stress and trauma throughout the world. The National Comorbidity Study reveals an incidence of exposure to traumatic events in 60.7 percent of the men, and 51.2 percent of the women.[50] Resnick and colleagues, in a national study of adult women in the United States, found a high incidence of exposure to trauma: 35.6 percent had experienced some type of crime, 14.3 percent a molestation or sexual assault, 13.4 percent a death of a relative or close friend by murder, 12.7 percent a completed rape, and 10.3 percent a physical assault.[51] Norris found a 69 percent incidence of exposure to a traumatic event in a sample of 1,000 adults in the United States.[52] Trauma is clearly part of the fabric of life.

Natural and manmade disasters are a worldwide norm. Between 1967 and 1991, disasters killed 7 million people and affected 3 billion.[53] The world's attention has been periodically riveted on episodes of genocide in Rwanda, Bosnia, and Kosovo, and more recently in Somalia and Sudan. The addition of suicidal terrorism in the late 1990s in Sri Lanka and Palestine, now spreading throughout the Middle East, has introduced a whole new concept to our sources of collective societal trauma. Although our culture in the United States has been shaken by a new threat to our children in the scattered but persistent homicidal assault by isolated peers within their schools, we have been spared the trauma of war or terrorism until the attack on the Twin Towers in New York City on 9/11/01. Although the incidence of PTSD in first-responders and citizens of New York City has been substantial, few statistics reflect the effects of this experience on the nation as a whole. Experienced observers of the behavior of the nation have noted a numbing of emotions, perhaps even a national lassitude, which would fit with the response to terror in a helpless state. Studying the incidence of certain diseases in the years since the attack would be a massive undertaking, but I suspect it would reflect an upsurge in many of the somatization disorders discussed previously. We have been confronted firsthand in what many other nations have known and experienced—that the world is a dangerous place, and neither economic development nor complex acculturation has changed that fact.

Of all of the forms of social trauma, sexual assault, particularly rape, has the greatest potential for leading to PTSD.[54,55] Breslau has documented that most forms of social trauma have a roughly similar potential to elicit symptoms of PTSD, with risk ranging from about 10 to 30 percent.[54] These include physical assault, serious accident or injury, sudden death of a close friend or relative, seeing someone seriously injured or killed, or a threat to one's life. But in Breslau's study, rape and sexual assault are associated with a subsequent incidence of PTSD of 60 percent or more. Koss and Burkhart note that the appearance of PTSD symptoms after rape may be delayed for years.[55] They also emphasize the unique implications of sexual assault with regard to the woman's sense of hopelessness and despair. As noted in Chapter 1, the magnitude of a traumatic event, and its threat to life, is directly proportional to the meaning of that threat within its societal frame of reference. Threats from primary caregivers are of the greatest magnitude, and physical and sexual assault of children by parents have the potential for the causing the greatest trauma and its subsequent symptoms. Trauma inflicted by another human being is high on the continuum of severity, and sexual trauma is at the top of that list.

The trauma of rape is predominantly experienced by women, with about 10 percent of rape victims being men, although that figure may be low based on the reluctance of men to report or seek counseling for rape.[56] The act of sexual intercourse in mammalian species is characterized by submission of the female to a variable degree, and the acceptance of a state of relative vulnerability, driven by deep-seated instinctual roles governing the survival of the species. In the human species, intercourse has taken on a deep interpersonal meaning in the form of trust, sharing, and accepted vulnerability on the part of the woman. It literally mimics a state of voluntary helplessness, one that almost ensures a state of trauma when that trust is violated. Violation of that state in the form of sexual assault thereafter destroys any sense of safe boundaries for that woman within human society, especially in relationship to males. The sense of degradation, guilt, and worthlessness that often accompanies rape is amplified by our society's tendency to doubt the credibility of the victim, to assume complicity in the act, or to imply provocation by the victim. An article in the international press in 1999 reported that a judge in an Italian court dismissed a rape conviction because the victim wore jeans, a presumed sexually provocative act. Rape myths of this sort in our society continue to perpetuate the fears of reporting the assault by the rape victim. The system of justice that accompanies sexual assault contributes greatly to the victims' sense of helplessness accompanying the event, and increases the likelihood of their developing PTSD.

Many cases of rape involve a man with whom the victim is familiar, either in the context of a consensual social event (date rape), or by a familiar acquaintance, friend, or family member. Familiarity with the perpetrator also enhances the sense of betrayal of trust and may increase the intensity of the trauma. Rape by an acquaintance is far more common than by a stranger. In a study of 6,100 undergraduate men and women, Warshaw noted that one out of four women had experienced rape or an attempted rape, 84 percent were acquainted with the rapist, and 57 percent of the rapes occurred on dates.[56] Comparison of the perception of the experience of rape by women who were victims of a stranger versus an acquaintance reveals remarkable differences. Victims of acquaintance rape were more likely not to consider the experience to be rape, and less likely to discuss it with someone, report it to the police, or seek crisis counseling.[57]

The event currently termed "date rape" illustrates this dilemma. In this circumstance, the woman has not only tacitly accepted at least a temporary relationship of trust, but has apparently entered willingly into a date, a presumably mutually pleasurable event. Current societal mores have probably contributed to problems with differentiating what constitutes rape and what constitutes consensual sex in this environment. The sexual revolution of the 1960s supposedly freed women from American society's unilateral expectations of feminine chastity. In reality, these new sexual mores also introduced a new set of expectations regarding the woman's role in friendships and dating relationships with men. The victim of date or acquaintance rape faces a greatly enhanced sense of shame, betrayal, and helplessness considering the fact that she has voluntarily entered a state of vulnerability, and that sexual intimacy may well be an acceptable outcome of the date experience. The sense of guilt resulting from this dilemma enhances her sense of helplessness, and often inhibits her access to therapy that might mitigate posttraumatic symptoms. In the confusion over the role she may have taken in the assault, the victim of acquaintance rape often will tend to assume some responsibility for the event. She may blame herself, have doubts about whether the event was indeed rape, and hesitate to file a police report or tell anyone about it. As one patient of mine put it, "I had sex lots of times in college when I didn't want to because I was too ashamed to refuse it. Now that I think back, a couple of times it was rape." Without the victim experiencing and expressing the normal rage associated with the assault under these circumstances, the dissociation so often reported by rape victims will continue to recur and to perpetuate the late emotional and somatic symptoms of trauma. Victims of acquaintance rape are often hesitant to report assaults. This probably contributes to a much higher rate of date/acquaintance rape and sexual assault than is reflected by current statistics.

In my experience with whiplash patients who have a past history of rape, delayed recovery with emotional and somatic symptoms from the MVA is common, often persisting for years after the accident. Myofascial pain, especially low back and pelvic, is typical. Piriformis syndrome, a form of sciatica due to spasm of one of the deep muscles of the buttock, is especially common, as it is in all patients with prior histories of sexual assault, rape, or incest (see Chapter 12). Gastrointestinal and menstrual symptoms frequently appear within a few months of the MVA.

Sleep disturbance with dreams involving a state of helplessness are typical, and initial dreams of the MVA often give way to dreams of personal assault. Arousal, rage, and a sense of injustice for being injured in the MVA reflect the suppressed rage generated by the original sexual assault. This sense of outrage after rape is often suppressed by the shame and guilt that have been perpetuated by the rape myths of our society. Remarkably, many of these women had never had counseling for their rape, and many have discounted the effect of their rape on their lives prior to the MVA. Under these circumstances, addressing the repressed and latent arousal, rage, and fear related to their rape experience in the context of the emotional and physical pain caused by the MVA affords an opportunity for real healing and transformation.

Medical Trauma

Anesthesia, Surgery, and Critical Medical Illness

Exposure to trauma within our current allopathic and technological system of medical care has been minimally addressed in the standard medical literature. Because the concept of PTSD has been around for less than twenty years, emotional responses to medical interventions in the past have been considered predictable and justified, and usually of no consequence. Emotional responses to medical experiences have often been attributed to neuroses, and blamed on defective personality traits. Several factors in the development of modem medical techniques appear to increase the potential for traumatic stress. The discovery of ether anesthesia in the early twentieth century introduced the rapid development of increasingly sophisticated surgical techniques. Many of these techniques were for the purpose of curing or relieving painful conditions, but most also presented the new dilemma of postsurgical pain. Anesthesia and surgery also introduced the cold, malodorous, and terrifying theater of the operating room, full of masked strangers, strange smells, and sounds that the patient entered in a state of primitive and helpless nakedness.

Surgeons have been concerned for a long time about preoperative anxiety and panic because of behavioral management, complications during the surgery, and postoperative outcomes. Fear of death, injury, postoperative pain, and even of helplessness and unconsciousness may be a source of preoperative anxiety in surgical patients.[58,59] Concern about the effects of preoperative anxiety on both the physical and emotional outcomes of surgical procedures has led to the routine use of preoperative psychological support and sedation to minimize these risks.[58,60–62] High levels of sympathetic arousal associated with marked preoperative anxiety often require a higher dose of thiopental for anesthetic induction, thereby increasing the risk of circulatory collapse. This anxiety may be modified by preoperative medication.[63,64]

Psychological and emotional responses to anesthesia and surgery have been documented, but the literature is remarkably sparse. Several studies have suggested that postoperative anxiety (A-State) is generally less than preoperative anxiety, and is unrelated to personality traits predisposing to anxiety (A-Trait), which may be predictive of preoperative anxiety.[65,66,67] This finding is in keeping with the logical explanation that preoperative anxiety may be heightened by fear of the unknown outcome and by the intrinsic threat of surgery, especially in predisposed patients, whereas postoperative anxiety is lessened by the gratifying awareness of having survived the ordeal.

Nevertheless, sleep disturbance and even nightmares have been reported fairly frequently in the postoperative days in surgical patients. Marked disruption of normal sleep patterns has been described in a group of patients during the early period of surgical convalescence.[68] A small group of twelve patients exhibited increased REM sleep, upsetting dreams, and nightmares beginning on the third postoperative night.[69] Delirium, sleep disturbance, and decreased REM sleep have been documented in patients after open-heart surgery, with no clear correlation with possible sources of lack of oxygen or circulation to the brain.[70] Long-term emotional and psychological morbidity, however, is more difficult to interpret because the effect of the passage of time obscures the direct relationship of the patient's distress to the surgery itself.

A number of studies demonstrate the long-term psychological effects of surgery and potentially catastrophic illness. The major areas of study have been in the uniquely threatening diseases of cancer and myocardial infarction (MI), both of which carry a high risk of pain, disability, and death. Coronary artery disease is a predominantly male affliction, and by far the majority of coronary artery bypass grafts (CABG) are performed on men. Males have approximately one-third the likelihood of developing PTSD as a result of a given traumatic experience as females, and one therefore would expect the risk of developing PTSD in MI and CABG to be quite low. Studies, however, reflect an incidence of PTSD in 5 to 10 percent of males experiencing MI and CABG.[71,72] Symptoms in these cases primarily represented those of an intrusive variety and often persisted for more than twelve months. Reexperiencing included both phobias of the illness itself with fears of recurrence, and intrusive memories and thoughts of particularly traumatic scenes from the acute hospital experience. Moderate to severe depression also occurred in another 8 percent.[72] Clearly both the patient's awareness of experiencing a life-threatening disease and an environment implying threat and helplessness contributed to the trauma.

One must consider in this context the physical environments of the operating room and intensive care unit (ICU), and what they represent to the terrified patient already burdened with the awareness of potential impending mortality. For reasons of safety, hygiene, staff comfort, and efficiency, these environments are cold, bright, sterile, noisy, and clogged with frightening technological paraphernalia. Equipment emitting rhythmic beeping sounds measures the life forces of the patient, and every variation in sound implies potential disaster. At some point, CABG patients experience the terror of the sensation and sounds of a respirator pumping air into their lungs through an endotracheal tube, a condition of ultimate helplessness. Postoperative pain can be severe following a CABG procedure, and many patients report severe pain during the days following surgery despite narcotic analgesia. In this context, uncontrolled pain alone as an independent variable has been reported to be a cause of PTSD.[73]

On the other hand, these studies also show that the majority of the subjects did not suffer significant or long-term psychological distress. This is not altogether surprising considering the relative resistance to development of PTSD in males, but it again illustrates the fact that traumatic stress is not necessarily traumatizing in all individuals. These studies, however, did not investigate the potentially traumatic premorbid life experiences of the subjects. Based on experience with PTSD in combat veterans, MVAs, and other sources of trauma, prior life traumatic experiences should also play a role in trauma associated with medical experiences.

Although studies addressing the development of PTSD in cancer patients are sparse, several shed light on the importance of prior life events and on the role of medical experiences themselves as a source of trauma. Studies addressing the significant occurrence of PTSD in cancer patients have appeared primarily in the past two decades.[74-79] A patient receiving the possible diagnosis of a potentially fatal disease is consistent with a criteria-based stressor for PTSD based on the DSM–IV.[3] Following the diagnosis of cancer, patients are well known to vacillate between states of arousal/anxiety and dissociation/denial, a state comparable to the period following exposure to any overwhelming traumatic stress. This emotional response had been documented in longitudinal studies of breast cancer patients that show that almost half of the patients diagnosed with cancer experienced high levels of intrusive anxiety prior to surgery, with significant reduction at six weeks after surgery.[78,79] One year after surgery, however, one-third still experienced insomnia due to intrusive thoughts or images from the illness, one-fifth experienced cancer-related nightmares, and more than half experienced dissociative symptoms, especially numbness and feelings of unreality. Twelve percent still had criteria-based PTSD.[80]

A number of premorbid factors were significantly predictive of development of symptoms of PTSD in this population. Prior impaired psychosocial functioning, negative life events, health problems, and especially a personality trait characterized by high emotional reactivity were all specifically noted to be risk factors for development of PTSD.[80] Of course, "high emotional reactivity" may well have reflected traumatic impairment of infant attunement in these patients. The patient cohort in breast cancer is composed almost exclusively of females. This factor logically explains the increased incidence of symptoms of PTSD in this group, based on the increased risk of PTSD in females, probably due to their increased tendency to dissociate at the moment of traumatic stress. The fact that more than half of the women experienced late symptoms of a dissociative nature is not surprising.

Although only a relatively small number of subjects developed criterion-based PTSD, the incidence and persistence of PTSD symptoms in these studies is still remarkable. These statistics again remind us that the presentation of the diagnosis of serious or life-threatening disease to a patient alone may have serious and even long-term emotional consequences. The period of maximum arousal and anxiety symptoms in women with breast cancer occurred between the making of the diagnosis and informing the patient, and the immediate postoperative period. The immediate reassurance that the patients experienced having survived the surgery was sufficient to allay further anxiety and symptoms of PTSD in many patients. On the other hand, a great many went on to develop significant long-term symptoms of dissociation, sleep disturbance, anxiety attacks, and intrusive thoughts and memories, even though they perceived that they had been cured. The experience of fear, threat, and helplessness associated with the early period of their contact with the medical care system seems to have played a critical role in their subsequent emotional health. As an anecdotal observation, I have had a number of female patients with symptoms of trauma after an MVA who with the passage of time realized that a prior successful bout with breast cancer was the underlying cause for their accident-related PTSD symptoms.

Patients accessing the complex and highly technical medical system of diagnosis are by definition exposed to a perceived life threat in many instances. This experience frequently occurs in a relative state of helplessness. Physicians face the potential risk of contributing to their patients' trauma many times each day. The importance of effective and caring communication with their patients is generally poorly understood and frequently ignored when it comes to the concepts of healing, or conversely, to trauma. The remarkable power that physicians possess in determining the health of their patients solely through their personal contacts with them and their empathic presence is addressed in books by holistic medical practitioners such as Larry Dossey[81] and Bernie Siegel.[82] Caring communication is often ignored in the education of physicians, and yet, emotional attachment and a trusting bond with the caregiver is probably the primary source of protection from being traumatized when facing serious disease.

An intact social support network in the face of overwhelming traumatic stress will often shield the victim from the late symptoms of trauma. This particularly applies to children, whose emotionally and physically available caregivers are the primary factors in protecting them from traumatic stress.[83] In the case of a serious illness, the physician may play the pivotal role in the patient's system of emotional and social support. Physicians assume too often that patients cannot understand the complexity of the process of their arriving at diagnostic and treatment decisions, and do not try to educate the patients and enlist them as partners in both the diagnostic and treatment processes. Telling a patient with back pain, "I really can't find anything seriously wrong, but I think we'd better get an MRI," means to the patient, "He's really more worried than he's willing to tell me; there must be something seriously wrong."

Approaching any diagnostic workup for potentially serious disease will inevitably engender anxiety on the part of most patients. Enlisting them as informed and educated partners in the diagnostic process, however, lessens their sense of helplessness and loss of control, the primary factors that may predispose them to long-term emotional distress in the face of subsequent serious disease. This is especially important in the face of pressures to perform complex tests because of concerns about medical-legal issues in our increasingly litigious medical system.

The Role of Past Trauma

The previous breast cancer studies also illustrate the importance of being aware of the patient's legacy of traumatic experience when approaching diagnosis and treatment for serious disease. Previous life trauma, psychiatric or physical illness, or recent negative life events are all predictors of impaired emotional adjustment after serious illness. Identification of these risk factors in presurgical patients is basically ignored in current medical practice. Studies of PTSD and other psychiatric disorders implicate the patient's past life trauma in the development of somatic and emotional disorders after medical procedures. The medical and surgical literature has largely ignored the predictable physical and emotional complications in these at-risk patients when confronted with diagnostic workup, surgery, or medical treatment for potentially life-threatening illness. The result is a large group of patients who develop delayed emotional symptoms, as well as a pattern of physical symptoms, especially chronic pain, which defy physiological and anatomical explanation. Failed back syndrome, persistent radicular pain (sciatica) attributed to arachnoiditis (inflammation of the spinal canal), variations of reflex sympathetic dystrophy (RSD), and complex regional pain syndrome (CRPS) are examples of this dilemma.

Many of these chronic pain problems involve dissociation and somatization disorders, well-known late manifestations of PTSD. The tendency for victims of trauma, especially children, who have experienced dissociation to dissociate again when traumatized, is well documented (see Chapter 7). Such patients are also inordinately sensitive to threatening events that would not be considered traumatic in other people. The sterile and alien environment of the surgical theater may be sufficient in this patient population to trigger a dissociative reaction, leading to persistence of somatic manifestations of the presenting complaint despite anatomically corrective surgery. The analogy is similar to that of the previously traumatized victim of a trivial MVA who develops a full-blown whiplash syndrome. Patients with these specific problems, as well as myofascial pain, constitute the majority of referrals to chronic pain programs. The high incidence of past life trauma, especially child abuse, in the chronic pain population suggests that identification of patients with these risk factors before elective surgical intervention might help to avoid subsequent emotional morbidity, and the perpetuation of "nonphysiological" pain. Incorporation of preventative emotional and social support systems to deal with the helplessness and trauma of life-threatening disease, especially involving surgery, may be critical to ultimate healthy recovery in patients with past histories of life trauma.

Awareness During Anesthesia

Since the introduction of ether anesthesia by Morton, the occurrence of awareness during anesthesia has been well recognized and documented. Morton himself documented such a case during his career.[84] The motor response of the patient awakening under ether anesthesia was usually sufficient to prompt the anesthetist to increase the depth of anesthesia and shorten the period of the pain experience. The later introduction of operative paralysis, initially with the paralytic agent curare, and then with succinylcholine, prevented patients from responding physically to inadequate levels of anesthesia. Scientific reports of anesthetic awareness subsequently began to address the issue of postsurgical neurosis in such patients.[85] Patient reports of awareness under anesthesia often addressed the overwhelming sense of helplessness that they experienced and the panic that it produced. Even in the absence of an experience of pain during the period of awareness, many patients developed symptoms of PTSD.[86] Typical symptoms in such patients include insomnia with avoidance of sleep, flashbacks of paralysis and terror, flashbacks of pain with light sleep, or with cues related to the operating theater. Panic or flashbacks with hospital-related cues, such as the color blue (scrub suits), medicinal smells, clinking silverware (surgical instruments), or hospital-related television shows are common in such patients.[87] In many cases, explicit recall of the events during the period of anesthetic awareness is remarkably clear and accurate, despite the fact that the anesthetic record did not reflect physiological changes that might give a clue to lightening of the depth of anesthesia.[88,89] Recall of negative comments by the operating team in these cases, especially when directed toward the patient, is noted to have particularly negative effects on emotional outcome. Clearly, accurate explicit memory for events occurring during surgical anesthesia occurs in many cases of anesthetic awareness.

The roles of explicit and implicit memory in trauma have been discussed. Explicit memory is verbal, semantic, conscious, and able to be elicited voluntarily. Implicit memory is not associated with conscious recall, but is represented by motor skills, conditioned responses, or memory linked to emotions. Some studies suggest that implicit memory still may be involved in the processing and storage of information under anesthesia.[90] If so, those experiences associated with emotionally charged events, such as pain, paralysis, helplessness, or derogatory remarks while supposedly under anesthesia may be expected to contribute to operative trauma even in the absence of subsequent explicit recall. The clinical features of memory in traumatic stress are characterized by their predominantly sensorimotor and emotional content, and by their relative lack of verbal or narrative content.[91]

This fact emphasizes the role of implicit memory in the retention of memory for traumatic experiences. Even in the absence of explicit recall, the occurrence of unexplained postoperative emotional responses, unpredictable problems with pain control, or persistence of preoperative pain experiences despite successful surgery, might be due to the lightening of anesthesia during the surgery sufficient to imprint implicit memory for the experience, again in the absence of explicit recall.

The appearance of even partial symptoms of PTSD after a surgical procedure should raise concerns about a degree of lightening of anesthesia during the surgery sufficient to reproduce the emotional content of implicit memory through partial awareness. Since there is no accurate way to measure depth of anesthesia, the experience of partial awareness should not be ruled out even in the absence of explicit memory for events of the surgery. In addition, typical symptoms of PTSD may be obscured by the occurrence of dissociation or numbing following a traumatic anesthetic experience. This scenario would predict that the primary symptoms of anesthetic awareness might well be solely somatic in nature.

Awareness of events during a surgical procedure while paralyzed represents an ultimate expression of a life threat in the face of helplessness, the prime condition for the development of PTSD. In the absence of any ability to exercise the fight/flight response, the inevitable response is the freeze or immobility response, the autonomic correlate of dissociation. Even if fragments of explicit memory for the events surrounding the awareness experience exist, they may be suppressed through dissociative amnesia. Reluctance by the patient to inform the surgeon or anesthesiologist of the episode of awareness has also been frequently documented, and may contribute to the physician's misunderstanding of supposedly unexplained postoperative distress.[84] Under such circumstances, emotional expression of the trauma may present in a delayed fashion in the form of chronic pain, bowel complaints, dissociative symptoms, panic disorder, obsessive-compulsive disorder, or depression.[9] Physicians frequently attribute such postsurgical behaviors to the stress of the underlying illness or to premorbid maladaptive neurotic personality traits.

With these considerations in mind, prevention of morbidity from episodes of anesthetic awareness needs to be addressed through postoperative evaluation and debriefing. If clues to the experiencing of awareness during surgery are present, even if only in the form of unexplained somatic and emotional symptoms, counseling should be initiated. The goals of this counseling should include validation of the experience, assistance in recovering explicit memories of the event, and integration of these memories into a meaningful narrative. Exposure-based therapy may be necessary to desensitize the experience and place it into a benign perspective. The somatically based therapies should offer a unique opportunity to extinguish the somatic elements of posttraumatic procedural memory.

Pediatric Medical Trauma

Fetal and Neonatal Trauma

The concept that children might be traumatized by their contact with our system of medical care was largely rejected for more than a century. This concept was primarily based on the unfounded opinion by most physicians that infants could not process information, remember, learn, or for that matter feel pain before myelination of the axons of frontal and limbic cerebral pathways has occurred. Myelination is the progressive covering of nerve pathways with the fatty sheath myelin, which in many nerve fibers is necessary for message conduction. It was not until 1988 that the American Medical Association declared in a report on the most recent research that infants could feel pain. Before that date, many surgical procedures on infants were performed with only curariform paralysis without the benefit of general or local anesthesia.

Until about 1986, surgery for the cardiac abnormality patent ductus arteriosus, involving insertion of arterial catheters and chest tubes, and thoracotomy with rib retraction, was performed in infants under only curariform paralysis. This traumatic experience involved one and one-half hours of exposure to complete helplessness and overwhelming pain without any concept of the effects of this trauma on the infant, who was felt to be impervious to pain, or at least would never remember the procedure.[92] Chamberlain documents the case of a boy, born at twenty-nine weeks gestation, who underwent brain surgery, with ventriculo-peritoneal shunting for hydrocephalus under curariform paralysis.[93] At fifteen, he was severely phobic about doctors, hospitals, medical procedures, and the sight of adhesive tape and bandages. He would not allow anyone to touch his head, neck, or abdomen, the site of his surgical incisions for the shunt operation. Clearly this neonate had experienced and processed his existential traumatic stress, even in the absence of explicit memory. Processing of traumatic memory takes place through implicit memory mechanisms and brain centers, many of which have achieved myelination during and even before the neonatal period. Clearly perception and processing of pain experiences in the neonate (and therefore in the fetus) are more than sufficient to be traumatizing.

There is also clear evidence for fetal and newborn sentience, the ability to interact with their environment. Newborns and even fetuses in utero have been shown to be capable of classical habituation and conditioning.[94,95] Fetuses confronted with an amniocentesis needle invading the uterus exhibit defensive motor behavior.[96] Intrauterine needling of the fetus causes a full-blown stress-related increase in plasma cortisol and B-endorphin levels, with modulation of the stress response slower than in the adult.[97] Fetuses can also learn to adapt their behavior to control the environment. When presented with a sequence of different voices through headphones, an infant will learn to access his mother's voice through regulating the frequency of sucking on a nipple.[98] The evidence for learning by the unborn fetus in utero, by the premature infant in the pediatric intensive care unit, and by the normal full-term newborn is overwhelming.[98] They learn through implicit conditioned memory. The assumption that infants in all stages of development do not experience pain, do not register arousal with threat, and do not process a response to traumatic stress is clearly outdated and invalid. The risks of induction of traumatic stress in the medical management of the premature newborn and unborn fetus cannot be underestimated. When one takes a history of childhood trauma from a patient one usually addresses psychological, physical, and sexual abuse in the first decade. Little if anything in the PTSD literature addresses the terrible trauma to which premature infants are exposed, or the long-term behavioral and emotional effects of that trauma.

Birth Trauma

The other major threat facing the newborn infant is the modern day obstetrical theater. Infants born in the hospital face a cold, brilliantly lit, noisy environment associated with fetal monitoring probes inserted in their scalps, metal forceps on their heads, the jabs of lancets in their heels, suction tubes in their noses, mouths, and tracheae, and caustic liquid instilled into their eyes. They also face separation and isolation from their mothers at the moment of birth, the most critical period for infant-maternal bonding, the period most important for early attunement. I personally viewed a "natural childbirth" video, developed for prenatal education classes, in which a mother gave birth to her infant in an unmedicated "natural" delivery with her husband in attendance. After the umbilical cord was cut, instead of placing the baby on her mother's breast, the nurse took the infant to a bassinet, where she began to perform vigorous nasotracheal suction (suctioning the lungs via a tube inserted in the nostril). The infant exhibited a vigorous Moro (startle) reflex, but after two or three assaultive suction sequences, the infant became limp and unresponsive. When the infant was finally placed on the mother's breast, he remained limp and immobile, locked into his very first freeze response in the face of needless and brutal trauma delivered by a supposed caregiver.

The current medical philosophy of birth appears to be driven by the pervasive fear of injury to the newborn infant that, unfortunately, is partly based on litigious concerns, as well as the increasing worship of the technology of medicine. Although overwhelming evidence indicates that fetal monitoring and a higher rate of cesarean sections has not lessened fetal mortality or morbidity, the standard use of these invasive procedures has now been established as a benchmark for obstetrical care, and the C-section rate now is approaching 30 percent of births in the United States. Injury to the newborn in the absence of these procedures is considered a red flag for litigation.

Birth is an inherently natural process. It provides the earliest opportunity for enhancement of infant brain development required to provide resiliency in the face of threat through early maternal bonding. Despite the impression of many physicians, the brain at this stage of life is at its most vulnerable state. Exposing the newborn to traumatic stress through thoughtless invasive and painful medical procedures is senseless and dangerous. Many child psychologists feel that the roots of societal violence, at least in part, relate to birth trauma.[93] A large study of 4,200 consecutive births revealed that the combination of birth complications and maternal separation were powerful predictors of violent crimes in later life.[99]

Circumcision

Male infant circumcision performed without anesthesia continues to be one of the most blindly accepted but inherently traumatic experiences of the neonate. While the male newborn is immobilized by wrapping it in a sheet, the penis is swabbed with alcohol to induce an erection, a clamp is placed over the penile fore-skin and painfully tightened, and the foreskin excised in a circular fashion with a scalpel. The procedure is so "simple" that most medical students, including myself, have been allowed to perform it. The infant will be observed to cry bitterly, often exhibit a series of Moro reflexes, and then lapse into immobility. Only recently have physicians begun to advocate local anesthesia when performing circumcisions. Recent studies reveal that circumcised boys show significantly more severe emotional response to vaccination injections at ages four and six months than boys who have not been circumcised.[99] More than 60 percent of American male infants continue to be circumcised.[100] In March 1999, the American Academy of Pediatrics established a policy recommending that newborn males receive pain relief for circumcision, admitting that the pain experienced by infants at circumcision could have long-lasting side effects.[100]

Childhood Medical Trauma

Both neonatal and pediatric stress responses, measured by the release of stress hormones, primarily cortisol, are significant in anesthesia and surgical settings and are relatively greater than adult responses to similar medical procedures.[101] The brains of young children, therefore, regulate arousal less efficiently than adults, and are more susceptible to trauma. Not surprisingly, emotional and behavioral problems have been reported often in children subjected to anesthesia and surgery. The procedure studied the most is childhood tonsillectomy. As always, the measures used to assess such responses affect interpretation of the outcomes. In general, phobic and disruptive behaviors seem to be the most common, and appear to be time limited and reduced by presurgical emotional support.[102] Responses indicating trauma in the child during medical procedures are by no means universal, but when present, may be quite dramatic.

Perhaps the most potent evidence lies in the stories themselves, in this case involving a number of my own medical colleagues who have undergone ether anesthesia and tonsillectomy in their first decade. One recalls that for many years thereafter, he could not spontaneously yawn without feeling panic and stifling the yawn. He recalls the operating room nurse encouraging him to inhale deeply during ether induction, an act that for years he found threatening when it involved yawning. I personally underwent five experiences of ether anesthesia before the age of eleven, and had a phobia of falling asleep throughout my childhood, primarily due to a fear of being unconscious. I also had a morbid childhood phobia of the smell of ether and other volatile chemicals. Finally, I had a host of stress-related respiratory tics. My pursuit of the medical profession can only be attributed to traumatic reenactment. Many of us in the medical profession recall being allowed to perform ether anesthesia induction on children for tonsillectomy under the supervision of an anesthetist. The event is characterized by wrapping the child in a sheet while a nurse attendant forcibly holds the child down to the gurney. A gauze-covered metal cone is clamped over the child's nose and mouth, and ether is dripped from a can onto the gauze while the child screams and thrashes. During the surgery, the mask must be removed for the surgical procedure itself, as well as for suctioning, and then placed back on the face to deepen anesthesia when the child begins to gag and cough due to the secretions and blood. The scene can only be described as barbaric, and the child exposed to it no doubt experiences the same horror. Fortunately more effective and humane techniques for anesthesia in children have replaced this archaic and brutal procedure.

The practice of immobilizing children by wrapping them in a sheet and isolating them from their mother when performing simple emergency room suturing for routine lacerations has all of the elements of threat and helplessness required to induce traumatic stress. One of my own children described the injection of local anesthetic for a scalp laceration as terrifying, and still recalls the certainty that the doctor was injecting his brain, and that he was going to die. Another of my children was separated from her mother for essentially the same procedure, demonstrated anger and rejection of her mother, and acting-out behavior for months thereafter. At that time early in my medical career, I assumed that this was to be expected, and not the significant trauma that it indeed was.

Unfortunately, more detailed or controlled studies of the effects of our technological system of medicine on children are not available at this time. Anecdotal medicine is uniformly rejected as a means of arriving at meaningful scientific conclusions, and for good reason. Using the words, "in my experience," to justify a medical conclusion is dismissed in the absence of controlled research studies. Yet catastrophic complications of medical procedures also merit immediate attempts to correct the fallacies in those procedures. Applying the concepts of traumatic stress to many current medical practices, reviewing the data from analogous sources of trauma in our society, and recognizing the results of that trauma should compel us to reassess some of our current standards of treatment for our patients, especially our children and infants. Anecdotal experience in medical practice does suggest that trauma with all of the features discussed previously occurs with shocking frequency, and undoubtedly, contributes significantly to the load-of-life trauma that ultimately may have devastating long-term effects on the individual.

Conclusion

I have only touched on the numerous sources of trauma in our world and society, neglecting entirely issues of torture, imprisonment, genocide, civilian experiences in war, and natural disasters to name but a few of the traumatic extremes of life experience. Rather, I have attempted to address relatively unappreciated, or ignored sources of trauma. I have previously addressed the role of motor vehicle accidents as a relatively unappreciated source of cultural trauma. I have also emphasized what I perceive to be a generally neglected source of trauma, our current system of medicine, because I am familiar with it, both as a childhood patient and a practitioner. I also see its influence on patients who suffer from chronic pain, often not because of an injury but because the tests and procedures used to diagnose and treat the pain were in fact the source of trauma that perpetuated the pain. Trauma will always be with us. Our bodies are designed to deal with it as an inevitable life occurrence. It certainly behooves us as the caregivers and healers who attempt to lessen the ravages of unresolved trauma not to contribute to its effects through procedures, institutions, traditions, and behaviors that unknowingly serve to initiate or perpetuate trauma.

Notes

1. American Psychiatric Association: *Diagnostic and Statistical Manual of Mental Disorders*, Third Edition (DSM–III). Washington, DC: American Psychiatric Association, 1980.
2. American Psychiatric Association: *Diagnostic and Statistical Manual of Mental Disorders*, Third Edition, Revised (DSM–III–R). Washington, DC: American Psychiatric Association, 1987.
3. American Psychiatric Association: *Diagnostic and Statistical Manual of Mental Disorders*, Third Edition (DSM–IV). Washington, DC: American Psychiatric Association, 1994.
4. Helzer, J. E., Robins, L. N., McEvoy, L.: Post-traumatic stress disorder in the general population: Findings of the Epidemiologic Catchment Area survey. *New England Journal of Medicine*, 1987; 317(26):1630–1634.
5. Zohar, J., Sasson, Y., Amital, D ., Iancu, J., Zinger, Y.: Current diagnostic and epidemiological insights in PTSD. *CNS Spectrums*, 1998; 3:7(2):11–14.
6. American Psychiatric Association: *Diagnostic and Statistical Manual of Mental Disorders*, Third Edition (DSM–I). Washington, DC: American Psychiatric Association, 1951.
7. American Psychiatric Association: *Diagnostic and Statistical Manual of Mental Disorders*, Third Edition (DSM–II). Washington, DC: American Psychiatric Association, 1968.
8. Blanchard, E., Hickling, E.: *After the Crash*. Washington, DC: American Psychological Association, 1997.
9. van der Kolk, B. Pelcovitz, D., Roth, S., Mandel, E., McFarlane, A., Herman, J.: Dissociation affect dysregulation and somatization: The complex nature of adaptation to trauma. *American Journal of Psychiatry*, 1996; 153(Supplement):83–93.
10. Levine, P.: *Waking the Tiger: Healing Trauma*. Berkeley, CA: North Atlantic Press, 1997. pp. 128–129.
11. Krystal, H.: Trauma and affect. *Psychoanalytic Study of the Child*, 1978; 33:81–116.
12. Hobfoll, S.: *The Ecology of Stress*. New York: Hemisphere, 1988.
13. Breslau, N., Davis, G.: Post-traumatic stress disorder: The stressor criterion. *Journal of Nervous and Mental Disease*, 1987; 175:255–264.
14. Solomon, S., Canino, G.: The appropriateness of DSM–III–R criteria for posttraumatic stress disorder. *Comprehensive Psychiatry*, 1990; 31:227–237.
15. Norris, F: Epidemiology of trauma: Frequency and impact of different potentially traumatic events on different demographic groups. *Journal of Consulting and Clinical Psychology*, 1992; 60(3):409–418.
16. Solomon, Z.: *Combat Stress Reaction: The Enduring Toll of War*. New York: Plenum Press, 1993.

17. Solomon, Z., Laor, N., McFarlane, A.: Acute posttraumatic reactions in soldiers and civilians. In van der Kolk, B., McFarlane, A., Weisaeth, L. (Eds.). *Traumatic Stress: The Effects of Overwhelming Experience on Mind, Body, and Society* (pp. 102–114). New York: Guilford Press, 1996.

18. Kulka, R., Schlenger, W., Fairbank, H., Hough, R., Jordan, B., Marmar, C., Weiss, D.: *Trauma and the Vietnam War Generation.* New York: Brunner/Mazel, 1990.

19. Kessler, R., Sonnega, A., Bromet, E., Hughes, M., Nelson, C.: Post-traumatic stress disorder in the national comorbidity survey. *Archives of General Psychiatry,* 1995; 52:1048–1060.

20. Solomon, Z.: Somatic complaints, stress reaction and post-traumatic stress disorder: A 3-year follow-up study. *Behavioral Medicine,* 1988; 14:179–186.

21. Solomon, Z., Mikulincer, M., Kotler, M.: A two-year follow-up of somatic complaints among Israeli combat stress reaction casualties. *Journal of Psychosomatic Research,* 1987; 31(4):463–469.

22. Solomon, Z.: The psychological aftermath of combat stress reaction: An 18-year follow-up. Technical report, Israeli Ministry of Defense, 1994.

23. Kiser, K., Moll, J., Rankin, J.: Unexplained illness among Persian Gulf war veterans in an Air National Guard unit: Preliminary report. August, 1990-March, 1995. *Journal of the American Medical Association,* 1995: 274:16–17, and *Morbidity Mortality Weekly Report,* 1995; 44:443–447.

24. NIH Technology Assessment Workshop Panel. The Persian Gulf experience and health. *Journal of the American Medical Association,* 1994; 272:391–396.

25. Persian Gulf Veterans Coordinating Board. Unexplained illnesses among Desert Storm veterans. *Archives of Internal Medicine,* 1995; 155:262–268.

26. Amato, A., McVey, A., Cha, C., Matthews, E., Jackson, C., Kleingunther, R., Worley, L., Cornman, E., Kagan-Hallet, K.: Evaluation of neuromuscular symptoms in veterans of the Persian Gulf War. *Neurology,* 1997; 48:4–12.

27. Bremner, J., Southwick, S., Johnson, D., Yehuda, R., Charney, D.: Childhood physical abuse and combat-related post-traumatic stress disorder in Vietnam veterans. *American Journal of Psychiatry,* 1993; 150(2):235–239.

28. Frye, J., Stockton, T.: Discriminant analysis of post-traumatic stress disorder among a group of Vietnam veterans: Analysis of premilitary, military and combat exposure influences. *American Journal of Psychiatry,* 1982; 139:52–56.

29. Solkoff, N., Gray, P., Keill, S.: Which Vietnam veterans develop posttraumatic stress disorder? *Journal of Clinical Psychology,* 1986; 42(5):687–698.

30. Keane, T., Scott, W., Chavoya, G., Lamparske, D., Fairbank, J.: Social support in Vietnam veterans with post-traumatic stress disorder: A comparative analysis. *Journal of Consulting and Clinical Psychology,* 1985; 53:95–102.

31. Foy, D., Sopprelle, K., Rueger, D., Carroll, E.: Etiology of post-traumatic stress disorder in Vietnam veterans: Analysis of premilitary, military and combat exposure influences. *Journal of Consulting and Clinical Psychology,* 1984; 52:79–87.

32. Snow, B., Stellman, J., Stellman, S., Sommer, J.: Post-traumatic stress disorder among American Legionnaires in relation to combat experience in Vietnam: Associated and contributing factors. *Environmental Research,* 1988; 47:175–192 .

33. Schore, A. *Affect Regulation and the Origin of the Self.* Hillsdale, NJ: Lawrence Erlbaum and Associates, 1994.

34. Perry, B., Pollard. R., Blakeley, L., Baker, M., Vigilante, D.: Childhood trauma. The neurobiology of adaptation, and "use-dependent" development of the brain: How "states" become "traits." *Infant Mental Health Journal,* 1995; 16(4):271–291.

35. Grigsby, J., Hartlaub, G.: Procedural learning and the development and stability of character. *Perceptual and Motor Skills*, 1994; 79:355–370.

36. Seghorn, L. Boucher, R., Prentky, R.: Childhood sexual abuse in the lives of sexually aggressive offenders. *Journal of the American Academy of Child and Adolescent Psychiatry*, 1987; 26:262–267.

37. Lewis, D., Pincus, J., Bard, B., Richardson, E., Pricep, L., Feldman, M., Yeager, C.: Neuropsychiatric, psychoeducational and family characteristics of 14 juveniles condemned to death in the United States. *American Journal of Psychiatry*, 1988; 145:584–589.

38. Perry, B.: Evolution of symptoms following traumatic events in children (Abstract). Proceedings of the 148th Annual Meeting of the American Psychiatric Association. Miami, FL, 1995.

39. Ford, J., Kidd, P.: Early childhood trauma and disorders of extreme stress as predictors of treatment outcome with chronic post-traumatic stress disorder. *Journal of Traumatic Stress*, 1998; 11(4):743–761.

40. McFarlane, A., van der Kolk, B.: Trauma and its challenge to society. In van der Kolk. B., McFarlane, A., Weisaeth, L. (Eds.) *Traumatic Stress: The Effects of Overwhelming Experience on Mind, Body, and Society* (pp. 36–19). New York: Guilford Press, 1996.

41. Springs, F., Friedrich, W.: Health risk behaviors and medical sequelae of childhood sexual abuse. *Mayo Clinic Proceedings*, 1992; 67:527.

42. Tennant, C.: Life events and psychological morbidity: The evidence from prospective studies. *Psychological Medicine*, 1983; 13:483–486.

43. Wood, C.: Sexual abuse during childhood and adolescence and its effects on the physical and emotional quality of life of the survivor: A review of the literature. *Military Medicine*, 1996; 161:582–587.

44. National Victim Center: *Crime and victimization in America: Statistical overview.* Arlington, VA, 1993.

45. Resnick, H., Kilpatrick, D., Best, C., Kramer, T.: Vulnerability-stress factors in development of post-traumatic stress disorder. *Journal of Nervous and Mental Disease*, 1992; 180:424–430.

46. McFarlane, A.: The aetiology of post-traumatic morbidity: Predisposing, precipitating and perpetuating factors. *British Journal of Psychiatry*, 1989; 154:221–228.

47. Breslau, N., Andreski, P., Peterson, E.: Post-traumatic stress disorder in an urban population of young adults: Risk factors for chronicity. *American Journal of Psychiatry*, 1992; 149:671–675.

48. Carlson, E., Rosser-Hogan, R.: Trauma experiences, posttraumatic stress, dissociation and depression in Cambodian refugees. *American Journal of Psychiatry*, 1991; 148:1548–1551.

49. Ramsey, R., Gorst-Unsworth, C., Turner, S.: Psychiatric morbidity in survivors of organized state violence including torture: A retrospective series. *The British Journal of Psychiatry*, 1993; 162:55–59.

50. Kessler, R., Sonnega, A., Bromet, E., Hughes, M., Nelson, C.: Post-traumatic stress disorder in the national comorbidity survey. *Archives of General Psychiatry*, 1995; 51:1048–1060.

51. Resnick, H., Kilpatrick, D., Dansky, B., Saunders, B., Best, C.: Prevalence of civilian trauma and post-traumatic stress disorder in a representative national sample of women. *Journal of Consulting and Clinical Psychology*, 1993; 61:984–991.

52. Norris, F.: Screening for traumatic stress: A scale for use in the general population. *Journal of Applied Social Psychology*, 1990; 20:1704–1718.

53. International Federation of Red Cross and Red Crescent Societies: *World Disaster Report. 1993*. Dordrecht, Netherlands: Martinus Nijhoff, 1993.

54. Breslau, N.: Epidemiology of trauma and post-traumatic stress disorder in psychological trauma. In Yehuda, R. (Ed.). *Psychological Trauma* (Review of Psychiatry, Vol. 17) (pp. 1–29). Washington, DC: American Psychiatric Association Press, 1998.

55. Koss, M., Burkhart, B.: A conceptual analysis of rape victimization. *Psychology of Women Quarterly*, 1989; 13:27–40.

56. Warshaw, R.: *I Never Called It Rape: The Ms. Report on Recognizing, Fighting, and Surviving Date and Acquaintance Rape*. New York: Harper and Row, 1988.

57. Koss, M., Dinero, T., Seibel, C.: Stranger and acquaintance rape: Are there differences in the victim's experience? *Psychology of Women Quarterly*, 1988; 12:1–24.

58. Bernstein, S., Small, S.: Psychodynamic factors in surgery. *Journal of Mount Sinai Hospital*, 1951; 17:938–958.

59. Deutsch, H.: Some psychoanalytic observations in surgery. *Psychosomatic Medicine*, 1942; 4:105–115.

60. Dumas, R.: Psychological preparation for surgery. *American Journal of Nursing*, 1963; 63:52–55.

61. Eckenoff, J.: Some preoperative warnings of operating room deaths. *New England Journal of Medicine*, 1956; 255:1075–1079.

62. Giller, D.: Some psychological factors in recovery from surgery. *Hospital Topics*, 1963; 41:83–85.

63. Williams, J., Jones, J.: Psychophysiological responses to anesthesia and operation. *Journal of the American Medical Association*, 1968; 203:415–417.

64. Williams, J., Jones, J., Williams, B.: A physiological measure of preoperative anxiety. *Psychosomatic Medicine*, 1969; 31:6:522–527.

65. Auerbach, S.: Trait-state anxiety and adjustment to surgery. *Journal of Consulting and Clinical Psychology*, 1973; 40:264–271.

66. Speilberger, S., Auerbach, S., Wadsworth, A., Dunn, T., Taulbee, E.: Emotional reactions to surgery. *Journal of Consulting and Clinical Psychology*, 1973; 40:33–38.

67. Martinez-Urrutia, A.: Anxiety and pain in surgical patients. *Journal of Consulting and Clinical Psychology*, 1975; 43:437–332.

68. Moote, S., Skinner, M., Grace, D., Knill, R.: Profound disruption of sleep in the first week after abdominal surgery. *Canadian Anesthetists' Society Journal*, 1986; 33:S105.

69. Knill, R., Moote, C., Skinner, M., Rose, E.: Anesthesia with abdominal surgery leads to intense REM sleep during the first postoperative week. *Anesthesiology*, 1990; 73:52–61.

70. Brimacombe, J., Macfie, M.: Peri-operative nightmares in surgical patients. *Anesthesia*, 1993; 38:527–529.

71. Kutz, L., Garb, R., David, D.: Post-traumatic stress disorder following myocardial infarction. *General Hospital Psychiatry*, 1998; 10:169–176.

72. Doerfler, L., Pbert, L., DeCosimo, D.: Symptoms of post-traumatic stress disorder following myocardial infarction and coronary artery bypass surgery. *General Hospital Psychiatry*, 1994; 16:193–194.

73. Schreiber, S., Galai-Gat, T.: Uncontrolled pain following physical injury as the core-trauma in post-traumatic stress disorder. *Pain*, 1993; 54:107–110.

74. Alter, C., Pelcovitz, D., Axelrod, A., Goldenberg, B., Harris, H., Meyers, B., Grofois, B., Mandel, F., Septimus, A., Kaplan, S.: Identification of PTSD in cancer survivors. *Psychosomatics*, 1996; 37:137–143.

75. Cella, D., Mahon, S., Donovan, M.: Cancer recurrence as a traumatic event. *Behavioral Medicine*, 1990; 16:15–22.

76. Cordova, M., Andryskowsky, M., Kenady, D., McGrath, P., Sloan, D., Redd, W.: Frequency and correlates of post-traumatic stress-disorder-like symptoms after treatment for breast cancer. *Journal of Consulting Clinical Psychology*, 1995; 63:981–986.

77. Kelly, B., Raphael, B., Smithers, M., Swanson, C., Reid, C., McLeod, R., Thomson, D., Walpole, E.: Psychological responses to malignant melanoma: An investigation traumatic stress reactions to life-threatening illness. *General Hospital Psychiatry*, 1995; 17:126–136.

78. Tjemsland, L., Soreide, L., Mall, U.: Traumatic distress symptoms in early breast cancer I: Acute response to diagnosis. *Psycho-Oncology*, 1996; 5:1–8.

79. Tjemsland, L., Soreide, L., Mall, U.: Traumatic distress symptoms in early breast cancer II: Outcome six weeks post surgery. *Psycho-Oncology*, 1996; 5:295–303.

80. Tjemsland, L., Soreide, L., Malt, U.: Traumatic distress symptoms in early breast cancer III: Breast cancer research and treatment. *Psycho-Oncology*, 1998; 47:141–151.

81. Dossey, L.: *Meaning and Medicine: Lessons from a Doctor's Tales of Breakthrough and Healing*. New York: Bantam Books, 1991.

82. Siegel, B.: *Love, Medicine and Miracles*. New York: Harper & Row, 1986.

83. van der Kolk, B., Perry, J., Herman, J.: Childhood origins of destructive behavior. *American Journal of Psychiatry*, 1991; 148:1665–1671.

84. Blacher, R.: On awakening during surgery: A syndrome of traumatic neurosis. *Journal of the American Medical Association*, 1975; 233:67–68.

85. Meyer, B., Blacher, R.: A traumatic neurotic reaction induced by succinylcholine chloride. *New York State Journal of Medicine*, 1961; 61:1255–1261.

86. Cheek, D.: Surgical memory and reaction to careless conversation. *American Journal of Clinical Hypnosis*, 1964; 6:237–240.

87. Osterman, J., van der Kolk, B.: Awareness during anesthesia and posttraumatic stress disorder. *General Hospital Psychiatry*, 1998; 20:274–281.

88. Schwendler, D, Kunze-Kronawitter, P., Dietrich, S., Klasing, H., Madler, C.: Conscious awareness during general anaesthesia: Patient's perceptions, emotions, cognition and reactions. *British Journal of Anaesthesia*, 1998; 80:133–139.

89. Moerman, N., Bonke, B., Oosting, J.: Awareness and recall during general anesthesia: Facts and feelings. *Anesthesiology*, 1993; 79:454–464.

90. Heneghan, C.: Clinical and medicolegal aspects of conscious awareness during anesthesia. *International Anesthesiology Clinics*, 1993; 31:1–11.

91. van der Kolk, B., Fisler, R.: Dissociation and the fragmentary nature of traumatic memories: Overview and exploratory study. *Journal of Traumatic Stress*, 1995; 8:505–525.

92. Pemick, M.: *A Calculus of Suffering: Pain, Professionalism, and Anesthesia in Nineteenth-Century America*. New York: Columbia University Press, 1985.

93. Chamberlain, D.: Birth and the origins of violence. *Journal of Pre- and Perinatal Psychology*, 1995; 10(2):57–74.

94. Leader, L., Baillie, P., Martin, B., Vermeulen, E.: The assessment and significance of habituation to a repeated stimulus by the human fetus. *Early Human Development*, 1982; 18:307–319.

95. Rovee-Collier, C., Lipsitt, L.: Learning, adaptation and memory in the newborn. In Stratton, P. (Ed.). *Psychobiology of the Human Newborn* (pp. 147–190). London: Wiley & Sons, 1982.

96. Iannirubito, A., Tajani, E.: Ultrasonographic study of fetal movements. *Seminars in Perinatology*, 1981; 5(2):175–181.

97. Giannakoulopoulos, X., Sepulveda, W., Kourtis, P., Glover, V., Fisk, N.: Fetal plasma cortisol and B-endorphin response to intrauterine needling. *Lancet*, 1994; 344:77–81.

98. DeCasper, A., Lecanuet, J., Busnel, M., Granier-Deferre, C., Mangeais, R.: Fetal reactions to recurrent maternal speech. *Infant Behavior and Development*, 1994; 17(2):159–164.

99. Taddio, A., Goldblach, M., Ipp, M., Stevens, B., Koren, G.: Effect of neonatal circumcision on pain responses during vaccination of boys. *Lancet*, 1995; 345:291–292.

100. American Academy of Pediatrics: Circumcision policy statement. *Pediatrics*, 1999; 103(3):686–693.

101. Anand, K., Phil, D., Ward-Platt, M.: Neonatal and pediatric stress responses to anesthesia and operation. *International Anesthesiology Clinics*, 1988; 26(3):218–225.

102. Jackson, K., Winkley, A., Fausl, O., Cermak, E., Burtt, M.: Behavior changes indicating emotional -trauma in tonsillectomy children. *Journal of the American Medical Association*, 1952; 149:1536.

eleven
Trauma Therapy: Essential Ingredients

Marge, at 50, awoke daily with the stiffness and dragging fatigue of fibromyalgia. She had been disabled for a decade by the pain, exhaustion, and intrusive and muddled thoughts associated with this puzzling condition, and despaired of any hope of recovery. I saw her for a friend, one of the therapists in town who practiced somatic experiencing, and who was not optimistic about her chances for healing with trauma therapy, since she clearly was markedly dissociated from normal perception of her body and had no clear-cut history of significant life trauma. Nevertheless, at his encouragement we enrolled her in pool therapy utilizing Watsu, a warm water-based form of shiatsu massage. We also incorporated body tracking of the "felt sense," part of the technique of somatic experiencing. With Marge's first exposure to this technique she had a severe dissociative episode in the form of a pseudoseizure. Using great caution, my friend and the Watsu therapist continued to treat her, stopping the pool therapy at the first sign of dissociation, and immediately taking her to a small room where she was allowed to recover, wrapped in blankets and resourced by the therapist. Invariably Marge would go through a stereotyped pattern of body trembling and deep breathing until she recovered, a process often taking more than an hour.

After several months of cautious weekly treatment, she began to show strange gulping and gasping behavior as part of her recovery from her Watsu sessions. For the first time, she recalled that her mother had told her about her very traumatic birth, with strangulation by the umbilical cord requiring intubation and assisted respiration for more than twenty-four hours. With the appearance of this unusual respiratory response to the Watsu sessions, her morning pain began to clear, her sleep became restorative, and her sense of cognitive slowing cleared. She continued to experience slow but remarkable remission of symptoms of fibromyalgia, but also remained extremely vulnerable to recurrence of symptoms when she encountered any life stress.

* * *

My goal in this chapter is to integrate existing opinions and data on the most accepted methods of therapy for PTSD into an approach to therapy based on somatic concepts of trauma. I strongly feel that new models of somatically based treatment for trauma need to be explored and tested in the light of emerging data concerning the neurophysiological basis for PTSD, and the theories presented in this book. Except for EMDR, few blind controlled studies have been done to support these frequently arcane techniques with scientific support, yet tens of thousands of anecdotal reports have documented their efficacy in individual cases. With this understanding in mind, I beg the forbearance of my psychology and psychiatry colleagues, and hope that the ideas presented may be applicable to some of their treatment paradigms.

With the addition to the DSM–III in 1980 of post-traumatic stress disorder as a diagnosis distinct from other anxiety-based disorders,[1] increasing attention has been given to specific treatment models for this common problem. Group therapy involving trauma victims has been a mainstay of treatment since combat-related trauma was again brought to the world's attention after World War II.[2] The impetus to explore treatment models was again revived by the Vietnam War experience, and by the designation of PTSD as a unique condition. Based on these experiences, enhancement of interpersonal connections through family and social support systems, including those involving fellow victims of trauma, has become a central thesis for therapeutic management of PTSD. This approach, together with other forms of cognitive therapy, falls under the category of re-sourcing the victim's own self-regulatory mechanisms for dealing with the intrusion of painful emotional and physical symptoms. Although limited in scope, these therapies provide a useful start to the process of traumatic healing.

Cognitive/Verbal Therapy

Conscious access to traumatic memories and their meanings in a verbal context may be difficult or impossible based on the memory mechanisms that operate in traumatic stress. As discussed in Chapter 4, traumatic memories tend to be stored in an emotional or somatic context, and the victim simply may not be able to express or experience them in words. Alexithymia, the inability to adequately express emotions or body sensations in words, undoubtedly relates to this problem. A review in Chapter 12 of personal case studies in trauma from my own practice documents a class of patients presenting with bizarre disorders of stuttering, speech blockage, and impairment of immediate verbal processing, clearly on a dissociative basis. From a psychiatric standpoint, dissociation is believed to be a fragmentation of conscious awareness. I have attempted to present dissociation as a measurable physiological event, both at the level of the central nervous system and at the dissociated end organ (see Chapter 7). The memory for the contents within the dissociative capsule also is primarily unconscious and procedural. This fact underlies the basic difficulties inherent in verbal/cognitive therapy in trauma.

A regional physiological basis for these verbal impairments in trauma victims, as well as for alexithymia, may well exist based on findings in trauma survivors in positron emission tomography, or PET scans. Impairment of verbal expression in trauma may have its roots in findings that, in states of arousal, trauma survivors show inhibition of metabolic function in portions of the left cerebral hemisphere. This especially involves Broca's area, the area that controls production of speech.[3] References to "speechless terror," and other metaphorical analogies reflect the well-recognized inhibition of verbal functions in trauma. Cognitive therapy involving verbal interaction, insight, and interpretation under these conditions of impairment of verbal expression would be predictably difficult. This dilemma is keeping with the conclusions of many trauma specialists that "talking about the trauma" is rarely sufficient to dissipate the kindled, self-perpetuating trauma cycle.[4]

Nevertheless, verbal cognitively based therapy appears to play an important part in initiating and ultimately completing the therapeutic process in trauma. The role of the therapist in providing guidance, interpretation, and education through verbal interaction is critical, especially early in the traumatic response. Stabilization through anxiety control skills and identification of the meaning of somatic sensations that represent uncomfortable feeling states enable the patient to cope with self-perpetuating states of arousal. Encouraging trauma victims to verbalize these somatic sensations may allow them to access and integrate intense feeling states into conscious awareness. Hopefully, doing so may help to diminish the dissociation that contributes to substitution of somatic discomfort for intense emotions. Since access to the underlying hyperarousal and anxiety associated with trauma is painful, the presence of the therapist is important in providing a safe and supportive environment for the process.

Patients with PTSD suffer from sensitivity to any arousal stimulus. Triggering of their fight/flight response has become generalized to a wide variety of nonspecific environmental trauma-related cues, in addition to nonspecific sources of arousal. As a result, a trusting environment is extremely important for trauma patients, based to a considerable extent on their predictably increased sensitivity to the nuances of the therapist's behavior and demeanor. Even the facial characteristics or behavioral quirks of the therapist may remind patients of threatening past experiences or perpetrators of their trauma. For example, a patient of mine on a follow-up visit confessed that the therapist I referred her to somehow made her anxious, despite the fact that my patient found her to be very supportive and empathic. I asked the patient to describe the therapist in detail, and when she related her red nail polish, she turned quite pale, and recalled that her sexually abusive grandmother had used similar colored polish.

As a result, great care must be taken to provide an environment of safety and trust to allow the patient to access painful and arousing memories in a form that is bearable and in a setting that is perceived as safe. Bringing these memories and feelings into consciousness, and providing a narrative verbal format for the experience is an important ingredient in beginning the process of integrating the memories into conscious experience, and presumably in inhibiting the patient's cue-related arousal recycling. By learning to apply words to these terrible feelings and memories, the patient may begin to attain skills in containing and to some extent controlling them, and in relegating them to past experience rather than to an ongoing traumatic experience within the present moment.[5]

Patient education is also an important therapeutic goal. Most patients can understand complexities of neurophysiological concepts that might surprise many therapists. Providing a logical cognitive format for the patient's somatic and emotional symptoms serves several important functions. Most patients with symptoms characteristic of somatization and affect dysregulation have been labeled and devalued by their medical providers because they are felt to show symptom magnification, psychosomatic symptoms, or behavior indicating secondary gain. Dismissal or shaming by the very people on whom trauma victims depend for support and care enhances and perpetuates the physiological trauma cycle. The pain and suffering that they experience with perceived rejection is greatly enhanced by their intrinsic vulnerability and is as real to them as acute surgical pain.

Most of my traumatized MVA patients experience a period of marked deterioration of both somatic and emotional symptoms when their insurance company begins to question provider reimbursement or begins the first round of independent medical examinations, and also when their legal case becomes active. Their response is usually one of helpless rage, self-doubt, and a sense of devaluation. This process continues to reinforce their state of helplessness, the very basis for their trauma. Under this environment of renewed threat, these patients often experience a recurrence of the entire constellation of physical, cognitive, and emotional symptoms of whiplash.

Detailed education and information about the very valid physiological basis for their physical and emotional symptoms is empowering and restores the sense of control needed for their recovery. Providing words for the meaning of these frightening sensations begins the process of integrating them into a narrative format and a logical cognitive structure. Knowledge and enlightenment in this environment are critical for reestablishing a sense of validity and restoring a sense of self in the trauma victim.

Enlightenment through education, however, attacks only one facet of the trauma edifice. Knowledge allows the patient to deal with the unbidden and recurrent symptoms of trauma at a higher level, to facilitate interpretation and understanding, and thereby to help the patient achieve some degree of control over painful sensations or memories when they arise. But knowledge and words do not alter the basic kindled cycle of arousal, recall, muscle bracing, and autonomic cycling that perpetuates trauma. Ultimately, one must gain access to the insidious conditioned trauma response from a physiological and unconscious reflexive approach in order to extinguish, desensitize, inhibit, or quench it. Since such a therapeutic process is likely to present substantial risks of flooding and further trauma, cognitive resourcing and empowerment is clearly indicated. Early limited cognitive therapy may therefore play an important role in preparing the patient for other, more confrontational, techniques such as exposure or desensitization, and for very important somatically based techniques.

Exposure and Desensitization Techniques

More confrontational and invasive techniques of therapy have evolved in an attempt to diminish the intrusive symptoms of PTSD. The technique with the best documentation is cognitive-behavioral therapy, a method designed to change the implications or meaning of intrusive symptoms. To some extent, the various techniques under this category share the process of extinction of a conditioned response by eliciting the response (memory, emotion) in an environment that does not contain a trigger (cues, threat) for that response. The meaning of the response in relation to the basic survival instinct is changed and diminished as exposure to the response occurs repeatedly in a benign environment. As a result, habituation through repeated exposure progressively diminishes the fear/arousal response in PTSD. Such techniques as imaginal exposure and systematic desensitization involve guided reexperiencing of traumatic memories and images in a controlled therapeutic setting. As we shall see, the use of imaging is almost universal in verbal and somatic trauma therapies.

Numerous studies suggest that these techniques have a substantial therapeutic effect on reducing intrusive and cue-related arousal symptoms in PTSD.[6–9] Exposure, however, may carry a significant risk of flooding. Intense arousal and reexperiencing may duplicate the original traumatic experience. Without a concomitant internal and external environment that incorporates a sense of safety and empowerment, the victim may move immediately into the freeze/dissociation response. Severe dissociative reactions and enduring negative emotional symptoms may complicate therapeutic techniques incorporating flooding.[10] In addition, most studies document that the primary PTSD symptoms that benefit from exposure techniques are those involving arousal, fear, and traumatic reexperiencing. Late symptoms of avoidance, dissociation, somatization, and depression may be less responsive to cognitive-behavioral techniques.

Many of the clinical studies in these techniques also suffer from methodological problems, often related to standard outcome measures. Also, the spectrum of expression of symptoms in PTSD varies greatly, with wide variation in manifestation of symptoms of arousal and avoidance. Gender differences in response to trauma play a significant role in efficacy of various techniques, as might be expected. Recall that women are more prone to freeze/dissociate in the face of a life threat, and are therefore more likely to flood with exposure techniques. The nature of the traumatic experience and the environment in which it occurred also produce variations in the resulting traumatic symptoms. Studies comparing the effectiveness of therapy for PTSD in female assault victims are therefore likely to show significantly different outcomes than similar therapy in Vietnam War veterans, both because of gender differences and the nature of the traumatic experience. These studies do not necessarily reflect the efficacy of a technique useful in one population but not useful in another. Indeed, studies of Vietnam veterans in general show resistance to many therapeutic techniques, including pharmacotherapy. This finding has been attributed at least in part to the association of guilt with the traumatic experience.[11]

Adverse responses to exposure techniques by Vietnam veterans have raised concerns that reinforcement of guilt in exposure techniques might substantiate rather than desensitize arousal and anxiety. Based on these concerns, Rothbaum and Foa advocate developing techniques for guilt reduction because of its prevalence in PTSD in general.[12] Meanwhile they recommend the use of exposure-based therapy for arousal-related symptoms, and cognitive techniques for issues related to guilt. The emotions of guilt and shame have many correlations with dissociation and the freeze response. The first experience of shame in the developing infant is in response to the first disapproving look by the mother, and is characterized by blushing and turning the head away from their mutual gaze, a parasympathetic state analogous to the freeze response. This association may in part explain the resistance to treatment of dissociative states and to guilt and shame.

Several mechanisms have been proposed to account for the apparent effectiveness of exposure-based therapies for PTSD.[13] Habituation through repetitive exposure to the precipitating internal or external cue for the traumatic response might lessen the arousal response. It might also correct the notion that anxiety is inevitable unless avoidance or dissociation is activated. Second, deliberate confrontation with the traumatic memories blocks or inhibits negative reinforcement associated with the repetitive arousal/avoidance cycle. Third, repeatedly reexperiencing the traumatic event through confrontation or memory in a safe and supportive setting incorporates the message of safety into the traumatic memory. This helps the patient realize that the memory itself is not dangerous. Fourth, focusing intently on the traumatic memory or cue for a prolonged period of time separates it from the nontraumatic portion of the patient's existence, thereby reducing the patient's tendency to generalize the trauma to any arousal cue. Fifth, reexperiencing through imagery assists the patient in restructuring the meaning of traumatic memories from representing states of helplessness and incompetence to states of mastery and control. Finally, repeated exposure to traumatic memories allows patients to focus on those portions of the experience that reflect negatively on themselves, and to modify those perceptions into a positive model.[13] All of these very logical rationales I believe relate to the basic process of extinction of a conditioned association, a memory that is stored in implicit procedural memory systems. Almost by definition, they will ultimately be insufficient to extinguish the more deep-seated somatic and emotional cues to the traumatic event that continue to perpetuate the cycle. I believe also that repeated exposure through imagery alone may repeatedly trigger dissociation and enhance its persistence, producing reduction in arousal without actually extinguishing traumatic cues. This fact may account for the relative lack of effectiveness of cognitively based and exposure techniques for the criteria of numbing and avoidance. Emotion-linked conscious memories may be suppressed, while conditioned somatic procedural memories continue to trigger states of dissociation.

Techniques directed toward anxiety management have also been employed extensively in PTSD treatment. These techniques are designed to develop coping skills in lessening arousal and anxiety, and generally involve body-training exercises, often supplemented with biofeedback. Examples include deep muscle relaxation, breathing exercises, thought stopping, cognitive restructuring, covert modeling, and stress inoculation. All of these techniques employ active intervention by the patient in diminishing painful somatic or emotional symptoms through learned techniques of self-regulation designed to control or diminish that part of the trauma cycle involving arousal. They do not address symptoms of avoidance and dissociation. Indeed, it is theoretically possible that a number of these techniques might enhance dissociative tendencies as an unwanted effect on relief from arousal symptoms, since the only objective measures for success are based on reduction of measures or symptoms of physiological arousal. In discussions with other therapists, I have noted a significant incidence of panic attacks in patients practicing intense meditation techniques. All of these patients had experienced significant childhood trauma and a tendency to dissociate. They very likely tended to dissociate under the guise of meditation, and experienced a rapid cycling into arousal after prolonged meditation practice. It is no surprise, however, that these techniques in general do show improvement in arousal symptoms after treatment that lasts as long as six months in cases, but studies testing them contain methodological flaws, including lack of confirmation of PTSD diagnostic criteria. Nevertheless, studies combining anxiety management and exposure techniques seem to show that a combination of these approaches might be useful supplemental treatment for chronic PTSD and complex trauma.[12]

Somatically Based Therapies

A varied, eclectic, largely unproven but intriguing body of somatically based trauma therapies has emerged in the past few decades, driven by a number of factors. These include the relative resistance in trauma victims to treatment of PTSD, the frustrating inadequacies of many psychological treatment models, the recognition of the neurophysiological base for PTSD, and the emergence of so-called mind/body and alternative medicine.

We have already noted previously that many of the treatment methods that have been used in the past focus extensively on reduction in symptoms of arousal, the most obvious sources of distress in this patient population. But cognitive/behavioral and exposure techniques do not appear to have a consistently measurable effect on reduction of avoidance or dissociation in published studies. In the model of PTSD and dissociation presented here, this relative deficiency represents a critical flaw in current accepted treatment methods for PTSD.

Some of the somatically based therapies are founded on solid theoretical but unproven physiological models of trauma. Some involve stereotyped visual, auditory, tactile, or vestibular stimulation in a variety of settings, usually with imaging of past traumatic events. These stimuli usually are bilateral and alternating, often with lateral eye movements. Some involve repetitive verbal incantations, generally involving self-realization and empowerment, sometimes associated with tapping of acupuncture meridian points. Others involve alternate humming of a tune and counting aloud. A number involve the practice of kinesiology, a technique also related to concepts of Eastern medicine, acupuncture meridians, and the flow of "energy" within the body. The founders of many of these techniques have experienced a revelatory therapeutic experience with one of their patients or even in themselves, often on a serendipitous basis. This sentient event is subsequently followed by a post hoc experiential definition and refinement of the practice of the technique, and the development of a theoretical physiological rationale for its effect. Theories explaining the mechanisms for the therapeutic effect are often couched in a vocabulary unique to the technique itself. Finally, a training workshop format with accreditation criteria for practitioners is established.

The clinical appeal of these therapies relates to their apparent relative simplicity and the quick results that are often reported, especially in clearing phobic and arousal symptoms. The enthusiastic response of many psychotherapists to these techniques is not surprising considering the resistance to therapy seen in chronic PTSD. The eclectic and largely unexplained rationale for effectiveness of these techniques and the skepticism of the behavioral science academic community is also not surprising. Most have not been exposed to appropriate rigorous scientific scrutiny. Nevertheless, the most publicized and studied of these techniques, EMDR, is clearly beginning to make inroads into the realm of acceptance as a valid treatment model for PTSD. EMDR has been subjected to significant scientific scrutiny using controlled trials, and is widely accepted as a valid therapy for trauma.

I have chosen to highlight and discuss these techniques because I feel that they represent a necessary ingredient for future treatment models for PTSD. They are intriguing because they represent a somatically based reflexive approach to a condition characterized by the predominantly unconscious perpetuation of conditioned neural responses that inevitably contain somatic cues. Decades of treatment techniques for PTSD that are based on cognitive intent have shown consistently positive results in subpopulations of PTSD victims, but they have also failed to break the underlying kindled somatic components of the dissociative capsule, and to dispel the dominance of dissociation in many patients. I think that it is likely that components of these somatic techniques may provide pathways to resolution of the physiological manifestations of trauma that remain a barrier to many of the existing accepted trauma therapies.

Eye Movement Desensitization and Reprocessing (EMDR)

In 1989, Shapiro discovered quite by chance that rapidly moving one's eyes while thinking of arousal-based memory lessened the anxiety associated with that memory for a prolonged time. The discovery was made as part of a personal experience, and as a psychotherapist, she began to apply a technique that she developed from this experience on her patients with PTSD.[14] Eye movement desensitization (EMD), as she called it, entailed the identification of a traumatic memory by the patient associated with the expression of a personal negative cognition ("I am shameful"), followed and replaced by a positive cognition ("I am honorable"). The therapist would then pass her fingers back and forth in front of the patient's face for ten to twelve cycles while the patient followed them visually and concentrated on the traumatic memory. Following each trial, the therapist would assess the status of the patient's distress in relationship to the memory, and the degree of incorporation of the positive cognition. In her 1989 early report, Shapiro claimed remarkable clearing of the negative affective component of the traumatic memory in all of her PTSD patients. As she developed the theoretical basis for her technique, she added the term "reprocessing" to its name (EMDR) based on her conclusion that the technique enhanced the speed of information processing and facilitated transformation within the traumatic memory.

The results of anecdotal studies documenting the apparent efficacy of EMDR began to spread throughout the psychotherapeutic community and hundreds of therapists have received training in the technique through workshops developed by Shapiro. The eclectic nature of the technique predictably has raised skepticism within the same community as well. Early studies attempting to validate the technique were primarily outcome studies using standardized measures of symptoms and the state of distress before and after treatment. Even large studies suggest universal short-term improvement in symptoms of hyperarousal, intrusion, and avoidance.[15] Follow-up studies suggest good retention of therapeutic benefits.[16] On the other hand, uncontrolled studies have been challenged with the assertion that results could well have been based solely on the placebo effect associated with patient contact, and that outcome studies do nothing to validate the unique therapeutic benefit of the eye movement process itself.

Controlled studies have now been done in EMDR, and give a mixed picture regarding patient benefit and validation of the technique. Several studies have been done comparing EMDR with nontreatment wait list patients with PTSD. Although comparison with a nontreatment group of patients does not negate the placebo effect, EMDR clearly appears to produce substantially more improvement than no treatment over a similar period of time.[16,17] Comparison of EMDR to a number of techniques that have not been validated in PTSD (relaxation, biofeedback, active listening, image habituation) suggests that there is either no difference among techniques[18] nor superiority of EMDR.[19,20] Only one randomized and controlled study compares EMDR with a validated treatment technique for PTSD. In comparison with cognitive-behavioral therapy (CBT), this study showed that

EMDR was less effective than CBT in reducing PTSD symptoms, both statistically and clinically, and that this disparity was actually more evident at a three-month follow up.[21]

Another concern raised about the specific technique of EMDR questions the relative roles of the eye movements themselves, the traumatic memory imagery, and the use of negative and positive cognitive processes. Shapiro has steadfastly maintained that the eye movements themselves remain the core element of the technique. As a result, researchers have attempted to "dismantle" the various components of EMDR in an attempt to discover the salient therapeutic elements. The results have been both startling and confusing. One study suggested that eye movements alone without the cognitive elements of EMDR produced therapeutic benefits comparable to those achieved by the standard treatment protocol.[22] Another study using alternate tapping on left and right fingers of the subject showed comparable clinical efficacy, but less change in measures of autonomic arousal.[23] A third demonstrated no difference between using the EMDR protocol with eye movement or with the eyes fixed, although compared to a past study by these investigators, EMDR was at least as effective as imaginal flooding.[24] Although these studies cast doubt on the critical nature of the eye movement component of EMDR as maintained by Shapiro, they by no means disprove the efficacy of the entire protocol in comparison to other generally accepted techniques.

Speculation about the physiological mode of action of such therapeutic modalities proves nothing, but it provides the basis for studies designed to validate it, to dissect its therapeutic elements, and to apply that knowledge to devising ancillary treatments. Shapiro presents the hypothesis that the traumatic event leading to the associated memory is isolated and static because it has never been integrated or processed into an adaptive level. EMDR is physiologically designed to allow that reprocessing to take place.[25] As we have noted, positron emission tomography (PET) studies in arousal activation in PTSD patients suggest a significant lack of physiological coherence between the cerebral hemispheres in patients with PTSD. Several studies using quantitative EEG (QEEG), and single photon emission computerized tomography (SPECT), also support this concept of impairment of cerebral hemispheric synchronicity in PTSD, and show preliminary evidence for integration and reactivation of metabolically inhibited regions in the left hemisphere by relatively brief treatment with EMDR.[26,27] Others have noted that alternate finger tapping and auditory stimuli seem to have an equivalent effect in diminishing symptoms of arousal in PTSD.[28]

All of these somatic techniques have the production of rhythmic alternating bilateral cerebral hemispheric stimulation in common. This has led several authors to suggest that this integrative effect on cerebral function may help to restore cortical control of sensitized and kindled limbic and brainstem structures. This process might occur from the top down through facilitation of cortical control of limbic structures,[26,27] or from the bottom up, through down-regulation of limbic and brainstem nuclei.[28]

"Positive cognition" in EMDR and a number of other techniques also appear to play an independent and important role in the therapeutic process. As noted, positive thinking may produce symptomatic improvement by itself. Activation of inhibited left hemispheric speech and language centers through repetitive verbalization, especially of a phrase with a positive emotional valence, might well facilitate bilateral cerebral coherence and integration, and enhance the effects of the accompanying somatic exercise. All of these hypotheses, of course, are speculative at this time. They do, however, point the way to avenues of investigation, both of the validity of EMDR and for the development of similar therapeutic techniques to achieve similar physiological goals. One of the most exciting aspects of this process is the attempt to view and conceptualize trauma therapy in terms of its brain pathophysiology and to approach that physiology as a benchmark for treatment. Another is the recognition that the body plays a critical role in the manifestation and perpetuation of trauma, and may be a potent avenue for accessing and extinguishing the core physiology and content of the dissociation capsule.

Somatic Experiencing (SE)

The technique of somatic experiencing developed by Levine[29] for the treatment of trauma led me to my interest in PTSD and, ultimately, to this book. Somatic experiencing has had far less application than EMDR, and has not been subjected to scientific scrutiny. SE is unique and intriguing in that it does not rely on specific cognitive elements to achieve its effects. Levine's theory of trauma uses the animal model of the fight/flight/freeze response in the wild. He notes that when animals can no longer escape a predator, they enter a freeze or immobility state, during which the high-level metabolic and neurochemical energy of the flight response continues despite the immobility of the freeze response. If the animal survives, the stored energy is dissipated through various stereotyped somatic and autonomic responses, including trembling, perspiring, and deep breathing. Human beings tend not to dissipate this energy, possibly through acculturated social restraint or neocortical inhibition, resulting in the storage of arousal-based energy. This phenomenon then leads to the complex physiological process of PTSD. Of interest is the fact that Levine links the late somatic manifestations and symptoms of complex trauma to this process, incorporating somatization, denial, affect dysregulation, and depression into the entire trauma response.

Although Levine addresses the process of traumatic memory in the generation of symptoms, he emphasizes the role of procedural or implicit memory in the storage of traumatic energy, and incorporates explicit cognitive processes to a limited extent in his therapy. He uses the "felt sense" to pursue and access the trauma response. Levine describes this somatic state of being primarily by example rather than by specific definition. A working definition of the felt sense might be the sum total of all sensations from all sense organs, both conscious and subliminal, at any given moment.

Since the brain rapidly filters and discards unnecessary sensory input, much of the felt sense is unconscious until one concentrates purposely on feeling the subtleties of somatic awareness. SE involves exploration of these sensations by the patient under the guidance of a therapist trained in the technique. When patients with PTSD or its late manifestations access the felt sense, they will eventually arrive at awareness of subtle somatic sensations that represent variants of sensory procedural memory for a traumatic experience. The patients will then be guided initially to experience the sensation more intensely, and then to retreat to a previously established imaginary "safe place" as they begin to experience arousal triggered by the developing link to the emotional portion of that memory, triggered by the trauma-linked sensation. By "pendulating" in and out of this "trauma vortex" with the guidance of the therapist, the patient will eventually undergo the stereotyped motor and autonomic "discharge" of traumatic energy typified in animals emerging from the freeze response. This response is remarkably stereotyped in human subjects, suggesting a common physiological response. It will usually involve an involuntary motor response that often reflects the movement patterns experienced in an unconscious and instinctual protective fashion during the traumatic event. "Completion" of that movement is felt to be an important event in dissipation of the procedural memory for the trauma and its link to arousal.

SE presents another interesting approach to what we know about the neurophysiology of trauma. Its primary appeal may lie in its non-cognitive approach to what is primarily a subcortical, limbic, and brainstem phenomenon. Accessing and eliciting a motor response linked to a kindled limbic event in a benign environment, and completing the response successfully, could exert a powerful effect on down-regulating these sensitized and kindled subcortical circuits, most specifically the amygdala. Levine believes that one does not need to access explicit memory for the core traumatic event for SE to successfully discharge the traumatic energy, although at times it may be a useful adjunct to facilitating the technique. The risk of flooding, including the recovery of unremembered traumatic events is moderate, hence the use of "pendulation" by the therapist. In general, SE appears to provide remarkable control of the therapeutic process.

My clinical impression based on experience with several hundred patients treated with both SE and EMDR is that SE tends to result in resolution of dissociative traits and behaviors more effectively than many techniques. I am also extremely impressed with the safety and efficacy of SE in the common problem of the traumatized patient with chronic pain. Myofascial pain is ubiquitous in the chronic pain population, and extremely resistant to treatment. Based on my theory that myofascial pain reflects procedural memory for regional muscular bracing patterns experienced at the moment of a life-threatening event, one might suspect that uncoupling of that memory from associated kindled arousal might mitigate the pain. I would prefer to use the term extinction to that of uncoupling, realizing that replication of the motor patterns of self-defense in the absence of arousal linked to the amygdala would extinguish the associated procedural memory for the movement pattern. This concept is in keeping with the theoretical basis for SE, and indeed, I have found in many patients that chronic pain, especially myofascial pain, may show striking improvement or even disappearance as part of the SE therapeutic process. Obviously SE needs to be scrutinized through controlled outcome and physiological studies before any conclusions regarding specific aspects of its efficacy can be validated.

Energy Psychology

A variety of unusual, mysterious therapeutic techniques have emerged in the past twenty years that have been designated for better or for worse as energy psychology. These techniques generally are associated with holding or tapping areas of the body that correspond with meridian-based acupuncture points. Stimulation of these points is believed to restore homeostasis, a state of autonomic stability that we have noted is uniquely dysregulated in trauma. They also usually involve ritualistic affirmative statements, repetitive verbalization of the trauma/conflict, eye rolling, humming a tune, and counting.

Thought field therapy (TFT), a technique devised by Callahan,[30] is based on a theory that "perturbations" in the "thought field"—i.e., any negative emotion, phobia, or anxiety—cause disruption in the body's energy system. This state of energy imbalance is measurable through a diagnostic process of strength testing based on the technique of applied kinesiology, which in turn is related to the concepts of meridian energy flow on which acupuncture is based. The treatment involves instructing the patient to tap strategic acupuncture meridian points determined by the diagnostic procedure, while simultaneously imaging or remembering a traumatic event, memory, phobia, or emotion. Frequently the process is blocked by "psychological reversals," a presumed reversal of a meridian polarity. These reversals are then corrected by tapping on the outside of the hand while saying three times, "I fully accept myself even though I have this problem." The patient then goes through a nine-step procedure involving a ritualized combination of eye movements, counting, and humming a few bars of a song while performing hand tapping. The primary measure of treatment success is the Subjective Unit of Distress Scale (SUDS), a self-reported symptom scale measured from 1 to 10 based on the severity of symptoms of distress. During this process, the patient's self-assessed SUDS rating is documented sequentially, with the goal being reduction of the scale to a 1 or 0.

The arcane nature of TFT, its radical departure from any standard concept of psychotherapy, and the supposed "quick fix" that it provides have predictably exposed it to the condemnation and ridicule of many research psychologists. These very features of rapidity and portability, however, have probably contributed to its remarkably widespread use by community-based psychotherapists frustrated by treatment failures with standard therapy for PTSD, and also to the success of Callahan's training seminars.

A derivative technique, EFT (emotional freedom technique) was developed from TFT by non-psychotherapist Gary Craig. EFT contains most of the elements of TFT, but is generally simpler and more accessible to the general public, making it theoretically useful as a self-help tool.[31] EFT incorporates the same basic principles and theoretical mode of action as TFT. Like SE, TFT, and EFT have not been subjected to rigorous scientific scrutiny at this time. This fact has not prevented them from achieving remarkably wide use in the trauma therapeutic community.

The basic outline for treatment in EFT involves determination of a SUD's rating on a scale of 1 to 10 for the specific phobia/emotion to be treated. While either repetitively tapping a specific point in the armpit, or tapping the outside of each hand together (the karate chop), the patient repeats an affirmation statement three times: "Even though I have this fear/anxiety, I deeply and completely accept myself." The patient then repeatedly taps the following points on the body while repeating the reminder phrase (" . . . this fear/anxiety."): above eyebrow, outside of eye, under eye, under nose, chin, collarbone, under arm, and top of head.

The patient then proceeds with the nine-gamut technique: While tapping on the gamut spot (the point between the fourth and fifth metacarpal of one hand) with the fingers of the other hand, the patient is instructed sequentially to close the eyes, open the eyes, look down right, down left, whirl eyes clockwise, whirl eyes counterclockwise, hum a few bars of a tune, count out loud from one to five, and hum again. A SUD's rating is again taken, and the process repeated until the SUD's scale is down to 0 or 1. There are many other nuances to this technique based on "reversals" of the emotion, secondary gain, dissociation, and other issues, to name a few.

Although many theories account for the efficacy of various psychotherapy techniques involving counseling and verbal interaction between therapist and patient, there really is no way to eliminate the effect of the placebo response in this relationship. In fact, the joint sharing of belief between therapist/physician and patient that they are working together to achieve healing is basically what constitutes the placebo response.[32] The power of suggestion in a therapeutic relationship can have powerful and measurable physical effects, both positive and negative.[33] By this definition, I would suggest that the placebo effect is an intrinsically desirable component of any treatment technique, and can only be achieved by the powerful empathic interaction between therapist and patient.

One must also consider that the clinical profile of the patient population likely to benefit from such techniques is highly weighted toward the dissociative and somatization disorders, both of which are common late expressions of PTSD. Patients with somatization disorders basically experience embodiment of emotions of distress through physical symptoms, are more likely to seek reassurance from the physician/therapist concerning the meaning of these symptoms ("effort after meaning"), and are more likely to benefit from their positive interaction, i.e., from the placebo effect. Dismissal of the efficacy of these techniques on this basis, therefore, is to criticize every psychotherapeutic technique ever devised.

Several other areas of major concern have been raised, especially with EMDR and TFT/EFT. These concerns relate to the peculiar nature of the concurrent physical stimuli (tapping, eye movements, sounds, touch) presented along with imaginal exposure, and with the basic concept of a rapid and dramatic therapeutic effect. Neither of these specific features of EMDR and TFT/EFT have any other historical precedents in methods of psychotherapy, except perhaps for the use of electroconvulsive therapy (ECT) for the treatment of major depression. They also do not relate to any treatment model for physical disease in the Western allopathic system of medicine. Rapid reversal of symptoms of disease through repetitive and somewhat ritualistic performance of prescribed motor activities by the therapist or the patient lends itself far more to folk or shamanic medicine than to anything to which allopathic therapists can relate. In other words, given our current paradigms, these exercises make no sense.

The performance of stylized rituals of healing in a primitive culture is based on generations of experience related to outcomes of treatment for specific symptoms and specific diseases, using very specific learned healing exercises. Not unlike EMDR and TFT, these ritualistic exercises are discovered and expanded through trial and error until a reasonable state of refinement is achieved. Since these treatments seem to be linked to a learned meaning of the procedure on a cultural basis, the brain and its effect on the stricken person almost certainly play a critical role in healing. If we continue to abide by the premise of the continuity of mind, brain, and body, then it is likely that this healing takes place through altered neurophysiology and neurochemistry, and very likely to the restoration of autonomic homeostasis. The very specific nature of such rituals also suggests that this brain/body effect cannot be achieved by any random nuance of behavior by the shaman, but only by those practices that have been found to alter the physiology of persons stricken with a curse.

Attempting to find the "active ingredients" in these unusual methods of treatment appears to be a worthwhile pursuit. However disparate they may appear to be, a common neurophysiological thread may connect them in theory and effect. The burgeoning application of psychotropic and anticonvulsant drugs to the treatment of PTSD certainly supports the widely accepted concept that PTSD is a "physioneurosis."[34]

All mental illness must no longer be considered solely on the basis of the psychodynamics that led to the aberrant symptom complex. Rather, one must consider the neurophysiological basis for the dysfunctional behavior due to experienced-induced changes in neural structure. The unconscious and conditioned nature of much of PTSD symptomatology remains a powerful impetus to the development of treatment models that incorporate basically unconscious methods of extinction, desensitization, and quenching.

The search for treatment tools that may alter dysfunctional behavior by changing reflex patterns and neuronal pathways through unconscious methods of access to procedural memory and arousal systems has great appeal. These considerations clearly call for validation of somatically based techniques through appropriate studies, including attempts at dismantling the peculiar physical tools used in TFT/EFT, EMDR, and other similar reflexive therapies. Arbitrary dismissal of a technique as being too strange to be real, however, presumes that we know more about the brain, body, and behavior than we probably do.

Brainspotting (BST)

Brainspotting is a unique, fairly complex therapy devised about ten years ago by David Grand, Ph.D., a psychotherapist and early student of Francine Shapiro, the founder of EMDR. In the process of treating one of his patients with EMDR, he drastically slowed down the rapidity of the side-to-side movements of his hand to diminish its intrusiveness because of the sensitivity of this patient. As he reached a certain point, the patient's eye's "wobbled," and he stopped to observe what was happening. The patient then experienced a rush of memories of old childhood traumas, and maintaining the gaze, processed them, leading to a remarkable emotional breakthrough in her treatment. Grand refined his approach to accessing these "brainspots," and developed a complex protocol for the technique, including nuanced exploration of the dimensions of these obvious procedural memories for old traumatic experiences. As he refined the technique, these dimensions included vertical, horizontal, and depth planes. With sustained maintenance of gaze within these dimensions, not only the arousal connected to these perceptual spaces diminished, but the pain, clumsiness, and emotions linked to them subsided as well. Since then, Grand has developed and refined protocols for the use of BSP. He has begun trainings that now are international in scope, and with a large and expanding cohort of trainers.

The theoretical basis for this technique is debatable, but many possibilities exist. It could involve extinction of procedural memories of a traumatic event that are linked to the visual perceptual space, or boundaries that I tested in my whiplash patients, noted in previous chapters. These "boundary ruptures" usually occurred in an area where the patient first saw the car, where the impact occurred and in a whiplash/rear-end impact, behind the patient, or in the upper right visual field where the rear view mirror was and where their eyes first traveled. I described these interruptions of one's perception of boundaries as "boundary ruptures," and found that having the patient follow my hand at a roughly ten-foot distance often elicited an arousal response in the area where the accident occurred, or where the patient first saw the other car.

These procedural memories could also be linked to the precise position of the eyes at the moment of trauma. This positioning would be produced by proprioceptive/movement-based signals from the extra-ocular muscles that move the eyes. You'll recall that the motor and sensory messages from muscles and sensory organs in the head and neck are uniquely attuned to threat, and provide the information to trigger the fight/flight response through the orienting response, the side-to-side head and neck movement that positions these sensory centers for optimal perception of danger. The extra-ocular muscles are part of this message system.

It could still be related to left/right cerebral hemisphere stimulation, with inhibition of the amygdala, as in EMDR. Having observed Grand in his treatment, it is also clear that the application of this technique requires profound attunement by the therapist, enlisting perhaps the most crucial element of trauma psychotherapy. Grand has also incorporated binaural alternating gentle auditory stimulation via headphones to modulate arousal, a technique also used in EMDR.

Finally, one researcher has invoked concepts of the axonal route of visual stimuli through the superior colliculus (SC), a brain center that provides a conduit to the visual cortex in the opposite posterior part of the brain. The superior colliculus has an intimate relationship with one of the brain's pleasure/reward centers, the periaqueductal gray matter (PAG), which is part of the brain's pleasure center, and also plays a role in development of what we call the "self." Complex trauma victims are universally noted to lack a "sense of self," verified in my case in most of my traumatized whiplash patients. Visual stimulation of these pathways could possibly mitigate the symptoms of trauma in this model through enhancement of one's sense of self/self-state.

As one of the newer somatically based trauma therapies, BST is still evolving, but appears to offer a new and theoretically appealing approach to healing trauma.

Neurofeedback

During the 1960s, a group of behavioral scientists began studying a method of training unconscious physiological processes by measuring these processes and feeding the data back to the patient.[34–37]

The term biofeedback was ultimately applied to these techniques, and the measures fed back to the patient included muscle contraction, hand skin temperature and galvanic skin response (a measure of perspiration), and brain waves. Auditory or visual measures of these processes were provided for the patient and provided documentation of the state of the body that they were trying to manipulate. With practice, they could learn to relax muscles, increase skin temperature, and reduce perspiration in the hands, all representing measures of relaxation, reduced arousal, and stress modulation. Similar feedback using the electroencephalogram frequency patterns allowed the patient to achieve increased states of alpha (8–12 Hz) or theta (5–8 Hz) frequencies in frontal regions, as well as coherence or commonality between both sides of the brain. Such brain states were felt to reflect calm alertness, presence, and optimal brain function.

Brain wave biofeedback was eventually called neurofeedback, which is accomplished by providing visual or auditory messages that correlate with specific brain wave frequencies that the therapist is trying to reproduce. Patients are trained through concentrating on reproducing the auditory and visual signals that represent desirable brain wave frequencies and distribution. In doing so, they theoretically train their own brain to achieve states of optimal function.[38,39] The development of computer-based analysis and representation of the EEG pattern greatly enhanced the specificity of its application. Computer-based images and graphic depiction of the brain wave distribution was called quantitative EEG, or QEEG. Computer analysis allowed fine-tuning of both the visual and auditory signals, and the accurate validation of the therapeutic response. It provided a real-time image of brain wave distributions that could be studied in detail. This assumes that restoring the optimal state of brain wave distribution and coherence will correct disorders of emotion, attention, or cognition that have disrupted brain waves. Early research in neurofeedback indeed suggested that normalizing brain waves was uniquely successful in improving or correcting such behavioral disorders.

Neurofeedback has been studied in a wide variety of conditions that have in common the disruption of cognitive function, behavior, mood and emotions, mental health in general, and physical symptoms, especially those complaints suggesting somatization. These conditions have included PTSD and anxiety disorder,[39] epilepsy,[40] attention deficit disorder (ADD/ADHD),[41] minor traumatic brain injury,[42] obsessive compulsive disorder,[43] depression and mood disorders,[44] autism,[45] migraine,[46] chronic fatigue syndrome,[47] stroke rehabilitation,[48] pseudoseizures,[49] criminal behavior,[50] fibromyalgia,[51] substance abuse/addiction,[52,53] and schizophrenhia.[54] Research testing the effectiveness of neurofeedback in the treatment of these conditions mostly consists of pilot, single case, and basic outcome studies.

The limited number of controlled studies in the success of neurofeedback reflects what appears to be a basic problem with most research in the behavioral sciences in which the control of variables is extremely difficult. However, the introduction of functional imaging of the brain through fMRI techniques has allowed us to identify more objectively the effect of neurofeedback on function in selected regions of the brain. fMRI studies generally display those part of the brain that are selectively using energy at any given time, a measure of which parts are "online." Since we know the general role and function of brain regions, we can get a general idea of how neurofeedback might improve brain function in conditions where it has been applied by documenting functional changes in specific brain areas with fMRI studies. It is of interest that the patterns of brainwave distribution in the QEEG correlate significantly with the findings of energy distribution on fMRI.

Levesque studied fMRIs of a group of children with ADD/ADHD, and found that the anterior cingulate cortex (ACC) did not come "online" during a task of attention, as it did with a control group of children without ADD/ADHD.[55] You may recall that the ACC acts as a brake on the arousal center of the brain, the amygdala (see Chapter 2). It tones down arousal triggered by the amygdala if the threat is not serious. Therefore, in the healthy person exposed to a threatening stimulus, you would expect the ACC to be activated to modulate the threat response. Children with ADD/ADHD tend to overreact to cognitive challenges, perhaps because they lack this inhibiting mechanism of the ACC on amygdala-induced arousal as shown in these fMRI studies. After a course of neurofeedback, however, the ACCs in these children now showed normal activation with tasks requiring attention, correlating with improvement in measures of attention in these children. So the use of fMRI provides strong support for the fact that neurofeedback not only improves performance, but also "normalizes" abnormal patterns of activation of strategic regions of the brain in ADD/ADHD.[55]

If neurofeedback is able to normalize the brain's response to threat/stress, one would expect that it would be specifically useful in PTSD. Larsen provides a variety of anecdotal case studies with the treatment of PTSD in Vietnam vets, showing the relative effectiveness of neurofeedback in these cases,[39] but other more comprehensive studies are rare. As noted, however, PTSD represents only the tip of the trauma iceberg. With time, the symptom criteria for PTSD generally subside, leaving a predominance of symptoms in the areas of complex trauma, or DESNOS (disorders of extreme stress not otherwise specified). These symptoms primarily consist of disordered control of mood or affect, dissociation, depression, substance abuse, cognitive impairment and attention deficit, and socialization and somatic complaints. If you review the previous list of conditions in which neurofeedback appears to have had significant benefit, you will find many of them relate to the symptoms that occur in complex trauma. Is it possible that, by normalizing healthy patterns of brain wave coherence and distribution, neurofeedback is contributing to the healing of trauma?

Neurofeedback optimally tends to enhance alpha and higher theta frequencies in frontal and central brain regions, as well as enhanced symmetry of wave frequencies on both sides, or what we call coherence. Not surprisingly, studies of brain wave patterns in persons skilled in the art of meditation show remarkably similar patterns of enhanced alpha and hemispheric coherence achieved through neurofeedback.[56,57] These patterns of enhanced alpha activity in meditation also appear to arise from the medial prefrontal cortex and anterior cingulate cortex, areas known to function as brakes, or inhibitors of the amygdala, suggesting that meditation moderates the stress response. Indeed, in another study, practitioners of meditation exhibited brain wave patterns that reflected better capabilities to moderate brain responses to stress than control subjects who did not meditate.[58] So meditation clearly appears to mimic the therapeutic effects of neurofeedback on brain function—increased alpha, brainwave coherence, inhibition of arousal, and enhanced resiliency to stress. Or could it be that neurofeedback by trial and error (and intent) has arrived at replicating the brain state and therapeutic effects of skilled meditation?

We have presented the concept of PTSD as being defined by a state of abnormal and exaggerated cycling of the autonomic nervous system (see Chapter 7). This process represents the antithesis of homeostasis, the smooth and rhythmic autonomic cycling between states of sympathetic and parasympathetic dominance that characterizes optimal health. One of the states that may be the most accurate measure of homeostasis is the normal respiratory sinus arrhythmia (RSA), or heart rate variability (HRV). When you inhale, you experience a slight but predictable increase in your heart rate, and when you exhale, your heart rate slightly decreases. The respiratory cycle probably is another example of the cyclical nature of all physiological processes of the body. The most important consideration here is that the higher the variation in heart rate during inhalation and exhalation, the healthier you are! A high HRV implies a healthy autonomic nervous system, and a lower HRV correlates with all manner of diseases and causes of death, especially cardiovascular disease.[59,60]

It is therefore no surprise that PTSD and panic attacks are characterized by a low HRV, a primary measure of an abnormally regulated autonomic nervous system.[61] And it should also be no surprise that a course of transcendental meditation (TM) resulted in significant improvement in HRV, not to mention hypertension and insulin resistance, in patients with coronary artery disease.[62] So many emotional and physical diseases are characterized by abnormal autonomic regulation, and restoring autonomic regulation by training the brain may improve or heal both disease states.

The more specific diseases and syndrome that I present as diseases of trauma in fact are characterized by abnormal autonomic regulation manifested by exaggerated cycling. As a result, they tend to be characterized by both sympathetic and parasympathetic symptoms and signs, for example, the initially trophic and later dystrophic signs of reflex sympathetic dystrophy, the alternating constipation and diarrhea of irritable bowel syndrome, the arousal and fatigue of fibromyalgia. This trait of diseases of trauma may explain in part why they are so difficult to pin down with standard medical testing that relies on a fixed state of pathology. But, if neurofeedback mimics the therapeutic effects of meditation, it also may explain its effectiveness in what appears to be some of the late manifestations of trauma, both emotional and physical, through the restoration of homeostasis. If it does so by down-regulating the amygdala through enhanced function of the anterior cingulate cortex (ACC) as noted previously, then I believe neurofeedback (along with meditation) is providing the essential ingredient for the healing of trauma.

The Search for the Essential Ingredient

If one accepts the premise that extinction of somatic forms of traumatic procedural memory is an absolute prerequisite to healing—admitting that many do not—then we need to address therapy from the standpoint of the unconscious, a state that defines implicit forms of memory. We know that the limbic nucleus—the amygdala—evaluates the emotional content of incoming sensory stimuli and triggers arousal if those stimuli imply threat. Antonio Damasio, in his book, *The Feeling of What Happens*, describes a woman with bilateral injury to the amygdale.[63] Although otherwise functionally normal, she showed no capacity for fear or rage. This case implies that without the amygdala functioning adequately, fear conditioning cannot be accomplished. One conclusion that we can make from this regarding trauma therapy is that we need to down-regulate or shut down the amygdala while the patient images, or otherwise accesses the somatic sensations linked to the traumatic event. Without the amygdala "online" the somatic feelings of arousal will not occur, and implicit procedural memories of the trauma—body sensations and emotionally linked declarative memories—will no longer have a meaning of threat in the present moment of their perception. They will be relegated to past memory, a prerequisite to dissolution of the dissociative capsule. Effectively down-regulating the amygdala in the face of experiencing the somatic perceptions of the trauma should extinguish this conditioned association in relatively few trials. This process may explain the seemingly inexplicable and sudden healing of traumatic memories seen in a number of the somatically based therapies, such as EMDR and TFT/EFT.

The following therapy processes should down-regulate the amygdala:

1. Rituals, especially those associated with intense social interaction, are often part of the healing process in non-Western and especially indigenous societies, sometimes as part of the cultural norms, sometimes as practiced by tribal healers or shaman. They may involve repetitive behaviors such as drumming, dancing, and/or singing, and frequently induce trance states that are hypnotic. The use of hypnosis in treating trauma may have its roots in this process. Ritual may well play a role in the eye movements of EMDR, the tapping of TFT/EFT and the repetitive affirmative statements of the latter two techniques. We know that brain centers that participate in social and maternal-infant bonding—the orbitofrontal cortex and the limbic cingulate gyrus—also inhibit and down-regulate the amygdala. It makes sense that social ritual would facilitate this process.

2. Integration of the cerebral hemispheres brings the left hemisphere online, a condition that is inhibited in arousal, where the left frontal cortex and Broca's speech area seem to be selectively inhibited on PET scans. Integration of the hemispheres would theoretically interfere with and inhibit the independent function of the right amygdala. Cerebral hemispheric integration may be achieved through alternating visual, tactile, and auditory stimulation, and might down-regulate the right amygdala while the patient images the traumatic event, removing the arousal charge. Bilateral hemispheric integration may be the desired effect in the alternating touch, auditory, and visual stimulation of EMDR. It also may occur with the eye rolling, counting (left hemisphere), and singing (right hemisphere) employed in TFT. The reprocessing of traumatic memory attributed to EMDR might well be relegation of traumatic memories to the past through extinction of their somatic components.

3. Empowerment is the ultimate goal of all trauma therapy—it removes the state of helplessness that is essential to the trauma experience. Empowerment may be accomplished in many ways, including intentional symbolic replication of the defensive movement patterns that accompanied the traumatic event but were truncated by the freeze. This is accomplished unconsciously through accessing the felt sense in somatic experiencing, and intentionally in a number of other somatic techniques, including dance, balance, equestrian, and art therapy. The ritualistic affirmative statements of TFT/EFT also may function as tools of empowerment. Finally, providing a conscious cognitive structure for the meaning of the contents of the dissociative capsule after its components have been extinguished empowers one with the knowledge that occasional recurrence of somatic symptoms reflecting the capsule is actually an event from the past, and not once again part of an imminent threat.

These hypotheses are clearly speculative at best. Nevertheless, the field of trauma has yet to solve the dilemma of the cascade of often-somatic posttraumatic symptoms that persist long after the criteria-based symptoms of PTSD have subsided. The concept of the dissociative capsule provides a holistic model that reflects the content of the late posttraumatic experience, and begs for a novel approach to its resolution through the use if techniques that address the feelings of the body. Although EMDR has achieved recognition after years of exhaustive study, the esoteric nature of most somatically based techniques has relegated them to the dustbin of accepted trauma therapy, despite their widespread use in many parts of the world and the many uncontrolled outcome studies that reflect positive results. We may have at our disposal therapeutic techniques that ultimately promise the quality of healing trauma that we have yet to achieve.

Pharmacotherapy of Post-Traumatic Stress Disorder

The compelling reemergence of Kardiner's concept of PTSD as a "physioneurosis"[64] might lead one to predict a flood of clinical studies examining the use of strategic pharmacological agents in the treatment of PTSD. Surprisingly, this has not been the case. Much of the research examining the use of medications for the arousal and avoidance symptoms of PTSD has been in the form of case studies and open-ended clinical drug trials. Randomized controlled trials (RCT) have been rare. Several factors have probably contributed to this problem. PTSD is a multifaceted biphasic disorder, characterized by a number of quite disparate criteria (arousal, avoidance/numbing, reexperiencing), and is associated with a group of equally varied late clinical expressions (dissociation, affect dysregulation, depression, somatization). Many studies predictably document that specific medications work for specific symptoms, but none work for the whole syndrome. This conundrum of drug/symptom specificity, however, is quite consistent with the probability that different neurotransmitters may contribute to each of the many expressions of this disorder. After all, we are dealing with a bipolar/biphasic syndrome. Although a given patient may fulfill the DSM–IV criteria for PTSD, his or her clinical manifestations may be strongly biased in the direction of one particular symptom complex, such as arousal or numbing. As a result, in a given treatment trial, the clinical response to a drug may vary considerably from other verified PTSD patients with differing symptom dominance.

Any physician attempting to manage the varied symptoms of PTSD is well aware of the problem of precipitating anxiety and arousal through the use of a serotonin reuptake inhibitor (SRI), or compounding numbing or depression with an anxiolytic agent. The kindled sensitivity to any ambient sensory stimulus and the tendency to experience arousal or anxiety through somatic symptoms also renders these patients exquisitely sensitive to medication side effect, whether real or actually related to other ambient environmental stimuli. Under these conditions, not only the treatment but also the valid scientific study of drug efficacy in PTSD is extremely difficult. Despite these constraints, many open-ended drug trials have demonstrated strikingly beneficial clinical effects by a variety of medications for specific PTSD symptoms. As one would expect, application of early trial use of a medication has usually involved the administration of that drug for a symptom of

PTSD that is similar to the symptom for which the drug is customarily prescribed. In general, the main medications studied and used in PTSD have fallen into the categories of anxiolytics, antidepressants, and mood modulators.

Anxiolytic medications have included the benzodiazepines and buspirone. Brain receptors that bind the benzodiazepines are linked to the receptors for the inhibitory neurotransmitter, gamma amino butyric acid (GABA). One role of GABA, and therefore of the benzodiazepines, appears to be the control and modulation of anxiety.[65] Benzodiazepines might also play a role in modulating kindling, a compelling model for PTSD, since increase in benzodiazepine receptor binding is noted in experimental models of kindling.[66] Although this class of drugs has been used extensively in PTSD, few RCT clinical studies have been done to document their efficacy. In addition, there is general concern among clinicians about withdrawal symptoms from benzodiazapines associated with rebound anxiety, insomnia, aggression, and exacerbation of PTSD symptoms.[67,68] This is especially true for the short-acting benzodiazepines such as alprazolam. On the other hand, several open-ended studies have indicated efficacy of alprazolam and clonazepam in PTSD.[68,69] Much of this success, however, is thought to represent only reduction in anxiety-related symptoms. Clonazepam may represent an optimal agent in this drug class because of its lower habituation potential and its antikindling role as a primary anticonvulsant. In general, however, benzodiazepines represent a group of drugs with numerous risks and side effects in this difficult syndrome.

Buspirone is an anxiolytic agent with serotonergic properties, acting primarily as a 5-HT-A partial agonist. It has a delayed onset of action, much like the SRI group of antidepressants. The limited research available concerning its efficacy suggests that it may improve symptoms of arousal, reexperiencing, and sleep impairment, but that it does not affect symptoms of avoidance or numbing.[70]

Tricyclic antidepressants (TCAs) have been subjected to the most utilization and clinical study in PTSD. Members of this class of drugs variably have both serotonergic and adrenergic actions, with suggestive evidence that those TCAs with the most serotonergic activity may be somewhat more effective. Consideration must also be given to the fact that, because of the frequent association of depression with PTSD, the major benefit of all of the antidepressant class of drugs may primarily be due to improvement in depression alone.[71] Randomized controlled trials (RCTs) with amitriptyline, a TCA with strong SRI effects, reveal moderate efficacy in improving symptoms of PTSD including depression and anxiety.[71,72]

Imipramine has also been shown to exhibit effectiveness in the treatment of PTSD in a number of RCTs, with its major area of benefit being reduction of symptoms of intrusion and reexperiencing, with less benefit observed in symptoms of avoidance.[73,74] Patients with major depression were excluded from the imipramine studies, lessening the likelihood that the therapeutic effects were primarily due to improvement in depression. Desipramine, a purely adrenergic TCA, was found to be little more effective than placebo in treatment of PTSD.[75]

The TCAs, of course, have a side effect spectrum and incidence that is diverse and common enough to limit their use in these highly sensitive patients. In my experience, weight gain is extremely common in those patients with substantial symptoms of PTSD after motor vehicle accidents. The common association of this weight gain with an acneiform rash suggests that early hypersecretion of cortisol as part of the hormonal modulation and adaptation to trauma may trigger both of these problems. As a result, the additional weight gain common to the TCAs compounds this problem and further limits their long-term use in PTSD. Perhaps the most useful application of the TCAs to this disorder is their use in extremely low doses as a medication promoting sleep maintenance, an extremely common problem in PTSD. Although widely used in this capacity, their efficacy in sleep maintenance has not been specifically documented by the results of adequate RCTs.

Monoamine oxidase inhibitors (MAOIs) have been used and studied in PTSD to a limited extent but have not been widely applied due to the serious nature of their side effects. One well-designed RCT compared imipramine, phenelzine (an MAOI), and placebo.[74] Phenelzine was the most effective of the three treatments, with significant improvement noted in symptoms of intrusion and avoidance. In general, however, most clinicians reserve the use of MAOIs in PTSD to cases that have proven refractory to other safer medications.

Anticonvulsant medications have been applied to the treatment of PTSD with a similar rationale and in much the same fashion as they are applied to the treatment of bipolar disorder. The neurophysiological model of kindling has been applied on a theoretical basis to both conditions, and has generated increasing use of the newer anticonvulsant medications as mood modulators. The most commonly used anticonvulsants in PTSD are carbamazepine and valproate, both of which have been studied in open trials. Carbamazepine-treated veterans showed reduction in the severity of symptoms of arousal and intrusion, with fewer flashback experiences and improved sleep quality.[76] Valproate-treated veterans also showed improvement in arousal and avoidant symptoms, but little in intrusion.[77] Other case studies generally showed comparable results but were marred by inclusion of patients with partial complex seizures, and by noting improvement in irritability and aggressive behavior without specifically addressing issues of PTSD symptoms. Newer anticonvulsant agents, including gabapentin and lamotrigine, have been used in PTSD with efficacy in anecdotal unpublished reports, but have not been subjected to formal study in open trials or RCTs. Gabapentin is unique in its remarkably benign side effect spectrum, its wide dose range and tolerance, and its freedom from apparent dependence or overdose risk. These features alone might raise skepticism about its actual effectiveness, but it appears to have achieved wide application in PTSD, chronic pain, and as a primary mood modulator. Its long-term efficacy as an antikindling agent in PTSD remains to be formally studied.

Alpha2- and beta-adrenergic blocking agents have demonstrated some degree of efficacy in reducing symptoms of arousal in selected PTSD patients. One would expect a reduction in the perception of the physical symptoms of arousal based on blocking of the somatic end organs affected by adrenaline release with this class of drugs, and this effect might reduce the anxiety cascade associated with panic. The beta-blocker propranolol has been found to reduce a wide spectrum of arousal-based symptoms (hypervigilence, aggression, enhanced startle, intrusion, nightmares) in a varied population of PTSD victims, including combat veterans[78] and abused children.[79] Clonidine, an alpha2-adrenergic antagonist, reduces adrenergic tone through a different mechanism than propranolol, but would be expected to have similar effects on arousal and anxiety. Like propranolol, clonidine has had some success in anxiety states. In a study with Vietnam veterans with PTSD, Kolb, Burris, and Griffiths[78] documented therapeutic effects with clonidine similar to those noted with propranolol. Improvement has been noted in arousal symptoms of PTSD with administration of clonidine in children,[80] and in combination with imipramine in open trials in Cambodian refugees. Side effects of both classes of drugs include bradycardia, hypotension, depression, and constipation, and are dose-limiting but usually manageable. Nevertheless, even open trial studies of this class of medicines have been rare despite promising results in the few published articles. Both classes of adrenergic blockers have clear application in PTSD patients who develop sustained elevation of blood pressure following trauma. Although sustained hypertension in these cases probably also stems from separate and additional risk factors, the use of adrenergic blockers as an approach to both problems has particular appeal.

Serotonin reuptake inhibitors (SRIs) have been studied and applied more extensively in PTSD than other agents, and appear to represent the most effective drugs for the treatment of this disorder. Although a number of open drug trials suggest that fluoxetine is effective in improving symptoms of intrusion, avoidance, and arousal, the most widely quoted RCT suggested that fluoxetine is uniquely effective in improving numbing, a symptom generally resistant to many of the other drugs studied.[81] This study by van der Kolk and colleagues also showed improvement in arousal, but less so in avoidant symptoms. In addition, fluoxetine improved associated symptoms of PTSD, including affect dysregulation and the distortion of interpersonal relationships. Depression, however, was not significantly improved, suggesting that fluoxetine possesses a specific anti-PTSD effect. Since serotonin is known to inhibit firing of the amygdala, the therapeutic effect of SRIs may depend on this property. FDA approval of sertraline as the first medication specifically indicated for the treatment of PTSD was based on two multicenter studies. Findings were reviewed in the PTSD Research Quarterly by Friedman, and reflected previous findings that the SRIs tend to positively affect all three categories of PTSD symptoms (numbing, hyperarousal, reexperiencing).[82]

As with all medications, the somatic side effects of SRIs may be incorporated as traumatic cues in the complex trauma victim, and may negate their effectiveness.

Narcotic antagonists have been applied to the treatment of PTSD in several studies based on the demonstration that arousal-induced analgesia was reversible by the narcotic antagonist, naloxone, when Vietnam veterans were exposed to combat scenes.[83] The emotional numbing of PTSD has been attributed to endorphin release associated with the traumatic experience.[84] This theory is consistent with theories of altered regulation of the endogenous opioid system in PTSD, and the role of opioid dysregulation in dissociation and the phenomenon of reenactment (see Chapters 6 and 8). However, an open study of the experimental opiate inhibitor nalmefene in Vietnam veterans produced improvement in numbing in less than half, and worsened anxiety and panic symptoms in a number of subjects.[85] A single case study also demonstrated reduction in traumatic flashbacks in two patients with the narcotic antagonist naltrexone.[86] These studies illustrate the dilemma in pharmacotherapy of PTSD related to the spectrum of symptoms at both extremes of arousal and freeze/dissociation. Although fluoxetine also has been shown to diminish numbing in a number of patients, it may also precipitate anxiety and hyperarousal. One would expect the same to be true of narcotic antagonists, since numbing and dissociation are defensive reflex responses to the arousal generated by any threat in the PTSD patient.

Conclusion

This chapter has been an admittedly brief and basic overview of therapy for PTSD as it exists at the present time. The basic principles of treatment have been addressed in many chapters and review articles.[9,12,87] Although our expanding knowledge of the neurophysiological substrates of this diverse syndrome has provided a variety of logical constructs for treatment, the remarkable variation in symptoms both within individual patients and among different patients with the disorder seems to limit consistent successful therapeutic approaches to the problem. One is often left with such terms as "processing," "consolidating," "controlling," and "anxiety management" as means of handling an out-of-control autonomic flood. Social and personal attachments provide means of resource and support and are meant, along with these other generic concepts, to keep a finger in the dike of the always threatening emotional deluge. Although researchers and clinicians who have devoted their lives to the study of PTSD recognize that emotional numbing remains the elusive white rabbit of trauma, the therapeutic key to dispelling dissociation and numbing remains an enigma. The theory of the dissociative capsule as a defined entity consisting of the specific procedural memories of a traumatic event suggests that refined techniques of extinction may provide more specific and precise means for healing trauma. Focus on methods for specifically inhibiting the amygdala may allow more rapid and complete clearing of traumatic procedural memory cues.

On the other hand, many victims of traumatic stress do respond to existing therapies, and many rise above their panic and pain and reconstitute a reasonable semblance of emotional stability. Hopefully, the increasing awareness of the fact that the mind and the emotions in PTSD, and for that matter in all mental illness, reflect an ultimately identifiable and measurable aberration of brain physiology may lead to more specific, comprehensive, and rational treatment paradigms. Optimally, increasing recognition of the neglected role of somatic symptoms in trauma will lead to integration of somatically based therapeutic techniques into the treatment mix.

Notes

1. American Psychiatric Association: *Diagnostic and Statistical Manual of Mental Disorders*. Third Edition (DSM–III). Washington, DC: American Psychiatric Association, 1980.

2. Grinker, R., Speigel, J.: *Men Under Stress*. Philadelphia: Blakiston, 1945.

3. Fischer, H., Wik, G., Fredrikson, M.: Functional neuroanatomy of robbery reexperience: Affective memories studied with PET. *Neuroreport*, 1996; 7(13):2081–2086.

4. van der Kolk, B., McFarlane, A., van der Hart, O.: A general approach to treatment of post-traumatic stress disorder. In van der Kolk, B., McFarlane, A., Weisaeth, L. (Eds.). *Traumatic Stress: The Effects of Overwhelming Experience on Mind, Body, and Society* (pp. 417–440). New York: Guilford Press, 1996.

5. van der Hart, O., Steele, K., Brown, P.: The treatment of traumatic memories: Synthesis, realization and integration. *Dissociation*, 1993; 6:162–180.

6. Cooper, N., Chum, G.: Imaginal flooding as a supplementary treatment for PTSD in combat veterans: A controlled study. *Behavioral Therapy*, 1989; 20(3):381–391.

7. Resick, P., Schnicke, M.: Cognitive processing therapy for sexual assault victims. *Journal of Consulting and Clinical Psychology*, 1992; 60(5):748–756.

8. Brom, D., Kleber, R.: Prevention of post-traumatic stress disorders. *Journal of Traumatic Stress*, 1989; 2(3)335–351.

9. Foa, E., Rothbaum, B., Molnar, C.: Cognitive-behavioral treatment of posttraumatic stress disorder. In Friedman, M., Chamey, D., Deutch, A. (Eds.). *Neurobiological and Clinical Consequences of Stress: From Normal Adaprmiol1 to Post-Traumatic Stress Disorder* (pp. 483–491). New York: Raven Press, 1995.

10. Pitman, R., Altman, B., Greenwald, E., Longpre, R., Macklin, M., Poire, R., Steketee, G.: Psychiatric complications during flooding therapy for post-traumatic stress disorder. *Journal of Clinical Psychiatry*, 1991; 52:17–20.

11. Foa, E., Davidson, J., Rothbaum, B.: Treatment of post-traumatic stress disorder. In Gabbard, O. (Ed.). *Treatment of Psychiatric Disorders: The DSM–IV Edition* (pp. 1499–1519). Washington, DC: American Psychiatric Press, 1995.

12. Rothbaum, B., Foa, E.: Cognitive-behavioral techniques for post-traumatic stress disorder. In van der Kolk, B., McFarlane, A., Weisaerh, L. (Eds.). *Traumatic Stress: The Effects of Overwhelming Experience on Mind, Body, and Society* (pp. 451–509). New York: Guilford Press, 1996.

13. Rothbaum, B., Foa, E.: Exposure therapy for PTSD. *PTSD Research Quarterly* (p. 3), The National Center for Post-Traumatic Stress Disorder: White River Junction, VT, Spring 1999.

14. Shapiro, F.: Efficacy of the eye movement desensitization procedure in the treatment of traumatic memories. *Journal of Traumatic Stress*, 1989; 2:199–223.

15. Wilson, S., Becker, L., Tinker, R.: Eye movement desensitization and reprocessing (EMDR) treatment for psychologically traumatized individuals. *Journal of Consulting and Clinical Psychology*, 1995; 63(6):928–937.

16. Wilson, S., Becker, L., Tinker, T.: Fifteen-month follow-up of eye movement desensitization and reprocessing (EMDR) treatment for post-traumatic stress disorder and psychological trauma. *Journal of Consulting and Clinical Psychology*, 1997; 65(6): 1047–1056.

17. Rothhaum, B.: A controlled study of eye movement desensitization and reprocessing in the treatment of post-traumatic stress disordered sexual assault victims. *Bulleting of the Menninger Clinic*, 1997; 61:317–334.

18. Jensen, J.: An investigation of eye movement desensitization and reprocessing (EMDR) as a treatment for post-traumatic stress disorder (PTSD) symptoms of Vietnam combat veterans. *Behavioral Therapy*, 1994; 25:311–325.

19. Carlson, J., Chemtob, C., Rusnak, K., Hedlund, N., Muraoka, M.: Eye movement desensitization and reprocessing (EMDR) treatment for combat-related posttraumatic stress disorder. *Journal of Traumatic Stress*, 1998; 11:3–24.

20. Vaughn, K., Armstrong, M., Gold, R., O'Connor, N., Jenneke, W., Tarrier, N.: A trial of eye movement desensitization compared to image habituation training and applied muscle relaxation in post-traumatic stress disorder. *Journal of Behavior Therapy and Experimental Psychiatry*, 1994; 25:283–291.

21. Devilly, G., Spence, S.: The relative efficacy and treatment distress of EMDR and a cognitive behavioral trauma treatment protocol in the amelioration of posttraumatic stress disorder. *Journal of Anxiety Disorders*, 1999; 13:131–157.

22. Cusack, K., Spates, C.: The cognitive dismantling of eye movement desensitization and reprocessing (EMDR) treatment of post-traumatic stress disorder (PTSD). *Journal of Anxiety Disorders*, 1999; 13:87–89.

23. Wilson, D., Silver, S., Cove, W., Foster, S.: Eye movement desensitization and reprocessing: Effectiveness and autonomic correlates. *Journal of Behavioral Therapy and Experimental Psychiatry*, 1996; 27:219–229.

24. Pitman, R., On, S., Altman, R., Longpre, R., Poire, R., Macklin, M.: Emotional processing during eye movement desensitization and reprocessing therapy of Vietnam veterans with chronic post-traumatic stress disorder. *Comprehensive Psychiatry*, 1996; 37:419–429.

25. Shapiro, F.: *Eye Movement Desensitization and Reprocessing: Basic Principles, Protocols and Procedures*. New York: Guilford Press, 1995.

26. Nicosia, G.: A mechanism for dissociation suggested by the quantitative analysis of electroencephalography. Paper presented at the International EMDR Annual Conference. Sunnyvale, CA, March, 1994.

27. van der Kolk, B.: Personal communication.

28. Bergmann, U.: Speculations on the neurobiology of EMDR. *Traumatology*, 1998; 4:1:Article 2.

29. Levine, P.: *Walking the Tiger: Healing Trauma*. Berkeley, CA: North Atlantic Press. 1997.

30. Callahan, R.: *The Five-Minute Phobia Cure*. Wilmington, DE: Enterprise, 1985.

31. Feinstein, D., Eden, D., Craig, G.: *The Promise of Energy Psychology*. New York: Penguin Group, 2005.

32. Rosenthal, D., Frank, J.: Psychotherapy and the placebo effect. *Psychological Bulleting*, 1956; 53(4):294–302.

33. Goleman, D.: *Vital Lies. Simple Truths: The Psychology of Self-Deception*. New York: Simon & Schuster, 1985.

34. Basmajian. J.: *Biofeedback: Principles and Practice for Clinicians*, Third Edition. Baltimore: Williams & Wilkins, 1989.

35. Brown, B.: Recognition of aspects of consciousness through association with EEG alpha activity represented by a light signal. *Psychophysiology*, 1970; 6:642.

36. Green, E., Green, A., Walters, D.: Voluntary control of internal states: Psychological and physiological. *Journal of Transpersonal Psychology*, 1970; 112:1–26.

37. Kamiya, J.: Conscious control of the EEG alpha rhythm: A program for the study of consciousness. In Peper, E., Ancoll, S., Quinn, M. (Eds.). *Mind and Body Integration: Essential Readings in Biofeedback* (pp. 239–298). New York: Plenum Press, 1979.

38. Demos, J.: *Getting Started with Neurofeedback.* New York: W.W. Norton & Company, 2005.
39. Larsen, S.: *The Healing Power of Neurofeedback.* Rochester, VT: Healing Arts Press, 2006.
40. Sterman, M.: EEG biofeedback training in the treatment of epilepsy. In Padnes, S., Budzinskl, T. (Eds.). *Roche Scientific Series.* NC 6. 1972.
41. Lubar, J. O., Lubar., J. E.: Electroencephalographic biofeedhack of SMR, and beta for treatment of attention deficit disorders in a clinical setting. *Biofeedback and Self-Regulation,* 1984; 9:1–23.
42. Ayers, M.: Electroencephalographic neurofeedback and closed head injury of 250 individuals. *National Head Injury Syllabus, Head Injury Frontiers,* 1987, pp. 380–392.
43. Hammond, D.: QEEG-guided neurofeedback in the treatment or obsessive compulsive disorder. *Journal of Neurotherapy,* 2003; 7(2):25–52.
44. Baehr, E., Rosenfeld, L., Baehr, R.: Clinical use of an alpha asymmetry neurofeedback protocol in the treatment of mood disorders: Follow-up study of one to five years post therapy. *Journal of Neurotherapy,* 2001; 4(4):11–18.
45. Jarusiewicz, B.: Efficacy of neurofeedback for children in the autistic spectrum: A pilot study. *Journal of Neurofeedback,* 2002; 6(4):39–49.
46. Kropp, P., Siniatchkin, M., Gerber, W.: On the pathophysiology of migraine links for empirically based treatment. *Applied Psychophysiology and Biofeedback,* 2002; 27(3):203–213.
47. Hammond, D.: Treatment of chronic fatigue with neurofeedback and self-hypnosis. *Neurorehabilitation,* 2001; 16(4):295–300.
48. Rozelle, G., Budzynskl, T.: Neurotherapy for stroke rehabilitation: A single case study. *Biofeedback and Self-Regulation,* 1995; 20(3):211–228.
49. Swingle, P., Neurofeedback treatment of pseudoseizure disorder. *Biological Psychiatry,* 1998; 44(11):1196–1199.
50. Smith, P., Sams, M.: Neurofeedback with juvenile offenders: A pilot study in the use of QEEG-based and analog-based remedial neurofeedback training. *Journal of Neurotherapy,* 2005; 9(3):83–99.
51. Mueller, H., Donaldson, C., Nelson, D., Lyman, M.: Treatment of fibromyalgia incorporating EEG-driven stimulation: A clinical outcome study. *Journal of Clinical Psychology,* 2001; 57:933–952.
52. Trudeau, D.: Applicability of brain wave biofeedback to substance use disorder in adolescents. *Childhood Adolescence Psychiatric Clinics of North America,* 2005; 14(1): 125–136.
53. Burdett, V., Cummins, J., Dickson, R., Skolnick, M.: An open clinical trial utilizing real-time EEG operant conditioning as an adjunctive therapy in the treatment of crack cocaine dependence. *Journal of Neurotherapy,* 2005; 9(2):27–47.
54. Peniston, E.: Evaluation of long-term therapeutic efficacy of behavior modification program with chronic male psychiatric inpatients. *Journal of Behavioral Therapy and Experimental Psychiatry,* 1988; 19(2):95–101.
55. Levesque, J., Beauregard, M., Mensour, B.: Effect of neurofeedback training on the neural substrates of selective attention in children with attention deficit/hyperactivity disorder: A functional magnet resonance imaging study. *Neuroscience Letter,* 2006; 394(3):216–221.
56. Yamamoto, S., Kitamura, Y., Yamada, N., Nakashima, Y., Kuroda, S.: Medical prefrontal cortex and anterior cingulated cortex in the generation of alpha activity induced by

transcendental meditation: A magnetoencepthalgraphic study. *Acta Medica Okayama*, 2006; 60(1):51–58.

57. Travis, F., Wallace, R.: Autonomic and EEG patterns during eyes-closed and transcendental meditation (TM) practice: The basis for a neural model of TM practice. *Consciousness & Cognition*, 1999; 8(3):302–318.

58. Aftanas, L., Golosheykin, S.: Impact of regular meditation practice on EEG activity at rest and during evoked negative emotions. *International Journal of Neuroscience*, 2005; 115(6):893–909.

59. Thayer, J., Lane, R.: The role of vagal function in the risk for cardiovascular disease and mortality. *Biological Psychology*, 2007: 74(2)224–242.

60. Sinski, M., Lewandowski, J., Abramczyk, P., Narkiewicz, K., Gaciong, Z.: Why study sympathetic nervous system? *Journal of Physiology & Pharmacology*, 2006; 57 Suppl. 11:79–92.

61. Cohen, H., Benjamin, J., Geva, A., Matar, M., Kaplan, Z., Kotler, M.: Autonomic dysregulation in panic disorder and in post-traumatic stress disorder: Application of power spectrum analysis of heart rate variability at rest and in response to recollection of trauma or panic attacks. *Psychiatry Research*, 2000; 96(1):1–13.

62. Paul-Labrador, M., Polk, D., Dwyer, J., Velasquez, J., Nidich, S., Rainforth, M., Schneider, R., Merz, C.: Effects of a randomized controlled trial of transcendental meditation on components of the metabolic syndrome in subjects with coronary heart disease. *Archives of Internal Medicine*, 2006; 1669(11):1218–1224.

63. Damasio, A.: *The Feeling of What Happens*. New York: Harcourt Brace, 1999.

64. Kardiner, A.: *The Traumatic Neurosis of War*. New York: Hoeber, 1941.

65. Guidotti, A., Baraldi, M., Leon, A., Costa, E.: Benzodiazepines: A tool to study the biochemical and neurophysiological basis of anxiety. *Federal Proceedings*, 1980; 39: 1039–1042.

66. Tietz, E., Gomaz, F., Berman, R.: Amygdala kindled seizure stage is related to altered benzodiazepine binding site density. *Life Science*, 1985; 36:183–190.

67. Risse, S., Whillers., A., Burke, J., Chen, S., Scurfield, R., Raskind, M.: Severe withdrawal symptoms after discontinuation of alprazolam in eight patients with combat-induced post-traumatic stress disorder. *Journal of Clinical Psychiatry*, 1990; 51(15):206–209.

68. Feldman, T.: Alprazolam in the treatment of post-traumatic stress disorder [letter]. *Journal of Clinical Psychiatry*, 1987; 48:216–217.

69. Lowenstein, R., Hornstein, N., Farber, B.: Open trial of clonazepam in the treatment of post-traumatic stress disorder. *Dissociation*, 1988; 1:3–12.

70. Wells, G., Chu, C., Johnson, T., Nasdahl, C., Ayuhl, M., Sewell, E., Statham, P.: Buspirone in the treatment of post-traumatic stress disorder. *Pharmacotherapy*, 1991; 11(4):340–343.

71. Davidson, L., Kudler, H., Smith, R., Mahoney, L., Lipper, S., Gammett, E., Saunders, W., Cavenar, J.: Treatment of post-traumatic stress disorder with amitriptyline and placebo. *Archives of General Psychiatry*, 1990; 47:259–266.

72. Davidson, L., Kudler, H., Saunders, W., Erickson, L., Smith, R., Stein, R., Lipper, S., Hammett, E., Mahoney, L., Cavenar, J.: Predicting response to amitriptyline in post-traumatic stress disorder. *American Journal of Psychiatry*, 1992; 150(7):1024–1029.

73. Frank, J., Kosten, T., Giller, E., Dan, E.: A randomized clinical trial of phenelzine and imipramine for post-traumatic stress disorder. *American Journal of Psychiatry*, 1988; 145:128–129.

74. Kosten, T., Frank, L., Dan, E., McDougle, C., Giller, E.: Pharmacotherapy for post-traumatic stress disorder using phenelzine or imipramine. *Journal of Nervous and Mental Disease*, 1991; 177(6):366–370.

75. Reist, C., Kauffmann, C., Haier, R., Sangdahl, C., Demel, E., Chicz-Demet, A., Nelson, J.: A controlled trail of desipramine in 18 men with post-traumatic stress disorder. *American Journal of Psychiatry*, 1989; 146:513–516.

76. Lipper, S., Davidson, J., Grady, T., Edingar, L., Hammett, E., Mahoney, S., Cavenar, J.: Preliminary study of carbamazepine in post-traumatic stress disorder. *Psychosomatics*, 1986; 27:849–854.

77. Fesler, F.: Valproate in combat-related post-traumatic stress disorder. *Journal of Clinical Psychiatry*, 1991; 52(9):361–364.

78. Kolb, L., Burris, B., Griffiths, S.: Propranolol and clonidine in the treatment of chronic posttraumatic stress of war. In van der Kolk, B. (Ed.). *Post-Traumatic Stress Disorder: Psychological and Biological Sequelae* (pp. 97–107). Washington, DC: American Psychiatric Press, 1984.

79. Famularo, R., Kinscherff, R., Fenton, T.: Propranolol treatment for childhood post-traumatic stress disorder, acute type. *American Journal of Diseases of Children*, 1988; 142:1244–1247.

80. Perry, B.: Neurobiological sequelae of childhood trauma: PTSD in children. In Murburg, M. (Ed.). *Catecholamine Function in Post-Traumatic Stress Disorder: Emerging Concepts* (pp. 233–255). Washington, DC: American Psychiatric Press, 1994.

81. van der Kolk, B., Dryfuss, D., Michaels, M., Berkowitz, R., Saxe, G., Goldenberg, I.: Fluoxitine in post-traumatic stress disorder. *Journal of Clinical Psychiatry*, 1994; 55:517–522.

82. Friedman, M.: A guide to the literature on pharmacotherapy for PTSD. *PTSD Research Quarterly*, Winter 2000; 11(1): 1–7.

83. Pitman, R., van der Kolk, B., Orr, S., Greenberg, M.: Naloxone-reversible analgesic response to combat-related stimuli in post-traumatic stress disorder. *Archives of General Psychiatry*, 1990; 47:541–544.

84. Glover, H.: Emotional numbing: A possible endorphin-mediated phenomenon associated with post-traumatic stress disorder and other allied psychopathologic states. *Journal of Traumatic Stress*, 1992; 5:643–675.

85. Glover, H.: A preliminary trial of nalmefene for the treatment of emotional numbing in combat veterans with post-traumatic stress disorder. *Israeli Journal of Psychiatry Related Sciences*, 1993; 30(4):255–263.

86. Billis, L., Kreisler. K.: Treatment of flashbacks with naltrexone. *American Journal of Psychiatry*, 1993; 150(9):1430.

87. van der Kolk, B., van der Hart, O., Burbridge, J.: Approaches to the treatment of PTSD. In Hobfall, S., De vries, W. (Eds.). *Extreme Stress and Communities: Impact and Intervention* (pp. 421–443). NATO Asi Series, Series D. Behavioral and Social Sciences. Volume 80, 1995.

twelve
Case Histories: The Somatic Spectrum of Trauma

I have already included a number of case studies in this book to illustrate several concepts of trauma in MVAs, especially related to the syndrome of somatic dissociation. I believe that a chapter devoted only to such stories will help to give a better picture of the wide range of symptoms of trauma, not only those categorized in the DSM–IV, but also those accompanying the late manifestations of trauma. The spectrum of unusual and varied symptoms in many of my patients paints a vivid and arresting portrait of trauma and the physical and emotional toll that it takes on the brains and bodies of its victims.

A State of Vulnerability

My first case history is that of a young man, injured in a most unusual accident in a grocery store, which in other circumstances would have been considered trivial. A six-foot-four-inch, thirty-year-old man, he had the bulky upper body of a weightlifter. Yet when he spoke, his voice was soft and tentative. He took great pride in his body and health, pursuing fitness through exercise, and health through an organic, vegetarian diet. He told his story of trauma with obvious great distress. While shopping at a local health food store, he passed a display of stacked boxes of crackers, piled to a height of almost eight feet. At that moment, a box of crackers probably weighing five to eight pounds fell off of the top of the stack, hitting him on the back of his shoulders and neck. He was immediately stunned, and felt shocked and confused. Store personnel assisted him to a chair, where he remained for almost two hours, unable to pull himself out of a sense of shock and detachment. An on-site massage therapist gave him a massage, and the store provided an ice pack and juice to drink. He was finally able to pull himself together and called a friend for a ride home. Although he had no bruising or other signs of injury, over the next weeks he developed a syndrome of headaches, neck pain and muscle spasm, panic attacks, flashbacks and nightmares, depression, and impairment of memory.

When I saw him four months after the accident, his symptoms were becoming worse, and he had begun to have flashback memories of childhood trauma. He was the child of a physically abusive father, the parents having separated when he was five years old. At age six, his father broke into their home, shot him and his mother, and critically wounded both. He had only vague and disjointed memories of that traumatic event, but previously absent memories emerged in the face of his new, seemingly trivial traumatic experience in his thirties. Further evidence of his pervasive traumatic amnesia was found in the numerous scars on his body, the causes of which he had no memory.

This patient's case illustrates several principles in understanding the experience of trauma. As in most cases of PTSD, distortions of memory in this patient were characterized by both traumatic amnesia and flashbacks. Flashbacks, nightmares, and intrusive thoughts represent exaggerated repetition of traumatic memory, and are part of the kindled cycle of arousal and memory seen in PTSD. Traumatic amnesia is dissociative in nature, and is typical of childhood trauma, in which dissociation is almost a universal response to trauma. Individuals traumatized in childhood continue to dissociate as adults when exposed to trauma, even when the trauma is relatively trivial, as in this case.

As perhaps the most potent predictor for the development of PTSD, dissociation in this case of unusual trauma led to full-blown PTSD that persisted for months, and was severe enough to resurrect old traumatic memories and PTSD related to childhood trauma. The patient's attempts to build personal resources through his compulsively health-oriented lifestyle were no match for the unstable autonomic and neurophysiological mechanisms for dealing with any new stress resulting from his horrible childhood experiences. In addition, the traumatic event that triggered PTSD in his case certainly did not constitute a criterion for traumatic stress as defined in the DSM–IV. Low-velocity MVAs also do not fulfill this criterion, but may result in severe trauma in selected cases. Clearly the meaning of the precipitating event must be considered when determining whether a person has been traumatized. In cases in which the victim has a past history of multiple or severe traumatic life events, especially in childhood, a seemingly trivial threat may be perceived as life-threatening. Individuals with childhood trauma lack the resiliency to deal with later traumatic stress, and easily decompensate under relatively minor stressful events. When confronted with a patient with a disproportionate emotional response to a stressful event, a careful history of life trauma will usually reveal past traumatic experiences that clearly explain the remarkable vulnerability exhibited by them.

Somatic Representations of Prior Trauma

A second case study also illustrates the role of past life trauma in establishing a meaning for subsequent life events which, although superficially trivial, may prove to be profoundly traumatizing. A female patient of mine in her twenties presented with a history of having visited a new chiropractor for an adjustment. The chiropractor took the patient's head between his hands and performed significant quick rotational adjustment more violent than she was used to. The patient immediately experienced a sense of shock and horror and told the therapist, who apologized and continued with a more gentle manipulation. That night the patient experienced increasing headache, nausea, and cervical muscle spasm. She returned the next day to the chiropractor, hoping for some relief from her pain. After examining her, the chiropractor indicated that he could "fix" her neck, and once again performed a ballistic adjustment. At this point, the patient experienced uncontrolled panic and left the office acutely agitated and in great pain.

Over the next two weeks she developed severe headaches, cervical spasm, blurred vision, photophobia, nausea, vertigo, confusion, and memory loss. She was hypervigilant with exaggerated startle, and experienced flashbacks of the therapy and of old childhood trauma. She experienced severe nightmares and sleep disturbance. Cognitive symptoms in the form of forgetfulness, distraction, and episodes of confusion soon appeared. At the time of her first visit to my office, the patient wore a cervical collar. She was able to move her head by herself to a limited degree, but when I attempted to test that motion by moving her head gently with my hands, her neck was completely rigid. Neck movement also caused nausea and vertigo. Nonphysiological give-away weakness, glove-distribution sensory loss, and dramatic pain behavior were prominent. Her syndrome could well have been consistent with a whiplash experience in a patient prone to somatization. Her psychosocial history, however, revealed that as a child of eight she had been subjected to repeated incest by a male relative who achieved compliance by partial strangulation with his arm around her neck as a means of control.

In many cases of seemingly trivial injuries leading to PTSD, the key to the puzzle is found in the somatic representations of both prior trauma and/or the precipitating traumatic event. The somatic association with the neck in this case is obvious. Once again, traumatic events incorporating the head or neck seem particularly potent with regard to trauma potential (see Chapter 4). This case also illustrates that the whiplash syndrome consists of a reproducible constellation of symptoms that may have nothing to do with an MVA. This syndrome includes not only regional myofascial pain, but also cognitive impairment typical of minor brain injury in the absence of any possible brain injury. A threat to one's life and resulting helplessness certainly occurred in this case, but only if one took into account the meaning of the presumed traumatic event in the form of the meaning of the region of the body involved in the experience.

Another simple example of the retention of procedural memory for prior trauma-induced pain concerned a middle-aged woman involved in a moderate velocity rear-end MVA. Months later, she presented to me with persistent pain underneath her left scapula. Examination revealed typical findings of taut, tender muscles in the area of her persistent pain. Upon palpating these painful muscles, she suddenly cried out in great distress. I apologized for apparently having been too vigorous in my examination. She, however, said that it was not my fault, but that she suddenly had a flash of insight that the area of pain was the spot that "the nuns used to hit me." As a child in a Catholic boarding school, the nuns supervising the students made it a habit to discipline their charges by confronting them unannounced while the students were in their evening bath, striking them with a switch for perceived misdeeds that day. Because of the position of the tub, my patient invariably received her punishing blows under the left scapula. Procedural memory for this frightening and dreaded experience remained stored for future reference in her survival brain, and was reactivated by the experience of a new life threat, her MVA. The location of the symptom, however, was determined by old procedural memory of her childhood trauma.

Medical and Forensic Trauma

Unfortunately, physical injuries that also cause emotional trauma often are associated with incorporation of the legal system in attempts to resolve issues of causation and validity. Such is the case in MVAs, athletic injuries, falls, and various types of assault, including rapes and muggings. Because patients with prior life trauma are disproportionately vulnerable to subsequent trauma, their overt emotional and somatic response to injury may appear inappropriately severe. These patients are often soon labeled by the medical profession as "overresponders," suffering from psychophysiological problems, or exhibiting secondary gain behavior. Personnel handling their case for their auto or health insurance company soon access this information and begin to question the validity of the injury. Feeling invalidated by their own physician and health care insurance provider, the traumatized patients soon seek legal advice. The cycle of mistrust, skepticism, invalidation, fear, and frustration thereafter serves to perpetuate the patient's symptoms as a self-fulfilling prophecy.

Many of my patients have experienced this dilemma to some extent. One in particular exemplifies this problem, as well as a number of other unusual features of trauma. A female accountant, she was driving a client home when an argument ensued. The client had a history of bipolar mental illness, became agitated and paranoid, and began to strike the woman on the right shoulder and head. Swerving to the left, the woman saw an oncoming truck, swerved to the right, and ran off the road into a ditch. The accident was at low velocity and did not damage the car or, apparently, its occupants. The assaultive client at that point left the car, and walked across the field to his home.

Although she appeared uninjured, the patient rapidly developed severe right neck, shoulder, and arm pain and underwent several years of therapy with limited improvement. She experienced the onset of severe cognitive symptoms after a delay of about six weeks, was diagnosed with a closed head injury, and received prolonged cognitive therapy. Anxiety and panic, flashbacks, intrusive thoughts of the attack and accident, and nightmares developed. She received psychotherapy and was given trials of many psychotropic medications. When I saw her, a trauma history revealed that throughout childhood her father had been physically abusive to the family to the extent that at age twenty-one, the patient was actually hospitalized after a beating. She had not seen or spoken to him since then.

Despite ongoing pain, weakness, and numbness of the right arm, as well as cognitive and emotional impairment, the patient had resumed working. I referred her for somatically based trauma therapy after interpreting her symptoms for her, and she had a remarkable resolution of virtually all of these symptoms. Especially notable was the clearing of most attention and memory deficits, i.e., her "brain injury." Symptoms of pain and PTSD largely subsided.

As her legal case progressed, however, she was subjected to a series of independent medical examinations (IMEs), including repeated neuropsychological test batteries. Faced once again with skepticism and challenges to the validity of her injury, some of her symptoms of arousal began to reemerge. After a confrontational and adversarial deposition by opposing lawyers, she returned to see me with a full-blown recurrence of all of her cognitive, emotional, and somatic symptoms. A repeat course of therapy and settlement of her case out of court for a trivial amount resulted in improvement of symptoms once again, and she has subsequently done well. Her recovery was clearly related to the cessation of hostilities with the legal and insurance industries, and not to secondary gain.

Had this patient been recognized from the start as a victim of trauma, with a valid and predictable syndrome based on the nature of the accident, and had appropriate trauma therapy been instituted early, medical cost savings would likely have been achieved. More important, however, the serial and repetitive trauma inflicted by medical, insurance, and legal systems would likely not have occurred, and her state of vulnerability to subsequent trauma would not have been enhanced. A careful history would have determined that the attack by her passenger, and not the MVA itself, was the source of trauma, based on her childhood physical abuse.

This patient represents dozens of my patients whose syndromes of trauma have been perpetuated or resurrected in this manner. My interactions with insurance adjustors and nurse case managers have revealed a deep-seated mistrust of patients who carry the diagnosis of "soft tissue injuries," "minor traumatic brain injury," or "whiplash." Understandably, this is based on the dilemmas posed earlier. Many physicians share this disdain for the validity of these symptoms and diagnoses. Some have chosen to take advantage of this bias and voluntarily seek the role of performing IMEs for automobile, disability and liability insurance companies, often at great profit. Predictably many such IME reports are demeaning and critical of the validity of the patient's complaints, and contribute to perpetuating sequential trauma for the patient. Because our system of jurisprudence is by definition adversarial, the prescribed sequence of legal events in an MVA insurance claim predictably enhances symptoms of trauma, prolongs the patient's illness, and jeopardizes the outcome. In virtually every case of delayed whiplash recovery due to this form of trauma, I eventually spend more time treating the patient for effects of stress from the insurance and legal systems than for the original accident.

Multiple Chemical Sensitivities

Another example of the appearance of cognitive and emotional symptoms in the absence of velocity-related injury occurred in a patient of mine who presented as a case of chronic carbon monoxide poisoning. Three months after moving into a new house, the patient, a middle-aged woman, developed a syndrome of intractable nausea, cramps, and urinary and fecal incontinence with subsequent negative medical evaluations. She then developed distal tingling of her hands, blurring of vision, impaired memory and attention, apathy, panic attacks, and depression. Diffuse muscular pain ensued, and one year after the onset of symptoms, elevated carbon monoxide levels were found in her house due to a defective furnace.

Despite correction of the defect, her emotional and cognitive symptoms worsened and she developed a peculiar slurred and stuttering speech pattern several months after the exposure. MRI of the brain and EEG were normal, as was her neurological examination except for a clearly nonphysiological stutter. All symptoms and signs fluctuated dramatically, in direct proportion to incidental life stress. The entire symptom complex nevertheless progressed to the point of complete disability, and she applied for Social Security disability.

Her past medical history included a long record of recurrent myofascial low back and neck pain, carpal tunnel, and thoracic outlet syndromes, the latter two conditions leading to surgery. She had been treated in a clinic for chronic pain. At age eight, she had experienced a prolonged hospitalization for pelvic and femoral fractures, and at age five, she suffered multiple episodes of sexual molestation by a babysitter. Her one marriage was associated with spousal abuse and ended in divorce.

This patient clearly demonstrates the typical pattern of symptoms of late effects of trauma, many of which are typical of delayed recovery in whiplash. Although it might be tempting to relate her neurological syndrome to brain injury from low-level exposure to carbon monoxide, injuries of this sort are unproven. In addition, appearance of neurological symptoms following acute exposure to toxic levels of carbon monoxide is usually severe and often fatal, usually involving brain white matter lesions on the MRI.

On the other hand, diffuse somatic, emotional, and cognitive symptoms, including those of PTSD, have been described in the syndrome of multiple chemical sensitivities (MCS).[1,2] Several investigators have postulated the role of neurosensitization or kindling in the etiology of MCS.[1,2] These theories relate the close association between olfactory and limbic pathways in precipitating neurosensitization in such patients. Sensitivity to olfactory stimulation in the kindled trauma patient may well be related to the fact that olfaction is the only primary sense that accesses the limbic system without the filter of the thalamus. The patient described here may represent a case of unique vulnerability to autonomic arousal triggered by what might be considered a trivial exposure to olfactory stimuli. Multiple episodes of prior life traumatic stress had already caused many of the symptoms of late effects of her new trauma, and led to an ongoing state of chronic neurosensitization, or kindling. Such a state typically is associated with increased sensitivity to arousal with even remotely negative environmental stimuli. Certainly the olfactory/limbic connection could lead to enhancement of kindling in such patients. An epidemiological study of the association of past life trauma with MCS certainly appears warranted.

The Mysterious Piriformis

Piriformis syndrome (PS) has been described and discussed for seventy years. It has been defined as buttock and back pain with a positive Lasègue (straight leg raising) sign, tenderness at the sciatic notch, absence of neurological signs, and improvement with conservative therapy.[3] The piriformis muscle arises from the ventrolateral surface of the sacrum and sacroiliac joint, passes out of the sciatic notch, and inserts on the greater trochanter of the femur. It forms part of the posterior boundary of the floor of the pelvis, and is intimately associated with the branches of the sciatic nerve. As a result, true sciatica, or neurogenic pain running down the posterior thigh and calf, is frequently associated with the piriformis syndrome. The syndrome often follows a minor low back strain or overuse injury of the back, but also often occurs without apparent injury. It is associated with myofascial tightness, spasm, and shortening of the piriformis muscle. Incidence is considerably higher in women, with a ratio of 6:1 compared to men.[3] In women, pelvic pain and dyspareunia (painful intercourse) often accompany piriformis syndrome. Treatment includes standard physical therapy measures, including modalities such as heat, ice, and ultrasound, as well as specific stretching exercises. Local injections with steroids and/or local anesthetics may be useful, but are difficult due to the muscle's relatively deep location. In women, however, close association of the piriformis with the posterior vaginal wall allows easy transvaginal injection.

In my clinical experience with piriformis syndrome, I have typically noted the significant female preponderance of cases, most occurring in the context of falls, MVAs, or nonspecific back injuries. One such case started me on the investigation of prior life trauma in the role of piriformis syndrome, with startling results.

A young woman suffering neck and low back injuries from a MVA came to see me with prolonged and recalcitrant left sciatica. Although she was married, another female invariably accompanied her when she came to see me. (In my long clinical experience, when an adult woman always brings another woman with her to see me, a male doctor, a high likelihood exists that she has experienced sexual trauma in her past.) The results of her examination, involving straight leg raising and strength testing, were consistent with the classic signs of piriformis syndrome, but remarkably the examination also caused her to become severely nauseated. She reported that this nausea often lasted for hours after she left my office, prompting me to discontinue my examinations at the time of her visits. Her past history was vague, but suggestive of some childhood trauma that I suspected was sexual in nature. The usual and appropriate physical therapy measures only made her worse, and she eventually did not return to see me.

Within the following year, I became interested in the role of trauma in the whip-lash syndrome and myofascial pain, and developed some of the theories on which this book is based. As I began to take trauma histories in all of my patients with myo-fascial pain, I discovered a shocking association in my next thirty female patients and one male patient who presented with clinically consistent piriformis syndrome. All of these patients without exception had suffered sexual trauma, including childhood incest, rape, or molestation with penetration, or rape as an adult.

Several conclusions can be made from this association of a myofascial pain syndrome involving the piriformis syndrome in women and forced sexual pen-etration. The anatomical and kinesiological function of the piriformis muscle is external rotation of the femur. It also results in clenching of the buttocks and compression of the posterior pelvic wall. Its contraction is involved in the Kegel maneuver, an exercise used for strengthening the vaginal wall after childbirth and for shutting off the stream of urine. In the case of forced vaginal penetration, the piriformis clearly will be involved in the unconscious and reflexive protective neuromuscular response to the traumatic event. Unconscious piriformis contrac-tion will, thereafter, be incorporated in the kindled circuitry of arousal, memory, and muscular bracing described in Chapter 4. Reminiscent life events, nonspecific stress or arousal, or repetitive use of piriformis in a variety of situations may pre-cipitate procedural memory for the defensive role of that muscle in past sexual trauma, and lead to its persistent contraction and spasm. In many cases, but obvi-ously not all, I believe that the piriformis syndrome in women is an unusual and dramatic example of the traumatic basis for regional myofascial pain involving a kindled neuromuscular reflex and incorporating the muscle used for a failed attempt at defense.

Disorders of Speech in Trauma

A number of my patients who have shown other signs of trauma after an MVA or other traumatic event have developed an unusual syndrome of delayed develop-ment of stereotyped disorders of articulation. The previously described patient with chronic carbon monoxide exposure manifested this symptom several months after she actually detected the smell of gas in her home. In virtually all of my other cases, the dysarthric speech disturbance also developed as a delayed event weeks or even months after the trauma. Onset of the speech disturbance was preceded by cognitive symptoms suggestive of a brain injury, as well as by criteria-based symptoms consistent with the diagnosis of post-traumatic stress disorder (PTSD). Most patients had a history of substantial prior life trauma.

One such patient, a middle-aged woman, was injured in a broadside MVA in which her husband was apparently unaffected. She may have experienced a brief period of unconsciousness, and was described by her husband as being confused on the way to the hospital. For several days she experienced only headache and stiff neck, but after several weeks, she developed increasing symptoms of dramatic stuttering, word blocking, and problems with attention and memory. Anxiety, photophobia, and sleep disturbance also appeared. She gradually developed right hand tremor, a right facial twitch, and squinting of her right eye. Her past history revealed a prior auto accident six years before characterized by prolonged spinal myofascial pain, with a prominent piriformis syndrome. She also had a history of cyclical depression.

Her initial physical examination by me six weeks after the accident revealed a dramatic stutter primarily with words starting with consonants. My impression was that the findings of my examination did not appear consistent with an organic pathological lesion of the brain. Indeed, MRI of the brain was normal.

The patient underwent a prolonged course of treatment, including cognitive therapy, physical therapy, and somatically based trauma therapy. Due to her stimulus sensitivity, she essentially remained confined to her house except for medical appointments. She experienced gradual improvement, with disappearance of the stutter, tremor, cognitive and emotional symptoms, and eventually was able to drive alone on side roads. Her agoraphobia related to being in public places when other people were present, however, remained disabling. Under such circumstances, all of her nonphysiological neurological symptoms, including her stutter, hand tremor, and facial twitch recurred.

Clinical features of speech abnormalities in the other patients have been remarkably similar to those described previously. Most speech impediments have appeared, disappeared, or fluctuated in direct proportion to incidental life stress and to fatigue. The disorder is most often described as a stutter, or blockage of speech, and is associated with independent word blocking as well. A scanning, slurred, and dysarthric pattern is common, with independent prolongation of vowels, consonants, and diphthongs without any consistency. In one case, the patient developed what could be described only as a foreign or regional accent, with a consistent and reproducible pattern of mispronunciation. Onset of the speech impairment is usually delayed and recovery incomplete. Imaging studies of the brain have been routinely negative. Neuropsychological test batteries all show significant cognitive impairment consistent with minor traumatic brain injury (MTBI), PTSD, or both. In most cases, the speech abnormalities have been extremely resistant to treatment, and have persisted for years, usually in association with residual late symptoms of trauma.

The impairment in speech in these patients is clearly dissociative in nature, and might well be classified under the conversion disorders. In many instances, forces involved in the MVAs were relatively minor and inconsistent with production of an MTBI. Evaluation by speech pathologists routinely led to the conclusion that the speech disturbances were nonphysiological, and not consistent with any clear pathological process. All of the patients were women, and most of them had a history of prior trauma before the precipitating event. Although many carried the clinical diagnosis of MTBI, and all had cognitive dysfunction, symptoms of PTSD were uniformly prominent. The cyclical periods of improvement in speech invariably correlated with reduction of life stress and improvement in symptoms of trauma.

In the case history described, the patient had a past history of piriformis syndrome following another auto accident. A history of childhood trauma could not be obtained, although her neurological symptoms were clearly dissociative in nature. Perhaps the most salient clinical feature in these patients is the similarity of the quality of the speech impediment among patients. This rare but consistent association with traumatic experiences suggests a common connection between areas of the brain linked to production of speech and the phenomenon of kindling involving the limbic amygdala. The frequent concomitant occurrence of a tremor of the right hand or right facial twitch in these patients obviously has raised concerns about a structural left hemispheric lesion, but imaging studies have invariably been negative.

A group of patients with PTSD were read stories of their traumatic experience while positron-emission tomography (PET) scans of their brains were done. Heightened brain activity was noted in the right hemisphere, an area predictably linked to arousal and memory mechanisms associated with their trauma.[4,5] Broca's area for speech in the left hemisphere, however, showed abnormally diminished activity in these patients. Van der Kolk, Rauch, and colleagues postulate that this finding may explain alexithymia in traumatized patients: the inability to put feelings into words, and the tendency to experience emotions as physical states. In our cases of rare but stereotyped dysarthria and stuttering in patients with PTSD, this phenomenon might also reflect changes in brain activity specific to the areas of the brain serving expressive speech that are inhibited by kindling and arousal activity in the right hemisphere. As we have noted, many patients with PTSD manifest simple word-finding difficulties. The dysarthric speech patterns observed in the patients described here may represent a further expression of the negative relationship between traumatic arousal and physiological suppression of metabolic function and circulatory patterns in Broca's area and related left hemispheric regions.

Spasmodic Torticollis: An Aberration of the Orienting Reflex

A woman came to see me for a second opinion regarding her long-standing involuntary head movements. At age three she broke her left clavicle, and at fourteen she suffered a broken nose and strained neck in a pool diving accident. During junior high school, she recalls having an occasional head twitch to the right without any change or worsening over the years. Then at age twenty-seven, she was involved in a catastrophic auto accident in which her husband was killed. For several hours, she was pinned in the car with her dead husband's head pinned against the left side of her head, forcing her head to the right.

Within months, she developed a persistent repetitive involuntary turning of her head to the right, diagnosed eventually by a neurologist as spasmodic torticollis. This head twitch was worsened by stress and emotion, and reduced by lightly touching the right side of her chin. Patching her left eye also partially corrected the head turning, a fact that she attributed to forcing her head to turn so that she could see straight ahead. The torticollis had not responded to a number of medications, and she was considering surgery, or possibly a trial of botulinum toxin injections. Her examination revealed spasmodic torsional movements of the head to the right, and the right ear to the right shoulder, quite typical of torticollis.

Because of the striking history of presumed traumatic origin of this patient's movement disorder, a course of somatic trauma therapy was instituted. After a fairly prolonged trial of therapy, the patient noted marked but incomplete improvement in the severity of her torticollis, with much of this improvement being due to the reduced effect of life stress on its severity. Pain due to the involuntary movement was substantially reduced.

Spasmodic torticollis is a focal dystonic movement disorder of unknown cause involving the head and neck, recognized for more than a century, and generally resistant to treatment of any sort. In many cases, the cause is believed to be due to psychogenic[6] or traumatic[7] factors, but psychotherapy and behavioral therapies have had mixed to poor results. Pain is common in up to 50 percent of cases and generally is associated with a poor prognosis.[7] Remission or improvement is common, but complete recovery is rare.[8] No pathology within the central nervous system has been demonstrated, and no specific cause has been found for torticollis.

The orientation response is a basic primitive sensorimotor reflexive response to perceived threat common to all animal species. Mobilization of the primary senses of smell, sight, and hearing for acquisition of potentially threatening sensory information involves orientation of those sensory end organs to the source of that information. This process involves neuromuscular control of the head and neck in order to position these organs for optimal sensory input. An animal perceiving a potential source of threat will exhibit immediate arrest of all movement, followed by a slow side-to-side scanning movement of the head associated with flaring of the nostrils, widening of the eyes, dilatation of the pupils, and forward rotation of the ears. These smooth turning movements of the head and neck in the direction of the threat orient the animal to the source of the arousal, and prepare it for defensive action. This reflexive sequence of movement is common to all species, and is triggered by the reflex process of arousal. The orienting response very likely is mediated by the influence of the brain stem ventral vagal complex (VVC) as part of the energy-conserving, early behavioral response to arousal.[9]

Careful observation of patients who have experienced trauma will often reveal altered and sustained positions of the head and neck that reflect muscle-holding patterns representative of procedural memory for that trauma. Thus, the patient who has suffered injuries in a broadside, or T-bone automobile impact will usually present with a subtle but quite obvious lateral shift and rotation of the head and neck in the direction away from the impact months, even years later. One may recall the patient described in Chapter 9 who had suffered severe injuries to the left arm, and whose posture was characterized by turning of the entire body away from the left side. These postures reflect orienting and defensive patterns of motor activity triggered by the threatening sensory input at the moment of a traumatic event, stored in procedural motor memory and linked to the arousal elicited by that event. Portions of these postures consist of the early orienting reflex involving scanning movements of the head as the initial response to possible threat. In the course of somatically based trauma therapy (such as eye movement desensitization and reprocessing, and somatic experiencing), subtle but at times dramatic involuntary turning movements of the head are elicited, presumably representing orienting movements from procedural memory for old trauma.

In the case of torticollis described previously, a series of traumatic experiences occurred in this patient that were specifically related to directional positioning of the head. The turning movements of the head in torticollis mimic in many respects those involved in the orientation response. Spasmodic torticollis, in fact, may be analogous to the bracing patterns of myofascial pain as a fixed reflex movement pattern associated with a traumatic event. That movement is then stored in procedural memory linked to the arousal based on absence of a freeze discharge. As such, it may reflect a stereotyped repetitive orienting response perpetuated by traumatic kindling.

Dissociation and Reflex Sympathetic Dystrophy

We have already discussed the syndrome of RSD in Chapters 8 and 9 in relationship to the concept of somatic dissociation, boundary rupture, and the role of the autonomic nervous system in its pathology. One of my patients presented to me with an uncanny validation of these concepts of the etiology of RSD. The patient herself had an intuition that her doctor's explanations did not make sense in relationship to her personal experience, and she had formed her own theory of how this process had taken place. As a psychotherapist with a holistic view of the mind–body relationship, she decided that the traumatic experience itself and the meaning of events surrounding it must be related to her disease process.

While driving at moderate speed, her car was hit head-on by another automobile, and although her seat belt restraints prevented more severe injury, she suffered a major fracture injury to her right foot. She anticipated the impact before it occurred, and experienced severe auto-related PTSD that required years of psychotherapy to partially resolve.

While in the hospital awaiting surgery on her foot, she experienced intolerable pain despite narcotic administration. Using her acquired skills in the area of self-modulation and pain management, she utilized imaginary distancing of herself from the painful foot, visualizing that it indeed was not part of her. This was quite successful in reducing the intolerable portion of the pain, and she went on to have uneventful surgical repair of the foot fractures. Postoperative pain was severe, however, and once again became resistant to narcotic analgesia. When the postoperative cast was removed, the foot was gray and cold, and soon progressed to full-blown RSD.

In the next few years she underwent extensive pharmacotherapy, and more than twenty-five sympathetic nerve blocks with only slight improvement in intractable burning foot pain. At some point in her recovery, she came to the conclusion that the act of her disowning the foot before surgery might indeed be related to her RSD. She then began an intensive program of imaging the blood vessels and temperature in her leg and foot, visualizing widening of the vessels, and an increase in blood flow and warmth. She also visualized the foot as belonging to her, since she realized that, despite the pain, it felt alien and strange to her. Although progress was slow, this practice began a gradual reversal of the dystrophy, pain, and exquisite sensitivity of the RSD, and without further medical intervention, she largely recovered a normal foot except for mild sensitivity and cold intolerance. Of interest is the fact that her pain syndrome also involved numbness and pain in the right jaw, face, arm, and hand, which gradually recovered.

Her physical examination at the time of her visit with me revealed no objective findings except for some residual tightness of muscles of the right shoulder girdle. With boundary testing, however, she experienced arousal and sudden pain in her right jaw when I passed my hand into her far right visual field at a distance of about four feet. This effect was quite startling to her, and reproducible on several trials. When I described to her my theory of RSD and how it exactly mimicked her process of intentional dissociation of her foot in the face of developing symptoms of trauma, she said that this actually was what she thought might have happened. She was afraid to tell her doctor, however, because the idea sounded so strange.

Since I have begun testing my patients for arousal symptoms within regions of their boundary perception, I have consistently found boundary rupture in RSD patients in the symptomatic region. Many of my RSD patients describe symptoms that might be interpreted as dissociation related to the initiating traumatic event. Many others develop RSD insidiously in the face of subtle injuries such as overuse of the hand, bumping part of the body, or suffering a minor sprain injury.

The aforementioned patient is obviously unique, not only in her powers of observation and self-control, but also in the 1:1 association of voluntary dissociation of the injured regions with subsequent development of RSD in the dissociated body part. A smoking gun at the scene of a crime is legal though not scientific proof, but it remains powerful evidence for an association.

Comments

These stories illustrate a spectrum of somatic responses to traumatic stress that hopefully reinforce the basic premise of this book: the presence of a direct link between the neurochemical and neurophysiological response of the brain to stress, and an explainable and measurable related somatic event. Using the symptoms and messages provided by apparent somatization as clues to the meaning of the patient's trauma may allow the clinician to trace that message back to its source and thereby achieve greater understanding of the roots of the patient's illness. Although it would be presumptuous to assert that the truth will actually free trauma victims from their autonomic bondage, self-knowledge through education and insight provided by the therapist remain powerful tools for providing resources for the patients throughout treatment. Understanding the links between their conditioned somatic and emotional response to internal and external sources of arousal may allow the patients to use self-regulatory skills attained through treatment to better advantage.

Establishing a relationship with a therapist that includes validation of the patient's physical symptoms as meaningful, measurable, and not "in one's head" lessens the ongoing stress of disbelief and devaluation by family, friends, health care providers, insurance personnel, and attorneys. Analysis of trauma-related postural changes, neurological symptoms, and boundary ruptures in relationship to the patient's trauma history may give valuable clues to which life trauma is the major perpetuating source of the patient's disability, and may provide valuable direction for the patient's treatment. Recognizing the true pathophysiological basis for the patient's symptoms may also facilitate treatment of the physical illnesses that may accompany and be attributable to traumatic stress.

Anecdotes such as these case histories do not make scientific fact. The role of coincidence and chance in the affairs of man and the universe have justifiably led to the role of the scientific method in determining truth in science. Unfortunately, medical science is among the least precise of sciences, and behavioral sciences are perhaps the least testable of all. The brief review of the history of PTSD in psychiatry would certainly confirm this. Freud based his theories on his experience with thousands of patients, seasoned by a formidable intellect. He was not able to apply blind controls to justify his conclusions. Nevertheless, before his views were warped by the need to succumb to the political pressures of his peers, he and Janet, through patient observation alone, had independently arrived at conclusions very close to our current neurophysiological theories of PTSD.

Similar to the anecdote of the four blind men and the elephant, we only believe in that part of the whole which we perceive, and what we perceive may be determined as much by secondary gain related to our role in the scientific community as by our search for the truth. The truth is actually out there in the brains and bodies of our patients. In our rush toward science, we at times have substituted technology for science. We tend to trust that what we see in numbers, images, and measurements constitutes reality and, therefore, the truth. We have in part abandoned and allowed the use of our own senses and perceptions as healers to atrophy, the attributes that in the early days of my training were valued as the essence of the true physician.

The greatest of these attributes is the spoken word expressed by the patient to his or her physician, in which we often find the truth that we so desperately seek. That truth lies not only in the simplistic description of a physical symptom of an obvious disease, but also in the convoluted, tangential complaints associated with somatization. Dismissing a symptom or physical complaint because it "doesn't make sense" or is "psychological," imprisons the patient in a web of misunderstanding, and the physician in the bonds of bias. Our patients who suffer from the physiological ravages of trauma exemplify this fact more than any other patient group. They constitute the least understood, most rejected, and most frustrating challenges to the medical profession only because they represent a threat to our jaded concepts of tangible physical disease and intangible psychology. Once we reject this dichotomy, we will begin to recognize the remarkable physiological basis for "functional," "hysterical," "nonphysiological," and "psychosomatic" symptoms and physical findings, and we may recognize them as a part of a definable and reproducible syndrome, and approach treatment with understanding, empathy, and a healing spirit.

Notes

1. Bell, I., Miller, C., Schwartz, G.: An olfactory-limbic model of multiple chemical sensitivity syndrome: Possible relationships to kindling and affective spectrum disorders. *Biological Psychiatry*, 1992; 32:218–242.
2. Miller, L.: Neurosensitization: A pathophysiological model for traumatization disability syndromes. *The Journal of Cognitive Rehabilitation*, 1997; November/December:12–23.
3. Pace, J., Nagle, D.: Piriform syndrome. *Western Journal of Medicine*, 1976; 124: 435–439.
4. van der Kolk, B.: The body keeps the score: Approaches to the psychobiology of posttraumatic stress disorder. In van der Kolk, B., McFarlane, A., Weisaeth, L. (Eds.). *Traumatic Stress: The Effects of Overwhelming Experience on Mind, Body, and Society* (pp. 214–241). New York: Guilford Press, 1996.
5. Rauch, S., van der Kolk, B., Fisler, R., Alpert, N., Orr, S., Savage, C., Fischman, A., Jenike, M., Pitman, R.: A symptom provocation study of posttraumatic stress disorder using positron emission tomography and script-driven imagery. *Archives of General Psychiatry*, 1996; 53:380–387.
6. Cleveland, S. E.: Personality dynamics in torticollis. *Journal of Nervous and Mental Disease*, 1961; 129:150–161.
7. Tibbets, R. W.: Spasmodic torticollis. *Journal of Nervous and Mental Disease*, 1971; 15:461–469.
8. Matthews, W. B., Beasley, P., Parry-Jones, W., Garland, G.: Spasmodic torticollis: A combined clinical study. *Journal of Neurology, Neurosurgery and Psychiatry*, 1978; 41:485–492.
9. Porges, S.: Orienting in a defensive world: Mammalian modifications of our evolutionary heritage. A polyvagal theory. *Psychophysiology*, 1995; 32:301–308.

Epilogue

We have arrived at a model of trauma that I suspect will be intriguing and even compelling to some and speculative at best to others. As our knowledge of the neurophysiological basis for PTSD expands, some elements of this theoretical model will undoubtedly change, and others I think will be validated. We have reemphasized the crucial role of dissociation in the perpetuation of the kindled autonomic cycle of PTSD. We have moved beyond the concept that the somatic sensations of somatization are simply imagined and exaggerated symptoms in the PTSD victim, to the concept that these sensations represent actual physiological changes in the body region encompassing messages of the old threat.

In this context, reexperiencing and dissociation driven by internal arousal cues have thrust the victim into a perceptual state locked in the past, incapable of experiencing the present, and blind to the future. Without the ability of the down-regulated frontal cortex to imagine "What if?" the future holds no other possibilities than existential threat. There can be no future while the unresolved procedural memories of the trauma continue to imply their ongoing and threatening presence. The ongoing cues of the present continue to trigger indiscriminate arousal and fear linked to the past. The present, therefore, serves only to thrust the victim back into instinctual and conditioned modes of self-preservation that by definition are based on past failed attempts at escape and completion of the survival effort, and that only serve to enhance their sense of helplessness. Perhaps the most poignant complaint of the trauma victim is the loss of the sense of "who I was," and "who I am now." One's sense of self is not only based on the internal historical narrative of one's life experiences and accomplishments, but also on the ability to apply these experiences to future efforts. The perception of helplessness by definition belies this capability. In this context, the conundrum of trauma is the corruption of the present by procedural and emotion-linked memories of the past.

In fact, the present moment is repeatedly invaded by the procedural memory contents of the dissociative capsules from past traumatic events. In the absence of the present moment, the trauma survivor's sense of self cannot grow and evolve, but remains frozen in the time warp of the traumatic event. The survivor lives in a perpetual "groundhog day" of reliving the trauma as if it were still happening.

The therapeutic implications of these concepts are that healing in trauma will not be achieved until empowerment occurs, and until the ongoing threats and cues to arousal have been removed from a state of ongoing imminence to a state of past and completed experience. Whether or not this experience encompasses a meaningful narrative may not be important, as long as the somatic correlates of the traumatic memory no longer contain messages of threat. If one no longer is able to experience the real-time somatic sensations of past traumatic emotional and autonomic states, those states cease to exist as threatening cues. Under this paradigm, the resolution of these somatic correlates may be the most important measure of successful trauma therapy.

* * *

During the preparation of this book, dramatic progress has been made in the study of the brain in PTSD. Among the most exciting areas of progress has been the use of imaging techniques to study brain metabolism and physiology in trauma victims. These studies have continued to demonstrate the selective facilitation and inhibition of areas of the brain known to participate in the cycle of traumatic kindling.

More attention has been directed at the role of childhood developmental experiences in the generation of personality, psychopathology, and vulnerability to trauma. Workers in the field of child development have begun to explore links between increasing childhood violence and more subtle issues of neglect and abandonment, such as the common use in the past decade of day care centers for children below the age of eighteen months. The association between issues of early childhood negative experience, including abandonment, impaired attachment, and the development of childhood attention deficit hyperactivity disorder (ADHD), bipolar disorder, autism, and its milder form, Asperger's syndrome is beginning to be addressed.

In the area of trauma therapy, more attention has been directed at somatically based trauma therapies, leading to a burgeoning growth of eclectic therapeutic approaches, many of them offshoots of existing therapies, and all of them as yet untested. Presentation of a variety of these techniques at conferences previously reserved for the more scientific exploration of PTSD has led to interest and excitement, as well as great controversy. At the same time, terrorism, war, ethnic cleansing, tribal genocide, and natural disasters throughout the world have continued to remind us of the inevitable presence of catastrophic trauma on our planet.

The theme of this book might appear to be overwhelmed by the enormity of the problem of pervasive life trauma, especially if one accepts the fact that even "trivial" trauma or negative life experiences in childhood has lifelong implications. The other side of this discouraging coin, however, implies that simple attention to these "trivial" traumatic life events in the therapeutic process may have disproportionately positive long-term effects. If we are able to conclude that many of the chronic, unexplained diseases that we treat so ineffectively may be based on a variation of autonomic dysregulation related to such cumulative life trauma, a whole new paradigm for prevention and management of these diseases may be developed.

In this perpetual and never-completed search for truth, I believe that one must combine the rigor and skepticism of the scientific with the wisdom and curiosity of the intuitive. Both approaches to the truth are subject to opportunism, bias, elitism, and financial secondary gain. But the blind application of science to the healing arts, by definition, limits our observations to the parameters for measurement that we have been able to standardize based on statistical limits that may miss the subtleties of clinical pathology. In this process of treading the fine line between art and science, the basic traditional diagnostic and intuitive skills of the physician-as-healer must never be allowed to fade and atrophy in the glare of technological advancement.

One must recognize that many legitimate techniques of the healing arts will never be adequately amenable to statistical validation by the scientific method. By the same token, diagnosis and treatment through intuitive techniques alone may open the way for opportunism and charlatanism. The only way that we may resolve this dilemma is for both sides of the issue—the intuitive and the scientific—to come together in recognition of the value of the other's position. Intuitive techniques, including untested somatically based trauma therapies, must be subjected to adequate, randomized controlled studies, and the scientific community responsible for funding of such rigorous studies must make a commitment to the more open process of investigation of novel but compelling therapies in the field of trauma.

Investigation of the role of brain development in the face of the subtleties of neglect must be pursued with open-minded but passionate intensity. Implication of neglect immediately casts a negative light on selected members of our society, and the pursuit of data in this area must be taken with compassion, understanding, and education. The rapidly evolving field of knowledge in the area of life trauma has opened a Pandora's box of information that has profound implications for the emotional and physical welfare of mankind. For the sake of mankind, further investigations in the field of the neurophysiology of trauma and the nuances of its treatment must not be impeded by personal bias or political or professional self-interest.

Index

Please note: page numbers in *italics* followed by an *f* indicate figures

multiple personality disorder *see*
dissociative identity disorder (DID)
MVAs *see* motor vehicle accidents;
post-traumatic stress disorder
myofascial pain 21, 24–5; head and neck
47–8; neuromuscular dysfunction and
45–7

nalmefene 185
naltrexone 185
narcotic antagonists 184–5
National Comorbidity Survey 136
National Vietnam Veterans Readjustment
Study (NVVRS) 135
natural killer cells 102
natural selection 103–4
neck and low back pain 22, 23, 24
negative feedback 3
negative feedback loop 99
neonatal trauma 149–50
neuroendocrine response to threat 68
neurofeedback (brain wave biofeedback)
176–9
neurological symptoms: of whiplash 22,
28; *see also* neurophysiology of trauma;
whiplash syndrome: brain trauma
model; whiplash syndrome: symptoms
neuromuscular dysfunction 45–7
neurophysiology of attunement:
developing brain and 51–3; *see also*
Social Engagement System
neurophysiology of trauma 7–8, 9f, 10, 11f,
38–49, 161, 166; binocular dysfunction
and 43–4; cognitive deficits in trauma
42–3; head and neck myofascial pain
47–8; kindling and trauma 39–40,
41f; neuromuscular dysfunction and
myofascial pain 45–7; post-concussion
syndrome and 43; summary of 207–9;
vestibular and autonomic dysfunction
44–5; *see also* kindling; neuroplasticity
and traumatic brain damage;
somatically-based therapies; somatic
dissociation; trauma sources; trauma
therapies; traumatic stress diseases;
whiplash syndrome: brain trauma
model
neuroplasticity and traumatic brain
damage 61–70; brain plasticity in
trauma 64–5; history of post-traumatic
stress disorder (PTSD) in psychiatry
62–4; objective measures in brain change
in trauma 65–6; permanence of PTSD
66–8

neuroplasticity model: character
development and 53–4;
see also brain plasticity
neurosensitization 48; *see also* kindling
neurotransmitters 12–13, 30, 35
nightmares 29, 62, 192
nociception (sense of pain) 3
nondeclarative (implicit) memory 34–5,
94, 104, 148
nonphysiological signs 88, 90; *see also*
somatic dissociation
noradrenergic arousal response *11f*
norepinephrine 10, 12, 13, 35, 42, 66, 99,
102, 121
nucleus ambiguus (ventral vagal nucleus)
56–8, 86, 201
nucleus tractus solitarius (solitary nucleus)
56
numbness 38, 73, 184

obsessive-compulsive behaviors
75–6, 82
OFC *see* right orbitofrontal cortex
opioid dysregulation 184
orienting reflex, aberration of 200–2
oscillatory phenomena, of the autonomic
nervous system in trauma 83, 84f, 85,
87, 90
"out of body" experiences 17, 38, 72
"overresponders" 194

pain 94; chronic 19, 103–5; infants
and 149–50, 151–2; phantom limb
pain 94, 104; sense of (nociception) 3;
soft tissue injuries and 29;
see also somatically-based therapies;
somatic dissociation; trauma therapies;
whiplash syndrome: brain trauma
model; whiplash syndrome:
symptoms
pain memory 108
pain threshold 12
panic attacks 29
parasympathetic nervous system 13, 15,
85–6, 100, 101
pathophysiology of stress 99–100; *see also*
neurophysiology of trauma; traumatic
stress diseases
pathophysiology of whiplash *see*
neurophysiology of trauma; whiplash
syndrome: brain trauma model;
whiplash syndrome: symptoms
patient education 163–4
Pavlov's dog experiments 14, 35

Printed in the United States
by Baker & Taylor Publisher Services